THE POSITIVE SIDE
OF NEGATIVE EMOTIONS

The Positive Side of Negative Emotions

Edited by
W. GERROD PARROTT

THE GUILFORD PRESS
New York   London

© 2014 The Guilford Press
A Division of Guilford Publications, Inc.
72 Spring Street, New York, NY 10012
www.guilford.com

All rights reserved

No part of this book may be reproduced, translated, stored in
a retrieval system, or transmitted, in any form or by any means,
electronic, mechanical, photocopying, microfilming, recording,
or otherwise, without written permission from the publisher.

Printed in the United States of America

This book is printed on acid-free paper.

Last digit is print number: 9   8   7   6   5   4   3   2   1

Library of Congress Cataloging-in-Publication Data

The positive side of negative emotions / edited by W. Gerrod Parrott.
    pages cm
  Includes bibliographical references and index.
  ISBN 978-1-4625-1333-8 (hardcover : alk. paper)
  1. Emotions.   I. Parrott, W. Gerrod.
  BF531.P67 2014
  152.4—dc23

                                                    2013041394

About the Editor

W. Gerrod Parrott, PhD, is Professor of Psychology at Georgetown University. His central interest is the nature of human emotion. His published work has focused on three areas: philosophical and historical approaches to the concept of emotion; emotion's social foundations and functions, including such social emotions as embarrassment, shame, guilt, envy, and jealousy; and the influence of emotion and emotional self-regulation on thought. Dr. Parrott is the author of over 75 scholarly chapters, articles, and books. He is past editor of the journal *Cognition and Emotion* and past president of the International Society for Research on Emotion.

Contributors

Levi R. Baker, MS, Department of Psychology, Florida State University, Tallahassee, Florida

Anne Bartsch, PhD, Department of Media, Knowledge, and Communication, University of Augsburg, Augsburg, Germany

Yochanan Bigman, BA, doctoral student, Department of Psychology, The Hebrew University, Jerusalem, Israel

Yulia E. Chentsova-Dutton, PhD, Department of Psychology, Georgetown University, Washington, DC

Philip J. Corr, PhD, Department of Psychology, City University London, London, United Kingdom

Stéphane Côté, PhD, Rotman School of Management, University of Toronto, Toronto, Ontario, Canada

Joseph P. Forgas, AM, DPhil, DSc, School of Psychology, University of New South Wales, Sydney, Australia

Christine R. Harris, PhD, Department of Psychology, University of California, San Diego, La Jolla, California

Tilo Hartmann, PhD, Department of Communication Science, VU University Amsterdam, Amsterdam, The Netherlands

Nicole E. Henniger, MA, Department of Psychology, University of California, San Diego, La Jolla, California

Ursula Hess, PhD, Institute for Psychology, Humboldt University, Berlin, Berlin, Germany

James K. McNulty, PhD, Department of Psychology, Florida State University, Tallahassee, Florida

Julie K. Norem, PhD, Department of Psychology, Wellesley College, Wellesley, Massachusetts

Mary Beth Oliver, PhD, Department of Film/Video and Media Studies, The Pennsylvania State University, University Park, Pennsylvania

Nickola C. Overall, PhD, Department of Psychology, University of Auckland, Auckland, New Zealand

W. Gerrod Parrott, PhD, Department of Psychology, Georgetown University, Washington, DC

Adam M. Perkins, PhD, Department of Psychological Medicine, Institute of Psychiatry, King's College London, London, United Kingdom

Andrew G. Ryder, PhD, Department of Psychology and Centre for Clinical Research in Health, Concordia University, and Culture and Mental Health Research Unit and the Lady Davis Institute, Jewish General Hospital, Montreal, Quebec, Canada

Nicole Senft, BA, doctoral student, Department of Psychology, Georgetown University, Washington, DC

Louise Sundararajan, PhD, private practice, Rochester, New York

Maya Tamir, PhD, Department of Psychology, The Hebrew University, Jerusalem, Israel

Gerben A. Van Kleef, PhD, Department of Social Psychology, University of Amsterdam, Amsterdam, The Netherlands

Preface

Bad weather is often used as a metaphor for negative emotions—that is why there is an image of dark rain clouds obscuring the sun on the cover of this book. That image provides a good way of introducing this volume, because bad weather and negative emotions are both underappreciated. In the case of bad weather, it is true that it can spoil picnics and destroy buildings, but that does not mean that people would be better off without it. If it never rained, most places would have no water and the plants and animals would die. Furthermore, not everyone prefers sunny weather, and even those who do benefit from the important functions served by changes of weather and seasons. Scientific study has greatly increased our understanding of these functions: that tropical storms redistribute heat around the planet, end droughts, and create barrier islands; that lightning adds fertilizing nitrogen to the soil; that strong winds cool the planet's surface, distribute seeds and pollen, and clear away old vegetation; that thunderstorms clean the air. When one thinks in terms of the complex dynamics of our planet and not merely in terms of picnics, one appreciates the storms along with the sunshine.

Like bad weather, negative emotions may also be unpleasant or destructive, yet people should no more wish for unremitting happiness than for continual clear skies. Happiness is not appropriate for every occasion, and negative emotions can focus the mind, send important signals to other people, and lend a seriousness and profundity to life. Research on emotion has surged over the past 30 years and has provided a much better understanding of what emotions are like and what they are for. Negative emotions, it turns out, have many important functions, and life would be

much the poorer without them. The purpose of this volume is to correct the misperception that negative emotions are without value by reviewing and integrating the tremendous variety of recent research that points to the opposite conclusion—that negative emotions *do* have value.

Any consideration of *negative emotions* must begin by clarifying what is meant by the term. The idea that some emotions are *negative,* whereas others are *positive,* has a long history (Colembetti, 2005). Throughout that history there has been reasonable agreement about which emotions are negative and which are positive. Negative emotions typically include fear, anxiety, loneliness, guilt, shame, embarrassment, regret, disappointment, sadness, envy, jealousy, disgust, scorn, anger, frustration, and irritation. Positive emotions, in contrast, typically include pride, contentment, relief, hope, exhilaration, delight, eagerness, amusement, cheerfulness, happiness, wonderment, desire, admiration, infatuation, and love (see, e.g., Shaver, Schwartz, Kirson, & O'Connor, 1987). Lists such as these provide one way to understand what the terms negative emotion and positive emotion refer to.

Despite the agreement about which emotions are positive and which are negative, there is disagreement and confusion about what makes an emotion positive or negative. In one analysis of this confusion, Solomon and Stone (2002) listed 18 ways in which positive and negative emotions have been distinguished. Some of the distinctions are ethical: virtue versus vice, right versus wrong, socially approved versus socially unacceptable. Other distinctions between positive and negative focus more on the emotions' effects: healthy or unhealthy, calming or upsetting, strengthening or weakening, satisfying or dissatisfying, motivating approach or motivating avoidance. Yet other interpretations focus on the various appraisals and judgments that are attached to the emotions: is the situation in accord with one's wishes or not; does one judge one's own actions or another person's actions to be praiseworthy or blameworthy; does one perceive oneself or another person as having high or low status; does one approve of one's self or of another person? Positive and negative have also been taken to refer to qualities of phenomenal experience: perhaps the former emotions are pleasant whereas the latter are painful.

The point of reviewing Solomon and Stone's (2002) analysis is not to reject the distinction between positive and negative emotions (as they did), but rather to highlight the vagueness of the terms positive and negative and to clarify what psychologists mean when they categorize emotions in this way. The problem with most of the 18 senses of positive and negative is that they do not categorize the same emotion consistently. For example, anger can be painful or pleasurable or both, depending on the circumstances, so phenomenal experience does not explain why anger is considered a negative emotion. Sometimes a classification simply seems irrelevant; for example,

most emotions do not seem to have consistent effects on health. What is wanted is a consistent basis for justifying why each emotion is classified as positive or negative. For the purposes of the present volume, the most useful criterion is the situation's perceived compatibility with a person's needs, goals, and values: negative emotions generally involve interpreting something as being against one's wishes (Gordon, 1987). More nuanced ways of classification have been devised (e.g., Shuman, Sander, & Scherer, 2013), but these refinements are beyond the scope of this Preface.

The present volume summarizes the progress that contemporary research has made in understanding the value of negative emotions. The chapters are divided into three parts. Part I focuses on particular negative emotions. Joseph P. Forgas, in Chapter 1, leads off by focusing on the effects of negative moods, particularly sad moods. Forgas points out that contemporary Western culture is anomalous in the extent to which it evaluates negative moods as undesirable. His findings about the beneficial effects of sad moods are therefore all the more surprising and important. In Chapter 2, Adam M. Perkins and Philip J. Corr discuss the adaptive nature of anxiety. Their chapter synthesizes research across species (both humans and rodents), and across biological, cognitive, personality, and social levels of analysis to demonstrate how anxiety promotes survival. In Chapter 3, Ursula Hess focuses on anger. Despite anger's reputation as a destructive force, Hess points out how it often serves the cause of justice and fairness. By motivating resolve and communicating strength, anger provides the personal and social means to promote people's values and goals. In Chapter 4, Nicole E. Henniger and Christine R. Harris survey research on five emotions that are especially social in nature: embarrassment, shame, guilt, jealousy, and envy. Henniger and Harris demonstrate how each of these emotions provide benefits in the context of social situations and relationships. Although these four chapters address only some of the many negative emotions, they include most of the major types and provide a sense of their similarities and differences.

Part II of the book follows from the increasingly social focus of Part I by considering the social and cultural aspects of negative emotions in general. Levi R. Baker, James K. McNulty, and Nickola C. Overall, in Chapter 5, consider how negative emotions function in close relationships. They show that negative emotions can be valuable by increasing intimacy, eliciting support, and resolving relationship problems. These authors are careful to note that negative emotions are not useful in all circumstances and that they must be expressed in the right way and at the right time for their potential adaptiveness to be realized. Chapter 6, by Gerben A. Van Kleef and Stéphane Côté, examines negative emotions' role in social interaction. Van Kleef and Côté survey numerous studies that demonstrate that expressions of emotion provide a powerful means of shaping other people's behavior.

This research, often conducted in settings that show the importance of emotions in the workplace, shows how negative emotions can elicit conformity, social support, better work, and more favorable negotiation offers.

The remaining two chapters in this part address the topic of culture. In Chapter 7, Yulia E. Chentsova-Dutton, Nicole Senft, and Andrew G. Ryder provide a broad theory of how culture affects the experience, expression, meaning, and regulation of negative emotions. They discuss a wide range of emotional and clinical topics, but their central example is sadness and how it is shaped by its very different valuation by Russian and European American cultures. Their integration of studies from a variety of disciplines makes a powerful case that human emotions are significantly shaped by their cultural context. In Chapter 8, Louise Sundararajan approaches the topic of culture and negative emotions by focusing on a single culture, China, and contrasting it with Western cultures. Sundararajan explores the Confucian tradition and how it fosters the development of empathy and a focus on one's relationship to others. One result is that the emotion the Chinese call *chi*—most similar to shame or embarrassment in English—is less aversive and more valuable as a means to the socialization of children.

The chapters in Part III build on the preceding topics to consider the reasons why negative emotions might be actively sought after and preferred to positive emotions. In Chapter 9, Maya Tamir and Yochanan Bigman develop a comprehensive taxonomy of motives for experiencing negative emotions or for avoiding positive emotions. When I first wrote about negative emotions over 20 years ago, psychologists routinely assumed that emotion regulation is restricted to two types: seeking and maintaining positive emotions and avoiding and inhibiting negative emotions. My proposal that there are occasions in which people are motivated to regulate in the opposite directions was unusual at the time (Parrott, 1993). Tamir and Bigman's impressive literature review demonstrates how extensively research and theory in this area have evolved over the past two decades. They list a multitude of motives for experiencing negative emotions and propose a scheme that organizes them. In Chapter 10, Mary Beth Oliver, Anne Bartsch, and Tilo Hartmann address the phenomenon of people choosing to experience art forms that they know will arouse negative emotions. People pay money and spend discretionary time watching tearjerkers, horror movies, tragic dramas, and other media that produce predominantly negative emotions. Oliver, Bartsch, and Hartmann survey explanations for why people spend their time and money this way. They conclude that the point of these experiences isn't their unpleasantness but rather their meaningfulness. Their conclusion agrees with that of other authors in this volume: It is a mistake to focus on unpleasantness in understanding negative emotions; significance, motivation, attention, relationships, and social influence must be considered as well.

The remaining two chapters in this part continue to develop these themes. In Chapter 11, Julie K. Norem discusses why some people prefer negative emotions more than others. In particular, anxious individuals may find that they can most successfully cope with stress by embracing pessimism and anxiety rather than by trying to inhibit these feelings. This strategy, known as "defensive pessimism," complicates the stereotype of the confident, optimistic, successful person because defensive pessimists achieve equal levels of success. Their pessimism helps them to prepare for possible problems while protecting them from disappointment. Norem broadens her analysis of defensive pessimism into a general functional analysis of positive and negative emotions: Emotions are tools; they must be chosen on the basis of the job at hand. Not everyone can use all the tools equally well, so the most useful emotion for one person may not be the most useful emotion for another.

I wrote the book's final chapter (Chapter 12) after reading all the others so I could underscore this book's themes and show how they apply to positive emotions as well as to negative emotions. One commonality is that both positive and negative emotions can be either functional or dysfunctional, so the chapter considers factors that help determine when an emotion will work adaptively in a particular context. It concludes by arguing that contemporary Western cultures find positive emotions attractive and negative emotions aversive because they focus on personal feelings and public cheerfulness at the cost of neglecting other, more meaningful and satisfying, aspects of life.

I want to express my gratitude to a number of individuals whose efforts contributed to making this book possible. First I want to thank Seymour Weingarten, Editor-in-Chief at The Guilford Press, who first had the idea for this volume and sought my advice about it. At every stage, Seymour contributed ideas and provided helpful feedback. I also am grateful to the authors of this book's individual chapters. They shared a commitment to this book's central message, and often collaborated generously by sharing ideas on how to improve the book. In addition, I want to thank two colleagues, Sarah McNamer and Laura Rosenthal, whose careful reading of my contributions to this volume improved their clarity in many places. Finally, I wish to thank the entire team at The Guilford Press for their professional work on this volume's production and marketing. I particularly want to thank Carolyn Graham and Anna Nelson, who were enormously supportive and patient at every turn.

W. GERROD PARROTT

REFERENCES

Colombetti, G. (2005). Appraising valence. *Journal of Consciousness Studies, 12,* 103–126.

Gordon, R. M. (1987). *The structure of emotions: Investigations in cognitive philosophy.* Cambridge, UK: Cambridge University Press.

Parrott, W. G. (1993). Beyond hedonism: Motives for inhibiting good moods and for maintaining bad moods. In D. M. Wegner & J. W. Pennebaker (Eds.), *Handbook of mental control* (pp. 278–305). Englewood Cliffs, NJ: Prentice-Hall.

Shaver, P., Schwartz, J., Kirson, D., & O'Connor, C. (1987). Emotion knowledge: Further exploration of a prototype approach. *Journal of Personality and Social Psychology, 52,* 1061–1086.

Shuman, V., Sander, D., & Scherer, K. R. (2013). Levels of valence. *Frontiers in Psychology, 3,* 380.

Solomon, R. C., & Stone, L. D. (2002). On "positive" and "negative" emotions. *Journal for the Theory of Social Behaviour, 32,* 417–435.

Contents

PART III. THE DESIRABILITY
OF NEGATIVE EMOTIONS

PART I

SPECIFIC NEGATIVE EMOTIONS

1

Can Sadness Be Good for You?

On the Cognitive, Motivational, and Interpersonal Benefits of Negative Affect

JOSEPH P. FORGAS

Homo sapiens is a remarkably moody species. Fluctuating affective states color and filter everything we think and do during our waking hours. What is the role of affective states in guiding our reactions to the manifold challenges of everyday life? And, in particular, are there any demonstrably adaptive benefits that flow from the temporary experience of negative mood states? Evolutionary theorists have long assumed that all affective reactions serve important adaptive functions, operating like functional "mind modules" that spontaneously spring into action in response to various environmental challenges (Forgas, Haselton, & von Hippel, 2007; Frijda, 1986; Tooby & Cosmides, 1992). This chapter surveys a number of experimental studies providing convergent and somewhat counterintuitive evidence for the often useful and adaptive consequences of mild negative affect for social cognition, judgments, motivation, and interpersonal behavior.

ON NEGATIVE AFFECT

Negative emotions have always been with us. Indeed, arguably, many of the greatest achievements of the human mind and spirit were born out of sadness, dysphoria, and even enduring depression. Many of the classic works

3

of Western culture and civilization also deal with the evocation and cultivation of negative feelings and emotions. There are more Greek tragedies than there are comedies, Shakespeare also wrote more numerous tragedies than comedies, and hilarity generally comes a distant second to seriousness in most great literature and art. It seems that dealing with negative affect and what it tells us about the human condition has long been the focus of many artists and writers.

Yet, remarkably, there is also another side to this tradition. The search for happiness has been an equally enduring theme in human affairs. Hedonism is sometimes considered as the most important simple and sovereign principle that can explain all human behavior (Allport, 1985), and utilitarian philosophers sought to explore the necessary and sufficient conditions for human happiness and the best ways to attain it. Our very own age is characterized by an incessant individual and cultural pursuit of happiness. So there is a strange duality about the way Western cultures, and modern industrial societies in particular, think about the costs and benefits of different affective states.

It is intriguing that despite the never-ending human quest for happiness, our emotional repertoire as a species is nevertheless also heavily skewed toward negative emotions. Four of the six basic emotions are negative—fear, anger, disgust, and sadness. These emotions were clearly adaptive in our ancestral environment, preparing the organism for flight, fight, or avoidance, and there is general agreement about their functional benefits. But what about sadness, perhaps the most ubiquitous of our negative emotions? What is the purpose or benefit of being sad? Although sadness is probably the most common of all our negative affective states, its possible adaptive functions remain puzzling and poorly understood (Ciarrochi, Forgas, & Mayer, 2006; Forgas, 2006).

Sadness in our culture is often considered an unnecessary and undesirable emotion. A plethora of self-help books promote the benefits of positive thinking, positive attitudes, and positive behaviors, consigning negative affect in general, and sadness in particular, to the category of "problem emotions" that need to be managed or eliminated if possible. Much of the psychology profession is employed in managing and alleviating sadness. Yet it seems that some degree of sadness and melancholia has been far more accepted in previous historical epochs than is the case today (Sedikides, Wildschut, Arndt, & Routledge, 2006). From the classic philosophers through Shakespeare to the works of Chekhov, Ibsen, and the great novels of the 19th century, exploring the landscape of sadness, longing, and melancholia has long been considered instructive and, indeed, ennobling. It is only in the last few decades that a veritable industry promoting the cult of positivity has managed to eliminate this earlier and more balanced view of the landscape of human affectivity.

The evidence reviewed here shows that negative affect in general, and sadness in particular, also have important adaptive consequences by spontaneously triggering cognitive, motivational, and behavioral strategies that are well suited to dealing with the requirements of demanding social situations (Frijda, 1986). This is not to suggest that positive affect has no beneficial consequences, such as promoting creativity, flexibility, cooperation, and life satisfaction (Forgas, 1994, 1998a, 1998b, 2002; Forgas & George, 2001). Rather, a number of empirical studies now demonstrate that negative moods such as sadness may often recruit a more attentive, accommodating thinking style that produces superior outcomes whenever detailed, externally oriented, inductive thinking is required (Bless & Fiedler, 2006; Forgas & Eich, 2012). This prediction is consistent with evolutionary, functionalist theories of affect that argue that affective states "exist for the sake of signalling states of the world that have to be responded to" (Frijda, 1988, p. 354).

It is the influence of moods rather than distinct emotions that is of interest here, as moods are more common and more enduring and typically produce more uniform and reliable cognitive and behavioral consequences than do more context-specific emotions (Forgas, 2002, 2007). Moods are low-intensity, diffuse, and relatively enduring affective states without a salient antecedent cause and therefore little conscious cognitive content. In contrast, emotions are more intense and short-lived, and they usually have a definite cause and conscious cognitive content (Forgas, 1995, 2002). This chapter begins with a brief review of theoretical approaches linking affect, motivation, and cognition. It then reviews a number of experiments demonstrating the beneficial effects of negative affective states for cognition, motivation, and interpersonal behavior. The role of different information-processing strategies in mediating these effects receives special attention.

AFFECT, COGNITION, AND BEHAVIOR

In empirical psychology, affect has long remained the most neglected member of the historical tripartite division of the human mind into cognition, affect, and conation. This may be partly due to the archaic idea that affect represents a more primitive, dangerous, and invasive force that is incompatible with rational thinking and behavior, a notion that can be traced back in Western philosophy to the works of Plato. Freud's psychoanalytic speculations gave further emphasis to this view of affect as a dangerous, invasive force that needs to be controlled. Fortunately, the past few decades saw a radical revision of this view. As a result of advances in physiology and neuroanatomy, we now know that affect is often an essential and adaptive component of responding adaptively to social situations (Adolphs & Damasio, 2001; Forgas, 1995, 2002; Zajonc, 2000).

Renewed psychological interest in affect emerged in the early 1980s, and Robert Zajonc (1980) was among the first to argue that affect often constitutes the primary and dominant dimension of responding to social situations (Unkelbach, Forgas, & Denson, 2008). Affect also plays a critical role in how people cognitively represent their everyday social experiences (Forgas, 1979, 1982), and many social "stimuli can cohere as a category even when they have nothing in common other than the emotional responses they elicit" (Niedenthal & Halberstadt, 2000, p. 381).

Only a few early experiments directly explored affective influences on cognition and behavior. For example, in one early study Feshbach and Singer (1957) found that attempts to suppress affect may paradoxically increase the "pressure" on affect to infuse unrelated attitudes and judgments. Their study showed that fearful persons were more likely to see "another person as fearful and anxious" (p. 286), especially when the fearful participants were trying to suppress their fear, indicating that the "suppression of fear facilitates the tendency to project fear onto another social object" (p. 286). In another early experiment, Razran (1940) showed that people who were made to feel good or bad (receiving a free lunch or being exposed to unpleasant smells) responded to sociopolitical messages in an affect-congruent manner. Similar conditioning experiments were subsequently reported by Clore and Byrne (1974), who explored affect infusion into interpersonal judgments and behaviors.

In contrast to earlier approaches, contemporary theories linking affect to cognition and behavior identify two kinds of affective influences: (1) *informational effects* (such as affect congruence), in which an affective state directly influences the valence of information that people access and use and (2) *processing effects*, in which affect influences the way information is processed.

Informational Effects

Affect can influence the valence of thinking and behavior according to two complementary theories of informational effects: *affect priming* and *affect-as-information* models. *The affect-priming* account (Bower, 1981) argues that affect is integrally linked to an associative network of memory representations. An affective state may thus selectively prime associated constructs previously linked to that affect, and such affect-congruent ideas are more likely to be used in subsequent constructive cognitive tasks. Early studies showed that people induced to feel good or bad tended to selectively remember more mood-congruent details from their childhoods and recalled more mood-congruent events from the recent past (Bower, 1981). Mood congruence can also influence how people interpret social behaviors (Forgas, Bower & Krantz, 1984) and form impressions of others (Forgas &

Bower, 1987). However, affect priming is also subject to several boundary conditions and is most reliably obtained when tasks require open, constructive processing, as is the case with many inferences and associations, with impression formation, and with interpersonal behaviors (e.g., Bower & Forgas, 2001; Forgas, 2002; Forgas & Eich, 2012).

A second, *affect-as-information* (AAI), model proposed by Schwarz and Clore (1988; Clore, Schwarz, & Conway, 1994; Clore, Gasper, & Garvin, 2001) suggests that "rather than computing a judgment on the basis of recalled features of a target, individuals may . . . ask themselves: "How do I feel about it? [and] in doing so, they may mistake feelings due to a pre-existing state as a reaction to the target" (Schwarz, 1990, p. 529). Thus affect congruence is due to an inferential error, as people misattribute a preexisting affective state to an unrelated social stimulus. The model makes very similar predictions to earlier conditioning theories (Clore & Byrne, 1974), emphasizing internal misattribution rather than temporal and spatial contiguity as responsible for affect infusion. Such affective misattribution is most probable when "the task is of little personal relevance, when little other information is available, when problems are too complex to be solved systematically, and when time or attentional resources are limited" (Fiedler, 2001, p. 175), as is the case, for example, when people are asked to perform personally uninvolving off-the-cuff judgments (Forgas & Moylan, 1987; Schwarz & Clore, 1988).

Processing Effects

Affect may also influence the *process* of cognition, that is, *how* people think (Clark & Isen, 1982; Fiedler & Forgas, 1988; Forgas, 2002). Early theories assumed that positive mood leads to less effortful processing (Clark & Isen, 1982; Sinclair & Mark, 1992), whereas negative mood promotes effortful and vigilant processing (Schwarz, 1990; Schwarz & Bless, 1991). Explanations of this effect at first emphasized either (1) *functional principles* suggesting that affective states signal the degree of effort and vigilance required in more or less demanding situations or (2) *motivational* principles, as happy people may seek to preserve their good moods by avoiding cognitive effort (mood maintenance) and dysphoric individuals increase cognitive effort to improve their moods (mood repair; Clark & Isen, 1982).

A more recent and comprehensive explanation for these processing effects by Bless and Fiedler (2006) suggests that rather than influencing processing effort, different moods have an evolutionary function recruiting qualitatively different processing *styles*. Following the processing dichotomy introduced by Piaget, they argue that negative moods call for *accommodative, bottom-up* processing, focused on the details of the external

world. In contrast, positive moods recruit *assimilative, top-down* process-ing and greater reliance on existing schematic knowledge and heuristics (Bless, 2000; Bless & Fiedler, 2006; Fiedler, 2001). Thus *assimilation* involves greater reliance on preexisting internal knowledge when respond-ing to a situation, greater use of heuristics and cognitive shortcuts, and more top-down, generative, and constructive processing strategies in gen-eral. *Accommodation,* in contrast, involves increased attention to new, external, and unfamiliar information, increased sensitivity to social norms and expectations, and a more concrete, piecemeal, and bottom-up process-ing style. This affectively induced assimilative–accommodative processing dichotomy has received extensive support in recent years, suggesting that moods perform an adaptive function, preparing us to respond to different environmental challenges.

Several studies suggest that such a processing dichotomy associated with good and bad moods can have significant consequences. For example, Fiedler, Asbeck, and Nickel (1991) found that people experiencing posi-tive moods were more likely to engage in constructive processing and were more influenced by prior priming manipulations when forming judgments about people, whereas negative mood reduced this tendency. Further, nega-tive affect, by facilitating the processing of new external information, can also reduce judgmental mistakes such as the fundamental attribution error (Forgas, 1998a), reduce halo effects and primacy effects in impression for-mation (Forgas, 2011a, 2011b), improve the quality and efficacy of per-suasive arguments (Forgas, 2007), and also improve eyewitness memory (Fiedler et al., 1991; Forgas, Vargas, & Laham, 2005), as I show later. The theory thus implies that *both* positive and negative moods can produce processing advantages, albeit in response to different situations that require different strategies. This model explicitly affirms that negative affect does have important adaptive functions, as several of the experiments reviewed here show.

Integrative Theories

As affect may influence both the *content* and the *process* of how people think, integrative theories such as the affect infusion model (AIM; For-gas, 1995, 2002) seek to link the informational and processing effects of mood and also to specify the circumstances that facilitate or inhibit affec-tive influences on cognition and behavior. The AIM predicts that affec-tive influences on cognition depend on the processing styles recruited in different situations that can differ in terms of two features: the degree of *effort* and the degree of *openness* of the information search strategy they recruit. By combining processing quantity (effort) and quality (open-ness, constructiveness), the model identifies four distinct processing styles:

direct-access processing (low effort, closed, not constructive), *motivated processing* (high effort, closed, not constructive), *heuristic processing* (low effort, open, constructive), and *substantive processing* (high effort, open, constructive).

Affect infusion into thinking and behavior is most likely when constructive processing is used, such as substantive or heuristic processing. In contrast, affect should not infuse thinking and behavior when motivated or direct-access processing is used. The AIM also recognizes that affect itself has a significant influence on information-processing strategies, consistent with the assimilative–accommodative distinctions proposed by Bless and Fiedler (2006).

There are thus good theoretical reasons to predict that affect has a significant influence on cognition, motivation, and interpersonal behavior in everyday life, including the likelihood that negative affect also has important beneficial effects in some situations. We now turn to reviewing a range of experiments demonstrating just such effects on cognition, motivation, and behavior. These experiments typically employ a two-stage procedure, as participants are first induced to experience an affective state (e.g., using exposure to happy or sad movies, music, autobiographical memories, or positive or negative feedback about performance). The effects of induced affect are then explored in subsequent tasks in what participants believe is a separate, unrelated experiment. Experimental evidence for the adaptive benefits of negative affect are summarized in four sections, discussing the benefits of negative affect for (1) memory, (2) judgments, (3) motivation, and (4) strategic interpersonal behaviors.

MEMORY BENEFITS: WHEN BAD MOOD IMPROVES MEMORY

Recent experiments showed that more accommodative processing triggered by negative affect can produce a variety of cognitive benefits, improving memory, reducing judgmental errors, and improving communications. Memory—the ability to access previously encoded knowledge—is perhaps the most fundamental cognitive faculty (Forgas & Eich, 2012). Accurately remembering mundane, everyday scenes is a difficult and demanding task, yet such memories can be of crucial importance in everyday life, as well as in forensic and legal practice (Loftus, 1979; Neisser, 1982). Negative mood, by recruiting a more accommodative and externally focused processing style, should result in improved memory performance. This expectation was investigated in a realistic field experiment in a small suburban shop (Forgas, Goldenberg & Unkelbach, 2009). We were curious as to whether happy and sad people might remember differently a number of

small unusual objects (little trinkets, toys, Matchbox cars, etc.) that we placed near the checkout counter.

Mood was induced naturally, by carrying out the experiment on both cold, rainy, and unpleasant days (negative affect) and bright, sunny, warm days (pleasant affect; Schwarz & Clore, 1988). The mood effects of the weather were further reinforced by playing sad and depressing or cheerful and upbeat tunes within the store. We surreptitiously observed customers to make sure that they did spend enough time in front of the checkout counter to get a chance to see the objects we displayed. After they left the shop, a young female research assistant approached them and asked them to try to remember as many of the little trinkets they saw in the store as possible (cued recall task), and they also completed a recognition measure (Forgas et al., 2009). As expected, people in a slightly negative mood (on rainy days and exposed to sad music) had significantly better memory for the objects they saw in the shop than did happy people questioned on a bright, sunny day (see Figure 1.1). Thus it seems that mild, natural moods indeed have an effect on memory accuracy, with negative mood improving memory, consistent with the assimilative–accommodative processing model.

Eyewitness Accuracy

Remembering the details of everyday scenes is a fragile process that is often influenced by what people pay attention to, as well as by contamination by subsequent incorrect information (Fiedler et al., 1991; Loftus, 1979; Wells & Loftus, 2003). For example, misleading information obtained after the event can produce a false memory later on, the so-called misinformation effect (Loftus, 1979; Schooler & Loftus, 1993). Affective influences on eyewitness memory have received relatively little attention in the past (cf. Eich & Schooler, 2000), even though Fiedler et al. (1991) identified more than 20 years ago a need to examine "the mediating role of mood in eyewitness testimony" (p. 376). For example, more constructive and assimilative processing in positive moods may impair eyewitness accuracy by increasing the likelihood that misleading information will be incorporated into memories (Fiedler et al., 1991). In contrast, negative mood may constrain such distortions by triggering more accommodative processing and reducing the tendency to assimilate misleading information into the original memory (Forgas & Eich, 2012).

We explored this prediction in one experiment by first showing participants photos of a car crash scene (negative event) or, alternatively, a wedding party scene (positive event; Forgas et al., 2005, Exp. 1). One hour later, they were induced into happy or sad moods (after recalling happy or sad memories from their past in an ostensibly unrelated study) and then received questions about the earlier target scenes that either did or did not

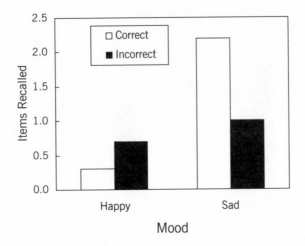

FIGURE 1.1. The effects of good or bad mood, induced by the weather, on correct and incorrect recall of items casually seen in a shop. After Forgas, Goldenberg, and Unkelbach (2009).

contain misleading, false information (e.g., "Did you see the stop sign at the scene?"—there was a yield sign, but no stop sign). After a further 45-minute interval, their memories for the target events were assessed. As expected, negative mood reduced and positive mood increased the tendency to assimilate misleading information into eyewitness memories. In fact, negative mood almost completely eliminated the common "misinformation effect" (Loftus, Doyle, & Dysert, 2008). A signal detection analysis confirmed that negative mood actually improved the ability to accurately discriminate between correct and false details.

We found a similar pattern in a subsequent experiment, in which students saw a staged but highly realistic 5-minute altercation between a lecturer and a female intruder (Forgas et al., 2005, Exp. 2). Misleading information was introduced 1 week later, when happy and sad eyewitnesses responded to questions about the incident that either did or did not contain false, planted information (e.g., "Did you see the young woman in a brown jacket approach the lecturer?"—the intruder wore a black jacket). We tested eyewitness memory after a further interval and found that those in negative mood while exposed to misleading information were less influenced by the planted details and retained more accurate eyewitness memory (see Figure 1.2), also confirmed by a signal detection analysis.

Interestingly, people seem unable to control this mood effect, even when explicitly instructed to do so. In a third study we showed participants videotapes of a robbery and a wedding scene. After a 45-minute interval,

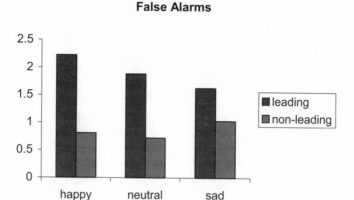

FIGURE 1.2. Mood effects on the tendency to incorporate misleading information into eyewitness memory (Experiment 2): Negative mood reduced and positive mood increased eyewitness distortions due to misleading information (false alarms). After Forgas, Vargas, and Laham (2005).

they were induced into happy or sad moods using films and then received questions that either did or did not contain misleading information about the events. Even though some participants were explicitly instructed to control their affective states, exposure to misleading information reduced eyewitness accuracy for happy participants but not for participants in negative moods. These results establish that negative affect can improve memory performance, consistent with the assimilative–accommodative theory (Bless, 2001; Fiedler & Bless, 2001; Forgas, 1995, 2002) that predicts that negative affect recruits more externally oriented accommodative processing.

THE JUDGMENTAL BENEFITS OF NEGATIVE MOOD

Reducing the Fundamental Attribution Error

More attentive processing in negative affect could also improve the accuracy of social judgments, such as people's tendency to succumb to the fundamental attribution error (FAE). This "dispositional bias" refers to the common tendency by judges to infer intentionality and internal causation in observed behaviors and ignore situational causes. By promoting more accommodative processing, negative affect should reduce the incidence of the FAE by directing attention to situational information (Forgas, 1998a). In one experiment happy or sad participants were asked to read and make inferences about the

writer of an essay advocating a popular or unpopular position (for or against nuclear testing), which they were told was either assigned or was freely chosen by the writer (e.g., Jones & Harris, 1967). Negative affect did reduce the FAE, a pattern also confirmed in a follow-up field study. Participants feeling good or bad after seeing happy or sad movies read and made attributions about the writers of popular and unpopular essays arguing for or against recycling. Once again, those in negative affective states were less likely to make incorrect, dispositional inferences based on assigned, coerced essays.

We also found direct evidence for the predicted processing differences using recall data. Happy or sad participants again made attributions about the writers of freely chosen or coerced essays (Forgas, 1998a, Exp. 3), and their recall memories of essay details were also assessed as an index of processing style. Negative affect decreased the incidence of the FAE, and those in negative moods also had better memory for essay details, consistent with their more accommodative processing style. A mediational analysis confirmed that processing style was a significant mediator of mood effects on judgmental accuracy.

Negative Affect Limits Halo Effects

Negative affect may also reduce some common judgmental biases such as halo effects and primacy effects in impression formation. Halo effects occur because judges tend to assume that a person having some positive features is likely to have others as well. For example, people judge a good-looking person as having a more desirable personality, or perhaps infer that a young unorthodox-looking female is less likely to be a competent philosopher than a middle-aged male. In a recent experiment we used just this manipulation (Forgas, 2011b), asking happy or sad judges to read a one-page philosophical essay about metaphysics. We also attached a photo of the writer showing either a casually dressed young female in one condition or a tweedy, bespectacled older male in the other condition, expecting that the appearance of the "writer" might exert a halo effect on judgments. Those in negative moods were indeed significantly less influenced by the appearance of the writer than were judges in positive moods. Happy judges showed a far greater halo effect and evaluated both the essay and the writer more positively when the photo showed an middle-aged male (typical philosopher) rather than a young female (Figure 1.3).

Negative Affect Reduces Primacy Effects

Primacy effects occur when judges place disproportionate emphasis on early information when forming impressions and pay less attention to later

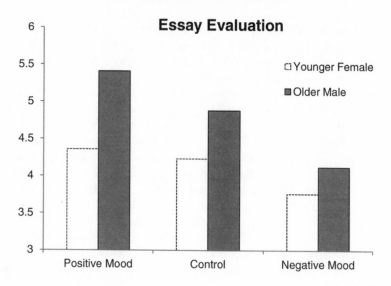

FIGURE 1.3. Mood moderates the incidence of halo effects on the evaluation of an essay: Positive mood increased and negative mood eliminated the halo effect associated with the appearance of the writer. After Forgas (2011b).

details (Asch, 1946; Luchins, 1958). First impressions are very important in many everyday situations, such as speed dating, job interviews, political communication, and marketing and advertising, yet little is known about how a judge's mood state influences primacy effects. Explanations of primacy effects emphasize cognitive mechanisms: People prematurely form a superficial impression based on early details and fail to process later stimulus information equally carefully and attentively. Primacy effects often disappear when every detail is processed equally carefully. As moods can play an important role in triggering qualitatively different processing strategies (Bless & Fiedler, 2006; Forgas, 2002, 2007), we predicted that primacy effects should be reduced by negative mood that recruits a more attentive, accommodative thinking style (Forgas, 2011a, 2011b).

Participants first received a mood induction (reminiscing about happy or sad events in their past) and then formed impressions about a target character, Jim, based on two descriptive paragraphs (Luchins, 1958). One paragraph described Jim as an extrovert, and the other paragraph described him as an introvert, and the order of presentation of the paragraphs was counterbalanced. We found a significant overall primacy effect, but negative mood completely eliminated this common judgmental bias. Conversely, primacy effects were consistently greater in those participants in positive moods (Figure 1.4).

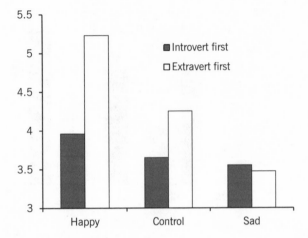

FIGURE 1.4. The effects of mood and primacy on the evaluation of a target person: Positive mood increased and negative mood reduced the primacy effect on evaluative judgments (vertical axis). After Forgas (2011a).

Negative Affect Improves People's Ability to Detect Deception

As negative affect seems to improve attention to stimulus details, it may also improve people's ability to detect deception (e.g., Lane & DePaulo, 1999). To explore this possibility, we asked happy or sad participants to detect deception in the videotaped statements of people accused of theft who were either guilty or not guilty (Forgas & East, 2008b). Those in negative moods were more likely to make guilty judgments, but they were also significantly better at correctly distinguishing between truthful and deceptive targets (Figure 1.5). Negative affect actually enhanced people's ability to correctly discriminate between deceptive and truthful targets according to a signal detection analysis, confirming the beneficial cognitive consequences of mild negative affect (Forgas & East, 2008b).

Negative Affect Reduces Gullibility and Increases Skepticism

Negative affect may well function as a general defense against excessive gullibility. Much of what we know about the social world is based on untested and potentially misleading information we receive from other people. How do we decide whether such secondhand information we receive in everyday life is trustworthy or not? Rejecting valid information as false (excessive skepticism) is just as dangerous as accepting invalid information as true

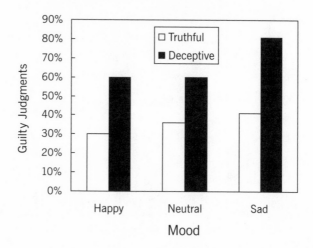

FIGURE 1.5. The effects of mood and the target's veracity (truthful, deceptive) on judgments of guilt of targets accused of committing a theft (average percentage of targets judged guilty in each condition). After Forgas and East (2008b).

(excessive gullibility). Several experiments suggest that negative affect has an overall beneficial influence on reducing gullibility and increasing skepticism. In one experiment happy or sad participants were asked to judge the likely truth of a number of urban legends and rumors, such as that power lines cause leukemia or that the CIA murdered John F. Kennedy (Forgas & East, 2008a). We found that negative mood increased skepticism and reduced gullibility, but only for new and unfamiliar claims. Presumably, judges already made up their minds about claims they were familiar with and simply retrieved those preformed judgments (direct-access processing), so their current moods had no influence on their judgments (Forgas, 2002). In a follow-up experiment we explicitly manipulated the familiarity of a variety of various ambiguous claims taken from trivia games. Positive mood increased gullibility, and negative mood again increased skepticism, consistent with a more externally focused and accommodative thinking style. In another experiment participants rated the likely truth of 25 true and 25 false general knowledge trivia statements and were also informed whether or not each claim was actually true. Two weeks later, after a positive or negative mood induction, only participants in negative moods were able to correctly distinguish between the true and false claims they had seen previously. Those in positive moods tended to rate all previously seen claims as true, confirming that happy mood increased and sad mood reduced their tendency to rely on the "what is familiar is true" heuristic. Thus negative mood confers a clear adaptive advantage by promoting a

more accommodative, systematic processing style (Fiedler & Bless, 2001) and more accurate discrimination between true and false claims.

Mood Effects on Truth Judgments

Evaluating the truth or falsity of information may also be subject to a number of heuristics, such as the "truth effect," in which cognitively fluent information is more likely to be judged as true than disfluent information. Subjective ease of processing, or *fluency*, is one of the most influential implicit cues people use in truth judgments. The experience of cognitive fluency itself is determined by a variety of factors, such as the familiarity, complexity, and clarity of the target information. Can positive affect increase and negative affect decrease the extent to which people rely on heuristic cues, such as fluency in their truth judgments? After an audiovisual mood induction (positive vs. neutral vs. negative films), participants judged the truth of 30 ambiguous statements presented with high or low visual fluency (against a high- or low-contrast background). Judges in neutral and positive moods rated fluent (presented with high contrast) claims as significantly more true than disfluent claims (presented with low visual contrast; Figure 1.6). However, negative affect completely eliminated this effect, demonstrating that affect can moderate people's reliance on fluency cues in truth judgments, consistent with Bless and Fiedler's (2006; Fiedler,

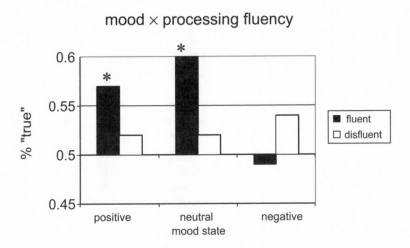

FIGURE 1.6. The interactive effects of mood and perceptual fluency on truth judgments: Negative mood significantly reduced the tendency for people to rely on visual fluency as a truth cue. Differences marked by an asterisk are statistically significant. After Koch and Forgas (2012).

2001) assimilative–accommodative processing dichotomy. Affective influences on truth judgments may be very important in real-life situations, as many such judgments (such as believing or disbelieving one's partner) occur in affect-rich contexts.

Judging Interpersonal Communication

One of the most difficult and demanding tasks in everyday social life is to decide whether a person is truthful or deceptive, and nonverbal expressions are notoriously hard to judge (Ekman & O'Sullivan, 1991; Jones, 1964). The same kinds of mood effects we identified previously may also influence people's tendency to accept or reject inherently ambiguous interpersonal communications as genuine or false. For example, when we asked happy or sad participants to judge the genuineness of positive, neutral, and negative facial expressions, those in negative moods were significantly less likely to accept facial expressions as genuine than were people in the neutral or happy condition. We also asked happy or sad judges to determine the genuineness of emotional facial expressions displaying the six basic emotions (i.e., anger, fear, disgust, happiness, surprise, and sadness). Once again, negative mood reduced and positive mood increased people's tendency to accept the facial displays as genuine, consistent with the more attentive and accommodative processing style associated with negative moods.

Negative Affect Reduces Stereotype Effects

Another common judgmental bias occurs when people rely on their preexisting stereotypes rather than valid individual information in responding to others (Bodenhausen, 1993). Can mood influence the implicit use of stereotypes? In one study we asked happy or sad people to generate rapid responses to targets who did or did not appear to be Muslims (visually identifiable by wearing a turban). Negative stereotypes about outgroups such as Muslims are difficult to assess using explicit measures, as people are unable or unwilling to reveal such prejudices. Implicit measures of prejudice, such as the Implicit Association Test (IAT), also suffer from serious shortcomings (Fiedler, Messner, & Bluemke, 2006). An alternative way to assess stereotype use is to employ disguised behavioral tasks that measure subliminal response tendencies (Forgas, 2003). For example, in the "shooter bias" paradigm (Correll, Park, Judd, & Wittenbrink, 2002) in which individuals have to shoot only at targets who carry a gun, U.S. participants show a strong implicit bias to shoot more at black than at white targets (Corell et al., 2002; Correll et al. 2007). We expected that Muslims might elicit a similar subliminal bias in a shooters' task and that positive mood should increase and negative mood reduce this reliance on their preexisting stereotypes.

We used a modified version of Correll et al.'s (2002) shooter game, asking happy or angry participants to shoot at targets appearing on a computer screen only when they were carrying a gun. We used morphing software to create targets who did or did not appear Muslim (wearing or not wearing a turban or the hijab) and who either held a gun or held a similar object (e.g., a coffee mug; see Figure 1.7). We found a significantly greater

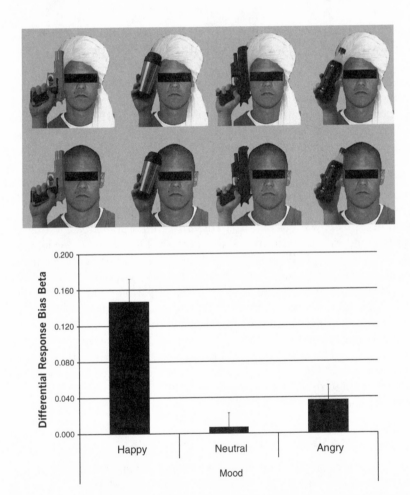

FIGURE 1.7. The turban effect: Stimulus figures used to assess the effects of mood and wearing or not wearing a turban on subliminal aggressive responses. Participants had to make rapid shoot–don't shoot decisions in response to targets who did or did not hold a gun and did or did not wear a Muslim headdress (a turban). Those in positive moods were more likely, and those in negative moods were less likely, to selectively shoot at targets wearing a turban.

tendency overall for participants to shoot more at Muslims rather than non-Muslims, but negative affect (induced anger) actually *reduced* this tendency. It was positive affect that increased a *selective* bias against Muslims, consistent with more top-down, assimilative processing that facilitates reliance on preexisting knowledge such as stereotypes in subliminal responses (Bless & Fiedler, 2006; Forgas, 1998a, 1998b, 2007).

MOTIVATIONAL BENEFITS: WHEN NEGATIVE MOOD INCREASES EFFORT AND MOTIVATION

To date we have looked at the cognitive benefits of negative affect. Considerable evidence now suggests that affect can also have a profound influence on motivation. In an influential paper, Clark and Isen (1982) suggested that positive affect can automatically trigger strategies designed to maintain and prolong a pleasant affective state: the *mood maintenance* hypothesis. In contrast, negative affect can serve as an evolutionary warning signal, automatically recruiting more effortful, attentive, and vigilant information processing and behavior, as a means of improving an unpleasant affective state: the *mood repair* hypothesis (Frijda, 1986). A similar idea was proposed by Schwarz (1990) in a *cognitive tuning* model suggesting that positive and negative affective states perform an automatic evolutionary signaling function indicating expected challenges and difficulties, motivating the organism to preserve or repair the affective state (Frijda, 1986). Thus feeling good can signal a safe, familiar situation requiring little effort and motivation to respond. In contrast, negative affect operates like a mild alarm signal, triggering more effort and motivation to deal with a more challenging environment. Thus negative mood, although unpleasant, may increase engagement and motivation. In contrast, positive affect may not only "feel good" but may also produce disengagement, reducing motivation and attention to the outside world (Forgas, 2007). Several experiments now provide support for such dichotomous motivational effects.

Negative Mood Can Increase Perseverance

There is a great deal of anecdotal and some scientific evidence suggesting that negative mood may sometimes trigger greater effort than positive affect (Clark & Isen, 1982). Any exertion of effort necessarily entails a fundamental psychological conflict. Although effort is costly and unpleasant in the short term, longer term success and gratification are unlikely to be achieved unless effort is extended. In one experiment we explored the possibility (Goldenberg & Forgas, 2013) that negative affect should produce beneficial motivational consequences and increase perseverance. In terms

of Atkinson's (1957) expectancy–value model, people should only engage in achievement-oriented actions if both the subjective probability of success (*expectancy*) and the incentive value of success (*value*) are high. As Feather (1992) suggested, the incentive value of the goal and the motivation to act depend mainly on the value attached to the desired end states, such as the anticipated hedonistic consequences of success or failure.

Hedonistic Discounting

If a person is already in a positive affective state, this may result in the *discounting* of the hedonistic value of expected future success, reducing perseverance and motivation (*hedonistic discounting*). In contrast, present negative affect may result in a higher evaluation of the expected hedonistic benefit of success on an achievement task, improving present effort and motivation. We decided to test the hypothesis that negative affect may actually increase the expected *value* of achievement and produce greater perseverance. Mood was induced by showing participants happy or sad films. Next, they were instructed to work on a demanding cognitive abilities task, comprising a number of difficult questions, for as long as they liked. Perseverance was assessed by measuring the total *time spent* on the task, total *number of questions attempted,* and total number of questions *correctly answered.* Expectancy-related and task-value beliefs were also assessed. As expected, participants in the positive-mood condition spent significantly less time working on the task compared with those in the negative-mood condition, attempted fewer items, and scored fewer correct answers (Figure 1.8). A mediational analysis supported the hedonistic discounting hypothesis, confirming that it was mood-induced differences in task-value beliefs that mediated mood effects on perseverance. These results are consistent with the theoretical prediction that negative mood may increase and positive mood decrease the motivation to persevere on effortful and demanding tasks.

Negative Affect Reduces Self-Handicapping

Negative affect may also improve motivation by reducing counterproductive strategies such as self-handicapping. Self-handicapping, first investigated by Jones and Berglas (1978), occurs when people create artificial handicaps for themselves as a means of protecting themselves from the damaging attributions they expect after failure. We hypothesized that self-handicapping might also serve a secondary purpose: to preserve a pleasant affective state. We investigated mood effects on people's tendency to *self-handicap* and create artificial hindrances for themselves (Alter & Forgas, 2007). Based on recent affect theories (Forgas & Eich, 2012), we predicted

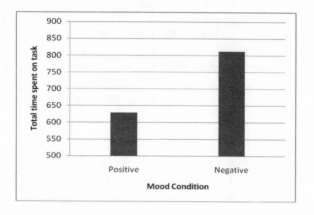

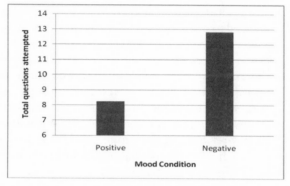

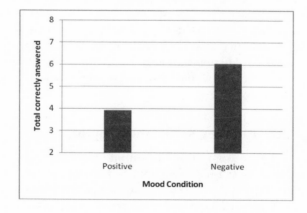

FIGURE 1.8. Positive affect reduces perseverance: The effects of induced mood on (top) the time spent (in seconds) on persevering with a cognitive abilities task, (middle) the number of tasks attempted, and (bottom) the number of questions correctly answered. After Goldenberg and Forgas (2013).

that positive mood should increase and negative mood decrease such defensive self-handicapping behaviors. Participants first received feedback about their performance on a task of "cognitive abilities," leading some of them to doubt their ability to do well on this task that they expected to perform again later in the experiment. They then underwent a positive, neutral, or negative mood induction using videos. Self-handicapping was assessed in terms of their subsequent decision in what they thought was an unrelated task to (1) drink a performance-enhancing or a performance-inhibiting herbal tea and (2) use the available time to engage or not engage in performance-enhancing cognitive practice.

When participants had reason to doubt their ability to perform well on a subsequent task, positive affect significantly increased their defensive tendency to self-handicap on *both* measures: Happy persons preferred the performance-inhibiting tea and engaged in less task-relevant practice (Figure 1.9). In contrast, negative affect reduced self-handicapping, consistent with those in a negative mood placing higher value on the expected hedonic benefits of succeeding in the task.

Given the pervasive role of affect in achievement outcomes, it is surprising that the influence of moods on perseverance and self-handicapping had received little prior attention. As predicted by the hedonistic discounting hypothesis, feeling happy may compromise the desire to work hard to obtain further hedonistic benefits. The beneficial consequences of negative affect on achievement may be particularly important in organizational settings, in which the presumed universal benefits of positive affect has

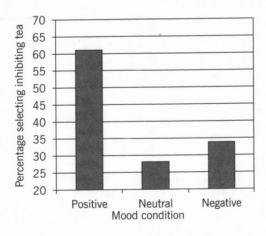

FIGURE 1.9. The effects of induced mood on self-handicapping: Percentage of participants who selected the performance-impairing tea as a function of mood condition. After Alter and Forgas (2007).

received almost exclusive emphasis in the past (Forgas & George, 2001). It now appears that in some circumstances, negative affect may deliver greater perseverance and a reduction in dysfunctional self-handicapping behaviors (Alter & Forgas, 2007; Goldenberg & Forgas, 2013).

INTERPERSONAL BENEFITS: CAN SAD MOOD MAKE YOU A NICER AND MORE EFFECTIVE PERSON?

One of the possible benefits of sad mood may have to do with its interpersonal functions. Evolutionary psychologists, puzzled by the ubiquity of dysphoria, have speculated that sad mood may provide hidden social benefits by possibly arousing interpersonal sympathy and reducing the likelihood of interpersonal challenges and competition (Forgas, Haselton, & von Hippel, 2007; Tooby & Cosmides, 1992). More recent work demonstrated a number of further interpersonal benefits. As *homo sapiens* is an extremely gregarious species, coordinating our interpersonal strategies presents a demanding cognitive task that requires open, constructive thinking. According to the AIM, affective states should have a mood-congruent influence on many interpersonal behaviors (Forgas, 1995a, 1999a, 1999b). Positive mood may selectively prime more optimistic, positive, but also more confident, assertive, and sometimes selfish behaviors. In contrast, sad mood should prime more pessimistic, negative interpretations and produce more cautious, polite, and considerate interpersonal strategies (Bower & Forgas, 2001; Forgas, 1995, 2002).

Thus, in situations calling for self-confidence and assertiveness (such as negotiation or self-disclosure), positive affect may confer distinct benefits (Forgas, 1994, 1998a, 2011c). We also found that female undergraduates who were feeling good after watching a happy film also communicated in a more positive way—they smiled more, disclosed more personal information, and generally acted in a more poised, skilled, and rewarding manner (Forgas, 2002). However, there is growing evidence that in other situations, in which more cautious and less assertive behavior is appropriate, it may be sad mood that produces real interpersonal benefits.

When Temporary Sadness Improves Politeness: Mood Effects on Request Strategies

Requesting is a complex communicative task that is characterized by uncertainty and typically requires open, elaborate processing. Requests must be formulated with just the right degree of assertiveness versus politeness so as to maximize compliance without risking giving offense. Whereas positive mood may prime a more optimistic and confident interpretation of the

request situation and thus produce a more assertive and less polite requesting style, sad mood should lead to more polite and considerate requests (Forgas, 1999a). This prediction is consistent with evidence suggesting robust mood-congruent effects on many social inferences and judgments (Forgas et al., 1984; Mayer & Hanson, 1995; Mayer, Gaschke, Braverman, & Evans, 1992). We found that when happy or sad persons were asked to select among more or less polite requests that they would use in easy or difficult social situations (Forgas, 1999a, Exp. 1), sad persons preferred more polite and happy participants preferred more assertive and impolite requests. Similar effects were found when happy and sad participants produced their own open-ended requests, rated for politeness and elaboration by trained judges. These mood effects on requesting were more powerful when requests were generated in a difficult rather than in an easy interpersonal situation and thus required more elaborate, substantive processing.

Similar mood effects on requesting also occur in real-life interactions. In one unobtrusive experiment (Forgas, 1999b, Exp. 2), participants first viewed happy or sad films. Next, the experimenter unexpectedly asked them to request a file from a person in a neighboring office. The participants' words when making the request were surreptitiously recorded by a concealed tape recorder. A subsequent analysis of their words showed that negative mood resulted in significantly more polite, elaborate, and hedging requests, whereas those in positive moods used more direct and less polite strategies (Figure 1.10).

Why do these effects occur? In uncertain and unpredictable interpersonal situations, people need to rely on open, constructive thinking to formulate their communicative strategies. Affect can selectively prime access

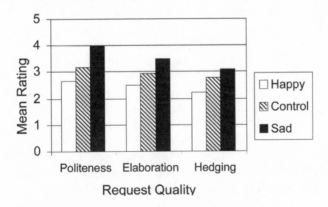

FIGURE 1.10. Mood effects on naturally produced requests: Positive mood increases and negative mood decreases the degree of politeness, elaboration, and hedging in strategic communications. After Forgas (1999b).

to more affect-congruent interpretations that will eventually influence behaviors. Of course, negative affect will not always result in more considerate and effective interpersonal strategies. Several experiments show that in some contexts, positive affect provides clear interpersonal benefits. For example, those in positive moods tend to be more effective and integrative negotiators (Forgas, 1998a), tend to respond more positively to requests directed at them in a natural setting (Forgas, 1998b), are better at managing interpersonal self-disclosure (Forgas, 2011c), and may be more effective in some organizational situations (Forgas & George, 2001). What I am arguing here is that these effects are not universal. In some situations in which more caution, tact, and consideration are required, it is negative rather than positive affect that seems to promote more effective interpersonal behaviors.

Negative Mood Can Increase Interpersonal Fairness

If somebody gave you a hundred dollars and your job was to divide the money between yourself and another person in any way you like, what would you do? How much would you keep for yourself? Selfishness versus fairness in situations such as these is a basic dimension of relating to others. A series of our experiments looked at mood effects on the levels of selfishness versus fairness that people display in strategic interactions such as the dictator game and the ultimatum game. Intriguingly, the possibility that affective states may influence interpersonal selfishness and fairness has received little attention in the past. Economic games offer a reliable and valid method to study interpersonal strategies such as fairness, selfishness, trust, and cooperation. These experiments predicted that negative mood might increase and positive mood reduce concern with the fairness of allocations.

In the *dictator game* the allocator has the power to allocate a scarce resource (e.g., money) between him- or herself and another person in any way he or she sees fit. In the *ultimatum game*, proposers face a responder who has veto power to accept or reject the offer. If rejected, neither side gets anything. According to classical economic and behavioral theories, rational actors should always maximize benefits to themselves as far as possible. Actual research suggests a far more intriguing and unexpected pattern. Instead of rational selfishness, proposers frequently offer a fair and sometimes an even split to others, suggesting that their interpersonal decisions are not simply driven by the desire to maximize benefits to themselves.

Affective state may influence such decisions in at least two ways. First, because those in negative moods tend to access more negative information, they might construct more careful, cautious, pessimistic, and

socially constrained responses. Thus positive affect should produce more confident, assertive, optimistic, and, ultimately, more selfish strategic decisions, and negative mood should result in more cautious and less self-ish allocations. Second, affect can also influence *processing tendencies.* As Bless and Fiedler (2006) suggested, negative affect may recruit more *accommodative,* externally focused processing, and positive affect tends to facilitate more internally focused, *assimilative* thinking. In terms of this model, negative affect should automatically promote *accommodation* to the external demands of fairness norms. In contrast, positive affect should recruit a more internally oriented, *assimilative* processing style, increasing selfishness in allocations.

In several experiments, we (Tan & Forgas, 2010) explored the effects of mood on the behavior of allocators in the dictator game, with happy or sad allocators dividing scarce resources (raffle tickets) between themselves and an ingroup or an outgroup partner. Happy players were significantly more selfish and kept more raffle tickets to themselves than did sad players. In a follow-up experiment, we used a different mood induction (affect-inducing films), and, rather than using a single allocation task, a series of 8 allocations were used to different partners, with the names and photos of partners displayed for each task to increase realism. Overall, those in sad moods were again fairer and less selfish and gave more points to their part-ners than did happy individuals, supporting our main hypothesis. Further, as the trials progressed, happy individuals actually became *more* selfish, and sad individuals became more *fair* (Figure 1.11).

Can such mood effects on fairness also endure in the more complex decisional environment faced by players in the ultimatum game, in which proposers must necessarily consider the willingness of responders to accept or reject their offers? We explored this question (Forgas & Tan, 2013) by ask-ing happy or sad participants to make allocations as proposers in the ultima-tum game. The latency of their decisions was also recorded as a measure of processing style. As hypothesized, those in negative moods allocated signifi-cantly more resources to others than did happy individuals, confirming the predicted mood effects on selfishness and fairness. These mood effects could also be directly linked to differences in processing style, as sad individuals took longer to make allocation decisions than did happy individuals, consis-tent with their expected more accommodative and attentive processing style.

If negative mood indeed promotes more accommodative and exter-nally oriented processing, we should find that responders in negative moods should also be more concerned with external fairness norms and therefore should be more likely to reject unfair offers. In the final experiment in this series (Forgas & Tan, 2013), the same procedure was employed as in the previous experiment, but this time all participants were "randomly" allocated to be *responders* rather than *proposers.* We found the predicted

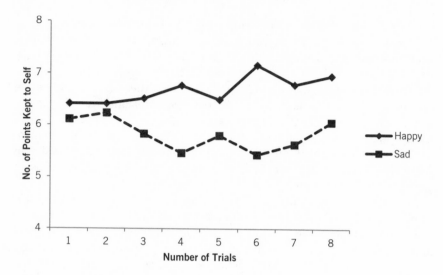

FIGURE 1.11. The effects of mood on selfishness versus fairness: Happy persons kept more rewards to themselves, and this effect is more pronounced in later trials.

significant mood main effect. Overall, 57% of those in negative moods rejected unfair offers compared with only 45% in the positive condition. Thus the tendency to reject unfair offers was consistently higher in negative than in positive moods, consistent with processing theories that predict that negative moods should increase and positive moods reduce attention to external fairness norms.

Paying greater attention to external information such as fairness norms when in a bad mood is also in line with recent findings showing that negative mood increases attention to external information and improves eyewitness memory, reduces stereotyping, increases politeness, and reduces judgmental errors (Forgas, 1998a, 1998b, 1999a, 1999b; Forgas et al., 2009; Unkelbach et al., 2008). These results further challenge the common assumption in much of applied, organizational, clinical, and health psychology that positive affect has universally desirable social and interpersonal consequences. Rather, our findings confirm that negative affect often produces adaptive and more socially sensitive outcomes.

Negative Affect Can Improve Persuasion and Interpersonal Strategies

Greater attention to external information in negative affect may also improve interpersonal effectiveness, such as social influence strategies.

One of the most ubiquitous influence strategies in everyday life is verbal persuasion. In order to get what we want from others, we typically rely on the medium of language to present as convincing a case as possible for a proposed view or action. Language represents a universal and highly flexible medium of social influence, allowing almost unlimited scope in producing an almost infinite variety of more or less effective persuasive strategies. Despite long-standing interest in how persuasive messages are processed by *recipients* (e.g., Bless, Mackie, & Schwarz, 1996; Eagly & Chaiken, 1993; Petty, DeSteno, & Rucker, 2001; Sinclair, Mark, & Clore, 1994), the question of how affect influences the *production* of persuasive messages has attracted far less attention (but see Bohner & Schwarz, 1993).

In a series of studies, I tested the prediction that accommodative processing promoted by negative affect should result in more concrete and factual thinking and better persuasive messages (Forgas, 2007). For example, participants received an audiovisual mood induction and were then asked to write persuasive arguments for or against an increase in student fees and for or against Aboriginal land rights. The arguments were rated by two raters for overall quality, persuasiveness, concreteness, and valence (positive–negative). Those in negative moods produced higher quality and more persuasive arguments on both issues than did happy participants. A mediational analysis showed that it was mood-induced variations in argument *concreteness* that influenced argument quality, with those in negative moods producing more concrete and informative arguments. In another study, happy or sad participants produced persuasive arguments for or against Australia becoming a republic and for or against a right-wing party. Negative affect again resulted in higher quality and more persuasive arguments (see Figure 1.12), consistent with negative mood promoting a more concrete processing style (Bless, 2001; Bless & Fiedler, 2006; Fiedler, 2001; Forgas, 2002).

In Experiment 3 the arguments produced by happy or sad participants were presented to a naive audience of undergraduate students whose attitudes on the target issues had been previously assessed. Arguments written by participants in negative moods were significantly more successful in producing a real change in attitudes than were arguments produced by happy participants. In a final experiment, happy and sad people directed persuasive arguments at a "partner" to volunteer for a boring experiment using e-mail exchanges (Forgas, 2007). Some persuaders were additionally motivated by the offer of a reward of movie passes if successful. Negative mood again resulted in higher quality persuasive arguments than did positive affect. However, offering a reward reduced mood effects, as predicted by the affect infusion model (AIM; Forgas, 1995, 2002). As the model suggested, mood effects on information processing—and subsequent social

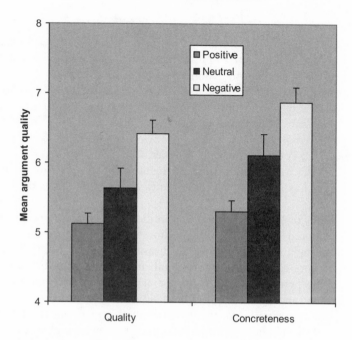

FIGURE 1.12. Mood effects on the quality and concreteness of the persuasive messages produced: Negative affect increases the degree of concreteness of the arguments produced, and arguments produced in negative moods were also rated as more persuasive. After Forgas (2007, Experiment 2).

influence strategies—were strongest in the absence of motivated processing. A mediational analysis again confirmed that negative mood induced more accommodative thinking and more concrete and specific arguments.

These experiments show that negative affect improved the quality and effectiveness of persuasive arguments because they contained more concrete details and more concrete and factual information. Such messages are seen by people as more interesting and more memorable. However, when motivation is already high, mood effects tended to diminish, as predicted by the AIM (Forgas, 2002). These results are consistent with negative affect promoting a more concrete, accommodative, externally focused information-processing style (Forgas, 1998a, 1998b; Forgas et al., 2005) that delivers marked benefits for the effectiveness of social influence strategies, such as persuasive arguments. Managing personal relationships involves a great deal of elaborate strategic information processing, and it is an intriguing possibility that mild negative affect may actually promote a more concrete, accommodative, and, ultimately, more successful communication style.

SUMMARY AND CONCLUSION

When considered jointly, the experiments reviewed here provide convergent evidence that negative affective states can provide distinct adaptive advantages in many everyday situations. These results are consistent with recent evolutionary theories that suggest that the affective repertoire of our species has been largely shaped by processes of natural selection and that all of our affective states—including the unpleasant ones—function as "mind modules" and can be shown to produce benefits in some circumstances (Tooby & Cosmides, 1992). These sets of findings stand in stark contrast with the overwhelming and unilateral emphasis on the benefits of positive affect in the recent literature, as well as in popular culture (Forgas & George, 2001). It is clear that positive affect is *not* universally desirable: People in negative moods are less prone to judgmental errors (Forgas, 1998b), are more resistant to eyewitness distortions (Forgas et al., 2005), are more motivated (Goldenberg & Forgas, 2013), are more sensitive to social norms (Forgas, 1999a, 1999b), and are better at producing high-quality and effective persuasive messages (Forgas, 2007). Given the consistency of the results across a number of different experiments, tasks, and mood inductions, the effects appear reliable.

Of course, we do not claim that negative affect is always beneficial or that positive affect does not have adaptive consequences in some settings. Clearly, intense, enduring, and debilitating negative affect such as depression has very negative consequences. We mostly looked here at the cognitive, motivational and interpersonal consequences of mild, temporary mood states of the kind that we all regularly experience in everyday life. Our findings are broadly consistent with the notion that over evolutionary time, affective states became adaptive, functional triggers to promote motivational and information-processing patterns that are appropriate in a given situation. Dealing with the demands of our social environment is necessarily a complex and demanding task that requires a high degree of elaborate processing (Forgas, 1995, 2002). The empirical studies presented here suggest that in many situations negative affect, such as sadness, may increase and positive affect decrease the quality and efficacy of cognitive processes and interpersonal behaviors. Much has been learned about the way affective states influence memory, thinking, and judgments in recent years, yet not enough is known about the evolutionary mechanisms that are responsible for the way we respond to various affective states.

ACKNOWLEDGMENTS AND NOTE

Support from the Australian Research Council is gratefully acknowledged. For further information on this research program, see the websites *http://forgas.social-psychology.org* and *www2.psy.unsw.edu.au/users/jforgas*.

REFERENCES

Adolphs, R., & Damasio, A. (2001). The interaction of affect and cognition: A neurobiological perspective. In J. P. Forgas (Ed.), *The handbook of affect and social cognition* (pp. 27–49). Mahwah, NJ: Erlbaum.

Allport, G. W. (1985). The historical background of social psychology. In G. Lindzey & E. Aronson (Eds.), *Handbook of social psychology* (Vol. 1, 3rd ed., pp. 1–46). New York: McGraw Hill.

Alter, A. L., & Forgas, J. P. (2007). On being happy but fearing failure: The effects of mood on self-handicapping strategies. *Journal of Experimental Social Psychology, 43,* 947–954.

Asch, S. E. (1946). Forming impressions of personality. *Journal of Abnormal and Social Psychology, 41,* 258–290.

Atkinson, J. W. (1957). Motivational determinants of risk-taking behaviour. *Psychological Review, 64*(6, Pt. 1), 359–372.

Bless, H. (2000). The interplay of affect and cognition: The mediating role of general knowledge structures. In J. P. Forgas (Ed.), *Feeling and thinking: The role of affect in social cognition* (pp. 201–222). New York: Cambridge University Press.

Bless, H. (2001). Mood and the use of general knowledge structures. In L. L. Martin (Ed.), *Theories of mood and cognition: A user's guidebook* (pp. 9–26). Mahwah, NJ: Erlbaum.

Bless, H., & Fiedler, K. (2006). Mood and the regulation of information processing and behavior. In J. P. Forgas (Ed.), *Affect in social thinking and behavior* (pp. 65–84). New York: Psychology Press.

Bless, H., Mackie, D., & Schwarz, N. (1996). Mood effects on encoding and judgmental processes in persuasion. *Journal of Personality and Social Psychology, 63,* 585–595.

Bodenhausen, G. V. (1993). Emotions, arousal, and stereotypic judgments: A heuristic model of affect and stereotyping. In D. M. Mackie & D. L. Hamilton (Eds.), *Affect, cognition, and stereotyping* (pp. 13–37). San Diego, CA: Academic Press.

Bohner, G., & Schwarz, N. (1993). Mood states influence the production of persuasive arguments. *Communication Research, 20,* 696–722.

Bower, G. H. (1981). Mood and memory. *American Psychologist, 36,* 129–148.

Bower, G. H., & Forgas, J. P. (2001). Mood and social memory. In J. P. Forgas (Ed.), *Handbook of affect and social cognition* (pp. 95–120). Mahwah, NJ: Erlbaum.

Ciarrochi, J. V., Forgas, J. P., & Mayer, J. D. (Eds.). (2006). *Emotional intelligence in everyday life* (2nd ed.). Philadelphia: Psychology Press.

Clark, M. S., & Isen, A. M. (1982). Towards understanding the relationship between feeling states and social behavior. In A. H. Hastorf & A. M. Isen (Eds.), *Cognitive social psychology* (pp. 73–108). New York: Elsevier-North Holland.

Clore, G. L., & Byrne, D. (1974). The reinforcement affect model of attraction. In T. L. Huston (Ed.), *Foundations of interpersonal attraction* (pp. 143–170). New York: Academic Press.

Clore, G. L., Gasper, K., & Garvin, E. (2001). Affect as information. In J. P. Forgas (Ed.), *Handbook of affect and social cognition* (pp. 121–144). Mahwah, NJ: Erlbaum.

Clore, G. L., Schwarz, N., & Conway, M. (1994). Affective causes and consequences of social information processing. In R. S. Wyer & T. K. Srull (Eds.), *Handbook of social cognition* (2nd ed., pp. 208–221). Mahwah, NJ: Erlbaum.

Correll, J., Park, B., Judd, C. M., & Wittenbrink, B. (2002). The police officer's dilemma: Using ethnicity to disambiguate potentially threatening individuals. *Journal of Personality and Social Psychology, 83*(6), 1314–1329.

Correll, J., Park, B., Judd, C. M., Wittenbrink, B., Sadler, M. S., & Keesee, T. (2007). Across the thin blue line: Police officers and racial bias in the decision to shoot. *Journal of Personality and Social Psychology, 92*(6), 1006–1023

Eagly, A. H., & Chaiken, S. (1993). *The psychology of attitudes.* New York: Harcourt Brace Jovanovich.

Eich, E. E., & Schooler, J. W. (2000). Cognition-emotion interactions. In E. E. Eich, J. F. Kihlstrom, G. H. Bower, J. P. Forgas, & P. Niedenthal (Eds.), *Cognition and emotion* (pp. 3–29). New York: Oxford University Press.

Ekman, P., & O'Sullivan, M. (1991). Who can catch a liar? *American Psychologist, 46*, 913–920.

Feather, N. T. (1992). Values, valences, expectations, and actions. *Journal of Social Issues, 48*(2), 109–124.

Feshbach, S., & Singer, R. D. (1957). The effects of fear arousal and suppression of fear upon social perception. *Journal of Abnormal and Social Psychology, 55*, 283–288.

Fiedler, K. (2001). Affective influences on social information processing. In J. P. Forgas (Ed.), *Handbook of affect and social cognition* (pp. 163–185). Mahwah, NJ: Erlbaum.

Fiedler, K., Asbeck, J., & Nickel, S. (1991). Mood and constructive memory effects on social judgment. *Cognition and Emotion, 5*, 363–378.

Fiedler, K., & Bless, H. (2001). The formation of beliefs in the interface of affective and cognitive processes. In N. Frijda, A. Manstead, & S. Bem (Eds.), *The influence of emotions on beliefs.* New York: Cambridge University Press.

Fiedler, K., & Forgas, J. P. (Eds.). (1988). *Affect, cognition and social behavior.* Toronto, Ontario, Canada: Hogrefe International.

Fiedler, K., Messner, C., & Bluemke, M. (2006). Unresolved problems with the "I," the "A," and the "T": Logical and psychometric critique of the Implicit Association Test. *European Review of Social Psychology, 17*, 74–147.

Forgas, J. P. (1979). *Social episodes: The study of interaction routines.* London/New York: Academic Press.

Forgas, J. P. (1982). Episode cognition: Internal representations of interaction routines. In L. Berkowitz (Ed.), *Advances in experimental social psychology* (pp. 59–104). New York: Academic Press

Forgas, J. P. (1994). Sad and guilty?: Affective influences on explanations of conflict episodes. *Journal of Personality and Social Psychology, 66*, 56–68.

Forgas, J. P. (1995). Mood and judgment: The Affect Infusion Model (AIM). *Psychological Bulletin, 116*, 39–66.

Forgas, J. P. (1998a). On feeling good and getting your way: Mood effects on negotiation strategies and outcomes. *Journal of Personality and Social Psychology, 74,* 565–577.

Forgas, J. P. (1998b). Happy and mistaken?: Mood effects on the fundamental attribution error. *Journal of Personality and Social Psychology, 75,* 318–331.

Forgas, J. P. (1999a). On feeling good and being rude: Affective influences on language use and requests. *Journal of Personality and Social Psychology, 76,* 928–939.

Forgas, J. P. (1999b). Feeling and speaking: Mood effects on verbal communication strategies. *Personality and Social Psychology Bulletin, 25,* 850–863.

Forgas, J. P. (2002). Feeling and doing: Affective influences on interpersonal behavior. *Psychological Inquiry, 13,* 1–28.

Forgas, J. P. (2003). Why don't we do it in the road . . . ? Stereotyping and prejudice in mundane situations. *Psychological Inquiry, 14,* 249–255.

Forgas, J. P. (Ed.). (2006). *Affect in social thinking and behavior.* New York: Psychology Press.

Forgas, J. P. (2007). When sad is better than happy: Negative affect can improve the quality and effectiveness of persuasive messages and social influence strategies. *Journal of Experimental Social Psychology, 43,* 513–528.

Forgas, J. P. (2011a). Can negative affect eliminate the power of first impressions?: Affective influences on primacy and recency effects in impression formation. *Journal of Experimental Social Psychology, 47,* 425–429.

Forgas, J. P. (2011b). She just doesn't look like a philosopher . . . : Affective influences on the halo effect in impression formation. *European Journal of Social Psychology, 41,* 812–817.

Forgas, J. P. (2011c). Affective influences on self-disclosure strategies. *Journal of Personality and Social Psychology, 100*(3), 449–461.

Forgas, J. P., & Bower, G. H. (1987). Mood effects on person perception judgements. *Journal of Personality and Social Psychology, 53,* 53–60.

Forgas, J. P., Bower, G. H., & Krantz, S. (1984). The influence of mood on perceptions of social interactions. *Journal of Experimental Social Psychology, 20,* 497–513.

Forgas, J. P., & East, R. (2008a). How real is that smile?: Mood effects on accepting or rejecting the veracity of emotional facial expressions. *Journal of Nonverbal Behavior, 32,* 157–170.

Forgas, J. P., & East, R. (2008b). On being happy and gullible: Mood effects on skepticism and the detection of deception. *Journal of Experimental Social Psychology, 44,* 1362–1367.

Forgas, J. P., & Eich, E. E. (2012). Affective influences on cognition: Mood congruence, mood dependence, and mood effects on processing strategies. In A. F. Healy & R. W. Proctor (Eds.), *Handbook of psychology: Vol. 4. Experimental psychology* (pp. 61–82). New York: Wiley

Forgas, J. P., & George, J. M. (2001). Affective influences on judgments and behavior in organizations: An information-processing perspective. *Organizational Behavior and Human Decision Processes, 86,* 3–34.

Forgas, J. P., Goldenberg, L., & Unkelbach, C. (2009). Can bad weather improve

your memory?: A field study of mood effects on memory in a real-life setting. *Journal of Experimental Social Psychology, 54,* 254–257.

Forgas, J. P., Haselton, M. G., & von Hippel, W. (Eds.). (2007). *Evolution and the social mind.* New York: Psychology Press.

Forgas, J. P., & Moylan, S. (1987). After the movies: The effects of transient mood states on social judgments. *Personality and Social Psychology Bulletin, 13,* 478–489.

Forgas, J. P., & Tan, H. B. (2013). To give or to keep?: Affective influences on selfishness and fairness in computer-mediated interactions in the dictator game and the ultimatum game. *Computers and Human Behavior, 29,* 64–74.

Forgas, J. P., Vargas, P., & Laham, S. (2005). Mood effects on eyewitness memory: Affective influences on susceptibility to misinformation. *Journal of Experimental Social Psychology, 41,* 574–588.

Frijda, N. (1986). *The emotions.* Cambridge, UK: Cambridge University Press.

Frijda, N. (1988). The laws of emotion. *American Psychologist, 43,* 349–358.

Goldenberg, L., & Forgas, J. P. (2013). *Mood effects on perseverance: Positive mood reduces motivation according to the hedonistic discounting hypothesis.* Unpublished manuscript, University of New South Wales, Sydney, Australia.

Jones, E. E. (1964). *Ingratiation.* New York: Appleton–Century–Crofts.

Jones, E. E., & Berglas, S. (1978). Control of attributions about the self through self-handicapping strategies: The appeal of alcohol and the role of underachievement. *Personality and Social Psychology Bulletin, 4,* 200–206.

Jones, E. E., & Harris, V. A. (1967). The attribution of attitudes. *Journal of Experimental Social Psychology, 3,* 1–24.

Koch, A. S., & Forgas, J. P. (2012). Feeling good and feeling truth: The interactive effects of mood and processing fluency on truth judgments. *Journal of Experimental Social Psychology, 48,* 481–485.

Lane, J. D., & DePaulo, B. M. (1999). Completing Coyne's cycle: Dysphorics' ability to detect deception. *Journal of Research in Personality, 33,* 311–329.

Loftus, E. F. (1979). *Eyewitness testimony.* Cambridge, MA: Harvard University Press.

Loftus, E. F., Doyle, J. M., & Dysert, J. (2008). *Eyewitness testimony: Civil and criminal* (4th ed.). Charlottesville, VA: Lexis Law.

Luchins, A. H. (1958). Definitiveness of impressions and primacy–recency in communications. *Journal of Social Psychology, 48,* 275–290.

Mayer, J., & Hanson, E. (1995). Mood-congruent judgment over time. *Personality and Social Psychology Bulletin, 21,* 237–244.

Mayer, J. D., Gaschke, Y. N., Braverman, D. L., & Evans, T. W. (1992). Mood-congruent judgment is a general effect. *Journal of Personality and Social Psychology, 63,* 119–132.

Neisser, U. (1982). *Memory observed: Remembering in natural contexts.* San Francisco: Freeman.

Niedenthal, P., & Halberstadt, J. (2000). Grounding categories in emotional response. In J. P. Forgas (Ed.), *Feeling and thinking: The role of affect in social cognition* (pp. 357–386). New York: Cambridge University Press.

Petty, R. E., DeSteno, D., & Rucker, D. (2001) The role of affect in attitude change.

In J. P. Forgas (Ed.), *Handbook of affect and social cognition* (pp. 212–236). Mahwah, NJ: Erlbaum.

Razran, G. H. S. (1940). Conditioned response changes in rating and appraising sociopolitical slogans. *Psychological Bulletin, 37,* 481.

Schooler, J. W., & Loftus, E. F. (1993). Multiple mechanisms mediate individual differences in eyewitness accuracy and suggestibility. In J. M. Puckett & H. W. Reese (Eds.), *Mechanisms of everyday cognition* (pp. 177–203). New York: Wiley.

Schwarz, N. (1990). Feelings as information: Informational and motivational functions of affective states. In E. T. Higgins & R. Sorrentino (Eds.), *Handbook of motivation and cognition* (Vol. 2, pp. 527–561). New York: Guilford Press.

Schwarz, N., & Bless, H. (1991). Happy and mindless, but sad and smart?: The impact of affective states on analytic reasoning. In J. P. Forgas (Ed.), *Emotion and social judgments* (pp. 55–71). Oxford, UK: Pergamon Press.

Schwarz, N., & Clore, G. L. (1988). How do I feel about it?: The informative function of affective states. In K. Fiedler & J. P. Forgas (Eds.), *Affect, cognition, and social behavior* (pp. 44–62). Toronto, Ontario, Canada: Hogrefe.

Sedikides, C., Wildschut, T., Arndt, J., & Routledge, C. (2006). Affect and the self. In J. P. Forgas (Ed.), *Affect in social thinking and behavior* (pp. 197–216). New York: Psychology Press.

Sinclair, R. C., & Mark, M. M. (1992). The influence of mood state on judgment and action. In L. L. Martin & A. Tesser (Eds.), *The construction of social judgments* (pp. 165–193). Mahwah, NJ: Erlbaum.

Sinclair, R. C., Mark, M. M., & Clore, G. L. (1994). Mood related persuasion depends on (mis)attributions. *Social Cognition, 12,* 309–326.

Tan, H. B., & Forgas, J. P. (2010). When happiness makes us selfish, but sadness makes us fair: Affective influences on interpersonal strategies in the dictator game. *Journal of Experimental Social Psychology, 46,* 571–576.

Tooby, J., & Cosmides, L. (1992). The psychological foundations of culture. In J. H. Barkow & L. Cosmides (Eds.), *The adapted mind: Evolutionary psychology and the generation of culture* (pp. 19–136). London: Oxford University Press.

Unkelbach, C., Forgas, J. P., & Denson, T. F. (2008). The turban effect: The influence of Muslim headgear and induced affect on aggressive responses in the shooter bias paradigm. *Journal of Experimental Social Psychology, 44,* 1409–1413.

Wells, G. L., & Loftus, E. F. (2003). Eyewitness memory for people and events. In A. M. Goldstein (Ed.), *Handbook of psychology: Forensic psychology* (Vol. 11, pp. 149–160). New York: Wiley.

Zajonc, R. B. (1980). Feeling and thinking: Preferences need no inferences. *American Psychologist, 35,* 151–175.

Zajonc, R. B. (2000). Feeling and thinking: Closing the debate over the independence of affect. In J. P. Forgas (Ed.), *Feeling and thinking: The role of affect in social cognition* (pp. 31–58). New York: Cambridge University Press.

2

Anxiety as an Adaptive Emotion

ADAM M. PERKINS
PHILIP J. CORR

Penetrating the mysteries of anxiety is a task that has challenged scientists and philosophers for centuries (Barlow, 2000; Corr, 2011). For example, in his book *The Concept of Anxiety*, the 19th-century philosopher Søren Kierkegaard portrayed anxiety as the root of humanity, informing us of our options and being central to self-knowledge and individual responsibility (Kierkegaard, 1844/1981). In recent decades, the discovery that anxiety disorders are the most prevalent of all psychiatric illnesses, affecting approximately 14% of the population at any one time (Wittchen, Jacobi, Rehm, Gustavsson, Svensson, Jonsson, et al., 2011), has lent new urgency to efforts aimed at understanding its causes. Although anxiety seems to have many paradoxical features (e.g., it often impairs performance), if Kierkegaard is correct, it is also useful, perhaps even crucial to human life.

Building on Darwin's (1859) hypothesis that our psychological attributes are shaped by natural selection in the same way as our anatomical characteristics, modern theorists have come to favor a functional account of anxiety as a phenomenon that evolved to facilitate avoidance of threat and the assessment of risk (Deakin & Graeff, 1991; Blanchard, Blanchard, & Rodgers, 1991). The purpose of this chapter is to assess the validity of this functional view of anxiety by reviewing findings from three domains of the scientific literature. First, we describe studies from applied psychology that

have explored the role of personality traits that reflect individual differences in anxiety proneness in influencing educational and occupational performance. Second, we describe the findings of studies that have attempted to explore a role for anxiety in human defensive reactions. Third, we evaluate a novel and emerging literature that investigates a possible role for anxiety in conscious awareness.

At the end of this chapter, based on our analysis of these three topic areas, we conclude that anxiety, once thought of as wholly negative and requiring "cure," instead evolved to serve useful adaptive, protective functions in humans, as in rodents. As a caveat, we caution that not all forms of human anxiety may be represented in rodents—there may well be truly human *angst*—but sufficient common ground is likely to exist between humans and rodents to make the study of basic, nonabstract, threat-related anxiety highly valuable in both species. Indeed, these more basic forms of anxiety probably form the necessary foundations of true human states of anxiety.

ANXIETY PRONENESS AND APPLIED PERFORMANCE

Study of the effects on applied performance of personality constructs that reflect individual differences in anxiety proneness has a long history in occupational and educational contexts. In correlational studies that examine the performance effects of anxiety proneness in isolation, results usually turn out to be inconclusive, showing either no effect or contradictory effects in which high levels of anxiety proneness appear to harm performance in some applied settings and benefit it in others (Barrick & Mount, 1991; Salgado, 1997). However, in studies that have examined the interaction of anxiety proneness and intelligence in determining performance, a clearer picture emerges. These studies show that a combination of high anxiety proneness and low intelligence typically leads to low performance but that high anxiety proneness combined with high intelligence usually allows performance to reach adequate levels, or even allows it to be boosted beyond the levels attained by equally intelligent but less anxiety-prone individuals. In this regard, there is an apparent strong complementarity between emotional and cognitive processes.

One of the first publications to examine systematically the possibility that anxiety proneness and intelligence combine to influence applied performance was Eliot Slater's (1943) article investigating the psychological makeup of 2,000 soldiers invalided out of the British Army for psychiatric reasons during the first 2 years of World War II. These soldiers were labeled as "neurotic," a personality profile characterized by Slater chiefly

as representing proneness to experiencing negative emotions, such as anxiety, hysteria, depression, and hypochondria. In this seminal work, Slater concluded that soldiers who combined the neurotic personality profile with inadequate intelligence were at especially high risk of psychological breakdown compared with soldiers who were neurotic but with adequate intelligence or those with low intelligence but an emotionally stable, nonneurotic personality type. In his 1947 book *The Dimensions of Personality*, also based on research with psychiatric invalids from the British Army, Hans Eysenck extended this work by outlining a hypothetical mechanism for the interaction between anxiety proneness and intelligence: "army training imposes a considerable stress on the dull person, who may find difficulties in understanding and following instructions; this strain may lead to breakdown in persons constitutionally disposed towards neuroticism" (Eysenck, 1947, p. 112).

Understanding of personality has advanced considerably since the 1940s, chiefly by replacing ideas of personality types with the notion that personality is best described by a small number of continua or dimensions, on which each person possesses a score. Consequently, older ideas of the neurotic type have been replaced in most modern personality models with a dimension that reflects proneness to anxiety. Arguments persist about the labeling and precise content of this personality dimension, and it is variously dubbed *trait anxiety, neuroticism,* or (in reverse) *emotional stability,* but regardless of semantics it can be accepted that people scoring at the upper end of the dimension tend, among other manifestations, to ruminate a lot (specifically about negative events: worry) and people at the low end do not. This is not simply cognitive overactivity but defensively oriented cognition (Ormel et al., 2013). This broad consensus has allowed the accumulation of research findings relating this construct to applied performance. For example, Spielberger (1966) found that although students scoring high on anxiety proneness tended, on average, to show lower academic performance than those who scored low on anxiety proneness, performance was not correlated with anxiety proneness in the students in the top 20% in intelligence. Moreover, in the students above the 95th percentile in intelligence, the best performers were those with high scores on anxiety proneness. (For other examples, see Norem, Chapter 11, this volume.)

This pattern of findings has since been replicated with varying degrees of fidelity in other applied settings. For example, Corr and Gray (1995) studied the effects of intelligence and personality on performance in 196 financial services salespeople, revealing that sales success correlated positively with a negative attributional style (an aspect of neuroticism linked to a pessimistic, depressive, self-critical attitude), but only in the more intelligent salespeople—presumably, they were better able to make sense of and use the critical feedback they received from potential customers (e.g., using

superior sales strategies to overcome objections). Similarly, Perkins and Corr (2005) investigated the effects of anxiety proneness and intelligence on job performance in 68 managers from a range of functional areas in a global securities company within a larger U.K. financial institution. This study revealed that, in the more intelligent managers, anxiety proneness was positively correlated with performance but that, as intelligence declined across the sample, this relationship disappeared. Mellanby and Zimdars (2011) obtained a partial replication of this interaction in an educational context, finding that, in 383 students, scores on anxiety proneness were higher in students obtaining the highest level of university degree compared with those obtaining the second highest level. However, this result reached statistical significance only in female undergraduates.

Applied studies outside an academic or office environment have further supported the notion that anxiety proneness interacts with intelligence to influence performance but have suggested a slightly different pattern for the interaction under these circumstances. For example, Perkins and Corr (2006a) studied the effects of personality and intelligence on the performance of 669 British military officer candidates as they underwent a 3-day officer-selection assessment. This assessment process is deliberately designed to be highly stressful and physically demanding in an effort to reveal those who could (or could not) cope with the demands of combat leadership. This investigation found that performance ratings were negatively correlated with neuroticism scores in the less intelligent officer candidates, whereas in the more intelligent individuals, neuroticism scores were uncorrelated with performance. Because the officer candidates were volunteers, not conscripts, and required relatively good high school grades in order to attend the assessment, a degree of range restriction with regard to both intelligence and personality would be expected to reduce the effects of this interaction.

In an effort to explore the combined effects of anxiety proneness and intelligence on military performance without problems of range restriction, Leikas, Mäkinen, Lönnqvist, and Verkasalo (2009) conducted a longitudinal study of 152 Finnish Army conscripts during a 1-year-long basic training period. Because these participants had no choice but to join the army, they could be viewed as providing a more representative sample of the human population than that used by Perkins and Corr (2006a). Despite the differences in nationality and psychological makeup of their sample compared with the earlier British study, the analysis by Leikas et al. (2009) revealed a similar pattern of results: An interaction of intelligence and neuroticism predicted adjustment among the conscripts. This interaction showed that lower levels of neuroticism were related to better adjustment to military life (as measured by self-evaluations, superior evaluations, military passport evaluations, and number of sick days), but only among individuals

with low intelligence scores. In contrast, in conscripts with high scores on intelligence, neuroticism was unrelated to adjustment.

Viewed together, these latter studies suggest that, at least in military settings, the performance boosting effects of anxiety proneness in highly intelligent individuals that were seen in academic or office jobs have vanished. This pattern of results raises the possibility that the more physically hazardous a job is, the more anxiety free the personalities of good performers must be, regardless of their intelligence. Some evidence exists to support this idea, as people employed in hazardous occupations (police officers, firefighters, electrical engineers, airline pilots, and flight attendants) have been found to be less apprehensive, less tense, less imaginative, and more emotionally stable than people employed in five nonhazardous occupations (janitors, nuns, priests, forepersons, and artists; Cattell, Eber, & Tatsuoka, 1970). In a study of 101 British Army officer cadets, it was found that fear proneness was negatively correlated with combat judgment in simulations of battle situations (Perkins, Kemp & Corr, 2007). Bomb disposal operators are significantly less neurotic than the general population, and the most successful operators are significantly less neurotic than their less successful colleagues (Hallam & Rachman, 1980). Moreover, military pilot applicants as a group score significantly lower on neuroticism than the general population, and those pilot cadets that pass training to become fully fledged combat aviators are even less neurotic than their peers already low in neuroticism (Bartram & Dale, 1982). This latter finding seems to be a product of the additional hazardousness specific to military aviation rather than of flying per se, as civilian amateur pilots are much closer to the general population norms in terms of average neuroticism scores than their military counterparts (Bartram, 1995).

In conclusion, these studies suggest that high levels of anxiety proneness do boost applied performance in intellectually demanding, desk-based activities, but only in relatively intelligent individuals. The more physically hazardous the situation, the more detrimental high levels of anxiety proneness become to applied performance, until a point of extreme dangerousness is reached (as with bomb disposal officer or military pilot roles) at which even high levels of intelligence cannot buffer the detrimental effects of high levels of anxiety proneness. Although the precise causal reason for these divergent patterns of effects has not been tested, one obvious possibility is that in cerebral, desk-based roles, with no element of physical hazard and in which employees have the luxury of making decisions over a period of hours, days, or even weeks, the high levels of rumination that are displayed by highly anxiety-prone individuals may increase the quality of decision making when combined with high intelligence. Additionally, in less frantic and/or dangerous roles, intelligent but highly anxiety-prone individuals may have the time to invent and apply anxiety management

co those taught in the cognitive-behavioral therapy clinic. self anxiety management process has been documented in cessful, intelligent but anxiety-prone individuals such as Sir urchill (Wilson, 1966; see Perkins & Corr, 2006a).

ively hazardous jobs, such as piloting a jet fighter plane, in which high. kes decisions must be made under extreme second-by-second time pressure (e.g., whether to destroy a target that may be friend or foe), the same rumination process is unlikely to be advantageous, as it would slow decision making to the point at which the job cannot be performed adequately. In addition, it is plausible that the time required to apply cognitive strategies that can reduce anxiety is not available when in a cockpit of a fighter jet on active duty.

ANXIETY AND HUMAN DEFENSIVE REACTIONS

The difficulty that highly anxiety-prone individuals, however intelligent they may be, have in performing adequately in highly hazardous jobs, such as bomb disposal or combat flying, suggests circumstantially that anxiety is elicited primarily by threat. Given that personality constructs reflecting individual differences in anxiety proneness have a substantial genetic basis (Bouchard, 1994; Plomin, DeFries, McClearn, & McGuffin, 2008), it would appear that the brain systems mediating anxiety are the products of natural selection and, therefore, that anxiety evolved as a threat response. This idea is widely supported by rodent findings (Blanchard & Blanchard, 2008) but has only begun to be explored scientifically in humans recently using paradigms that index responses to threat.

The origins of these human defense studies lie in rodent experiments that show that drugs with clinical effectiveness against anxiety disorders systematically alter the innate defensive reactions of rodents (e.g., Blanchard, Blanchard, Tom, & Rodgers 1990). The use of threat-naive rodent subjects in these experiments verifies the idea that anxiety is an evolved reaction to threat that serves as a psychological prompt to avoid harm, as it suggests that behavior is innate and not learned (Blanchard & Blanchard, 2008). In the case of humans, this adaptive defensive explanation for anxiety has considerable heuristic promise, as it allows anxiety-related illness to be viewed as reflecting alterations in defensive brain systems. Similarly, personality traits associated with anxiety proneness can be readily explained as reflecting individual differences in the reactivity of these defensive brain systems. However, there are long-standing concerns that rodent models of psychological processes are too simple to apply in humans (Matthews, 2008): For example, there is no evidence that rodents experience anxiety of an abstract type related to existential issues, whereas

historical and literary accounts abundantly point to the existence of such angst in humans. Concerns of this type have raised a need for studies of human defense that can test the validity of the defensive explanation for anxiety in humans.

The first step toward the experimental study of human defense was made using a threat scenario questionnaire (Blanchard, Hynd, Minke, Minemoto, & Blanchard, 2001) in which participants were presented with 12 situations containing different types of threat (modeled on typical animal paradigms) and were asked to choose a response from a list of 10 plausible options (modeled on typical animal defensive reactions). This study showed that human responses to threat are patterned in a similar manner to those of rodents, with ambiguously threatening stimuli, such as suspicious noises, eliciting risk assessment and clear threats, such as the presence of a predator, eliciting more explosive or intense responses (e.g., fight and flight). This finding was replicated and extended by a study examining the effect of human personality on threat responses (Perkins & Corr, 2006b), which revealed that the tendency to select a flight response was positively correlated with scores on the Fear Survey Schedule (FSS; Wolpe & Lang, 1977).

This latter questionnaire was originally created to measure phobic change under therapy but has been recognized subsequently as a useful measure of trait individual differences in sensitivity to aversive or threatening stimuli (e.g., Cook, Davis, Hawk, Spence, & Gautier, 1992). The value of this questionnaire has been demonstrated in a human defense context by a recent study using the threat scenario questionnaire, in which participants were asked to rate each scenario for threat intensity before then selecting which defensive reaction they would deploy in real life (Perkins, Cooper, Abdelall, Smillie, & Corr, 2010). It was found that perceptions of threat intensity mediated the association between FSS scores and the tendency to select flight responses. This result indicates that the reason that high scorers on the FSS tend to select flight responses is that they perceive the threat scenarios as more intensely threatening than do average participants. Because scores on this same questionnaire have already been found to be correlated positively with neuroticism (e.g., Abdel-Khalek, 1988) and negatively with combat judgment in British Army officer cadets (Perkins et al., 2007), it appears that the FSS captures individual differences in responsivity to threat that plausibly make up one facet of human neuroticism.

These findings also touch on an interesting issue in the study of anxiety, namely, how it relates to fear. Correlational studies show that scores on questionnaire measures of fear proneness are typically only modestly correlated with scores on questionnaires measuring anxiety proneness, suggesting that, psychometrically at least, fear proneness and anxiety proneness may be separable (Gray & McNaughton, 2000; Perkins et al.,

2007). A distinction between fear and anxiety has also been found in facial expressions: Using an actor–observer paradigm, a facial expression posed in response to ambiguously threatening scenarios (Figure 2.1, image 1) was preferentially labeled by naive observers as representing anxiety, whereas a facial expression posed in response to clear threat scenarios (Figure 2.1, image 6) was preferentially labeled as representing fear (Perkins, Inchley-Mort, Pickering, Corr, & Burgess, 2012). This split of fear and anxiety depending on the clarity of the threat stimulus closely echoes rodent findings and the results of threat scenario studies (Blanchard et al., 2001), suggesting that fear and anxiety are functionally separable phenomena in both rodents and humans.

The nature of these functional differences between facial expressions for anxiety and fear plausibly relates to the difference in information gathering required by a situation that *might* contain a threat versus a situation in which the threat is already apparent. Thus the facial expression of anxiety contains environmental scanning behavior that is likely to aid the localization of an ambiguous threat. Based on this analysis, it is plausible that the anxious facial expression initially evolved by natural selection because it conferred a survival advantage in situations that contained ambiguous or potential threats and only subsequently became a social signal of anxiety. In contrast, it seems plausible that the fixed-gaze facial expression for fear might have evolved by natural selection as a response to situations containing a clear threat because it conferred a survival advantage by allowing the individual displaying it to gather a maximal amount of information about the threat so that an appropriate counterattack or other defensive maneuver can be launched. The fixed pattern of defensive reactions in relation to clear versus ambiguous threats is detailed by Gray and McNaughton (2000).

However, actual threats activate whole-body reactions, not just facial expressions, creating a need for human defense studies that investigate associations between anxiety and avoidance behavior as expressed by integrated bodily action—in this important regard, defensive reactions are "embodied." The systematic measurement of human defensive behavior is acknowledged to be ethically and practically difficult (e.g., Blanchard & Blanchard, 2008); however, some recent studies suggest that these problems can be substantially overcome by the use of computer-based measures of active avoidance behavior that use relatively innocuous, yet unpleasant, threat stimuli. The hand movements used to operate these computer tasks differ physically from archetypal mammalian avoidance behaviors, such as running, but appear to be mediated by the same defensive brain systems owing to their functional equivalence (i.e., both types of behavior serve to reduce threat). For example, Mobbs et al. (2007) examined the effects of threat proximity on brain activity by means of a task in which a cursor was pursued around an onscreen maze by a computer-controlled threat stimulus

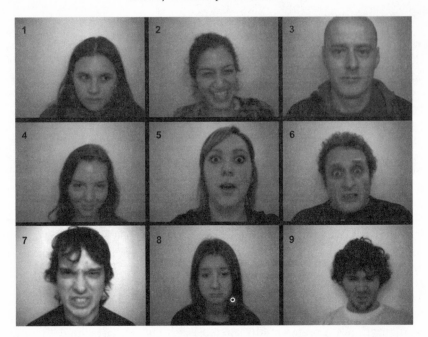

FIGURE 2.1. Facial expressions posed in response to emotive scenarios. Images 1 and 6 were posed in response to scenarios describing ambiguous threat and clear threat, respectively. Image 3 was intended to be an expressionless control stimulus. The remaining images were posed in response to scenarios intended to convey happiness (image 2), interest (image 4), surprise (image 5), anger (image 7), sadness (image 8), and disgust (image 9). Image 1 was preferentially labeled as representing anxiety, not fear or any other major emotion. Image 6 was preferentially labeled as representing fear, not anxiety or any other major emotion. From Perkins et al. (2012). Copyright 2012 by the American Psychological Association. Reprinted by permission.

that inflicted a mild but unpleasant electric shock to the participant if it caught up. The participants controlled the cursor by tapping direction keys with their fingers while their brains were scanned by functional magnetic resonance imaging (fMRI). Mobbs et al. (2007) found that, as the threat stimulus neared the cursor (i.e., threat intensity increased), brain activity shifted from the ventromedial prefrontal cortex to the periaqueductal gray. Because this pattern of change in brain activity was predicted on the basis of studies in nonhuman mammals (e.g., Fanselow, 1994), this finding suggests that, in humans, computerized active avoidance tasks engage the same brain systems that govern mammalian defensive behavior.

In order to conduct pharmacological tests in humans of associations

between anxiety and threat avoidance behavior, the joystick-operated runway task (JORT) was created, a computer-based translation of the mouse defense test battery (MDTB; Griebel, Sanger, & Perrault, 1997). The MDTB allows the systematic on-demand elicitation and measurement of defensive behaviors in mice and consists of two straight sections of runway each 2 m long, joined at each end by curved sections and surrounded by walls 0.30 m high (Figure 2.2A). A mouse is placed in the runway and exposed to an anesthetized rat held in the experimenter's hand, with its behavior being video recorded for subsequent scoring (in the wild rats are predators of mice, and so mice respond to the anesthetized rat as if it were a lethal threat; Nikulina, 1991). By fitting or removing a pair of temporary doors, the MDTB can be configured so that the mouse is either trapped in a closed section of straight runway or free to move along an endless runway.

In the closed-runway configuration of the MDTB, forward–backward oscillations are part of risk assessment and are conceptualized as indicating anxiety, and flight behavior in the endless runway configuration is conceptualized as indicating fear (Blanchard, Griebel, & Blanchard, 2003). These hypothetical behavior–emotion associations have been validated by drug studies: Forward–backward oscillations in the closed-runway configuration are preferentially altered by drugs that are clinically effective against generalized anxiety disorder (e.g., Stemmelin et al., 2008). In the endless-runway configuration, flight intensity (i.e., running speed) is preferentially reduced by drugs that are clinically effective against panic disorder, suggesting that this behavior indicates fear (Griebel, Blanchard, Agnes, & Blanchard, 1995). The JORT was specifically designed to retain the dual configuration of the MDTB (Figure 2B, 2C), so that the intensity of responses to threats of different threat situations could be separately measured, rendering it a plausible means of conducting a pharmacological dissection of human defense.

Pharmacological tests of the JORT have not supported the same clean distinction between anxiety and fear that appears to exist in rodents: Contrary to rodent results, the anti-panic drug citalopram exerted no significant effect on flight intensity in 30 human males (Perkins et al., 2009), but in line with rodent results, the same study found that 1 mg of the anti-anxiety drug lorazepam altered forward–backward oscillation during conflict. However, in a more detailed, multidose follow-up study, a higher dose of lorazepam progressively altered flight intensity, as well as oscillation, in a dose-dependent manner during goal conflict (Perkins et al., 2013). The capacity of lorazepam to alter human defensive behavior in two separate studies nevertheless suggests that anxiety and defensiveness are linked in humans and that activity in the brain systems that control perceptions of threat intensity are damped by this anti-anxiety drug. A genetic study of JORT responses provides additional support for a link between anxiety disorders and defense, as a candidate genetic risk factor for panic

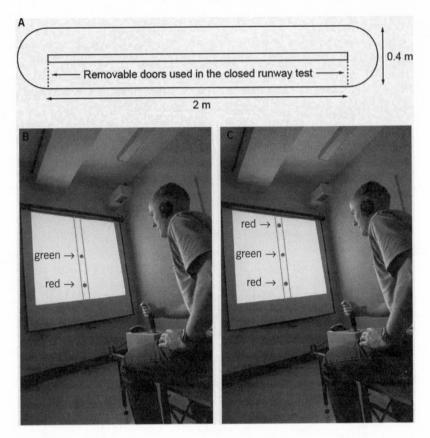

FIGURE 2.2. (A) The mouse defense test battery (MDTB). (B, C) The human translation of the MDTB, the joystick-operated runway task (JORT). A force-sensing joystick apparatus (PH-JS1; Psyal, London) controls the speed of a cursor (green dot) in an onscreen runway; the harder the joystick is pushed, the faster the cursor travels. In the one-way active-avoidance phase, this cursor is pursued by a single threat stimulus (red dot; B). Participants receive an unpleasant but harmless 115-dB white noise burst if the red dot collides with the green dot. The two-way active-avoidance phase (C) is identical, except that a second red dot travels ahead of the green dot at a constant velocity, causing a goal conflict whereby the participant has to travel fast enough to avoid the pursuing threat, but not so fast that he or she collides with the leading threat stimulus. From Perkins et al. (2013). Copyright 2013 by Macmillian Publishing Limited. Reprinted by permission.

disorder was found to intensify flight behavior in 200 healthy adult volunteers (Perkins et al., 2011).

The reason for the broader responsivity of human defensive behavior to this anxiety-reducing drug may have to do with the greater cognitive elaboration in human experimental volunteers: In this specific context,

participants know they will receive punishment at some point, and this may be enough to elicit mild anxiety that floods the whole testing session, regardless of the specific stage of the task (Davis, Walker, Miles, & Grillon, 2010). Thus the human defense findings, so far, suggest that the JORT may be viewed as a general measure of threat sensitivity rather than a tool for clean behavioral dissection of fear and anxiety—indeed, in the absence of a high intensity of fear elicited by an unambiguous threat, anxiety may always prevail in typical human experiments. Interestingly, the defense state of rodents modulates the effects of anti-anxiety drugs: When the animal is in a state of mild defensiveness and is already showing risk assessment behavior (such as when exposed to the odor of a predator), anti-anxiety drugs reduce risk assessment behavior, but when the animal is in a state of severe threat (such as when exposed to a predator), anti-anxiety drugs increase risk assessment behavior (Blanchard et al., 1991). As risk assessment is typically deployed at lower levels of perceived threat intensity than other defensive behaviors, such as flight, freezing, or defensive attack (Blanchard et al., 2003), this pattern of drug effects has been interpreted as suggesting that anti-anxiety drugs cause threats, in general, to appear less intense, moving the animal down the perceived threat intensity gradient that has prethreat behaviors at the bottom, risk assessment in the middle, and more intensely defensive behaviors, such as freezing, fleeing, or fighting, at the top (Blanchard et al., 2003). This analysis gives rise to the construct of perceived "defensive distance" (Blanchard et al., 1990). Different states of threat in rodents have been likened to personality differences in humans—a drugged rat being portrayed as analogous to a human with an anxiety-resistant personality (McNaughton & Corr, 2004).

ANXIETY IN CONSCIOUS AWARENESS

We can learn much about the adaptive value of anxiety by examining its pathological expression. This is especially true if we assume that anxiety has an evolutionary function. However, one of the main, but by no means exclusive, features of anxiety is its subjective nature—its experiential angst as represented in conscious awareness. Indeed, we could not say that someone was anxious unless he or she made a verbal complaint of it. In an attempt to explore the subjective experience of anxiety, Corr (2011) proposed a conceptual model of the different neural–behavioral levels of control seen in anxiety. This model sought to answer two questions: (1) What is the content of subjective awareness? (2) What might be its functions? It was noted that people with anxiety report ruminating about, specifically, bad events; their focus of attention is on possible bad outcomes, and they find themselves easily distracted. These features are often said to characterize

the person with anxiety as someone who is hypervigilant for threat with a negative cognitive bias. Though the target for treatment in patients with anxiety, these features highlight some of the positive aspects of anxiety, which, especially in nonpathological states, may be adaptive.

Corr's (2011) model, which builds on a more general model of consciousness by Corr (2010), argues that all behaviors (and thoughts, feelings, etc.) are automatically organized and executed without the immediate control of consciousness, which simply takes too long to be generated by the brain to have control over the events it represents. When everything is "going to plan," then we are not generally aware of events; it is only at critical junctures that psychological events enter conscious awareness, and these events tend to be ones that involve error, usually in the form of actual states of the world departing from expected states. For example, while driving a car we may brake suddenly and only *then* realize why this happened—that is, we are conscious of the error only *after* it has occurred and only after the brain has automatically organized the appropriate response. Corr's (2011) model assumes that stimuli associated with error signals enter conscious awareness and that they are replayed there for detailed analysis; and, after this analysis, the automatic neural–behavioral machinery that controls behavior at any given moment can be adjusted so that future behavior is more appropriate when the same set of stimuli, which led to the error signal, are encountered again. By this means, we learn from experience. This model is shown in Figure 2.3.

The model is built on an elaboration of the behavioral inhibition system (BIS; Gray & McNaughton, 2000). The BIS is responsible for the resolution of goal conflict in general (e.g., between approach and avoidance, as in foraging situations). Once activated, it generates the "watch out for danger" emotion of anxiety, which entails the inhibition of prepotent conflicting behaviors, the engagement of risk assessment processes, and the scanning of memory and the environment to help resolve concurrent goal conflict. The BIS resolves conflicts by increasing, by recursive loops, the negative valence of stimuli until behavioral resolution occurs in favor of approach or avoidance. Subjectively, this state is experienced as worry and rumination. The person with the associated personality factor is worry prone and anxious constantly on the lookout for possible signs of danger, a state that clinically maps onto such conditions as generalized anxiety, depression, and obsessive–compulsive disorder (OCD). In everyday life, we are comparing the actual state of the world against the predicted state, in which we are crossing a busy road, preparing to speak to someone, or simply walking down the street; thus the opportunities for detecting conflicts between goals, and thus the generation of related anxiety, are numerous.

This extended BIS model assumes that anxiety results from the

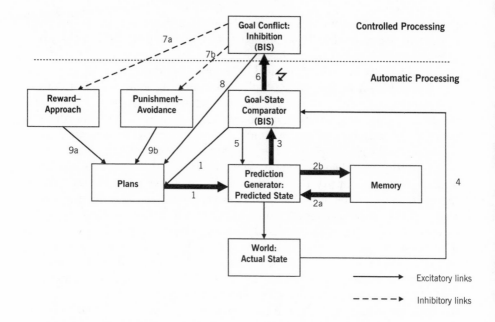

FIGURE 2.3. Information-processing diagram of the functioning of the behavioral inhibition system (BIS) in automatic and controlled modes, containing basic reward–approach and punishment–avoidance factors. Behavioral plans (Plans) lead to predictions (Prediction Generator; path 1) of future states of the world; the Prediction Generator receives input from path 2a and sends output to path 2b, stored previous experience (Memory). The BIS (Goal-State Comparator) receives input from the Prediction Generator (path 3) and then compares the response-reinforcement outcomes (World: Actual State) with predictions (path 4). Then one of two things happens: (1) "everything is going to plan," and the BIS Goal-State Comparator sends input to the Prediction Generator to continue the motor program ("just checking" mode; path 5); or (2) the BIS Goal-State Generator detects a mismatch between prediction and outcome and generates an error signal (path 6), which leads to activation of the BIS and controlled processes.

Once the BIS is activated, there is inhibition of the reward–approach system (path 7a) and the punishment–avoidance system (path 7b); and at this time the BIS initiates cautious behavior and risk assessment, which then inform Plans (path 8), which simultaneously receives input about current states from the Reward–Approach and Punishment–Avoidance systems (paths 9a, 9b), as well as input about the nature of the conflict from the BIS Goal-State Comparator (path 10). Plans initiate appropriate behavior, and the cycle is repeated until behavioral resolution is achieved in the form of avoidance or approach. To illustrate in relation to BIS and anxiety, bold lines highlight possible sources of dysfunction seen in anxiety states/conditions, which may include: (1) inappropriate plans (path 1); (2) inadequate prediction generation (path 3); (3) inappropriate retrieval/storage of information from/to memory (paths 2a, 2b); or (4) overactive BIS comparator (path 6).

detection of goal conflict, often involving aversive stimuli, which attract conscious, attentional, and controlled cognitive processing. In everyday life, this is highly valuable, but when extreme it leads to clinical anxiety. In the normal course of the day, the BIS works effortlessly and resolves conflicts without engaging conscious awareness; but where tried-and-tested strategies do not work, the full toolkit of cognitive analysis is brought to bear on the problem, and anxiety-related outputs are experienced. These processes might account for the interaction of anxiety and cognitive ability: A low capacity to analyze the stimuli associated with the generation of error signals will be less likely to resolve them, and future goal conflicts may result. In contrast, the more cognitively able individual has a larger cognitive toolkit and, therefore, is better equipped to resolve the goal-conflict problem.

Corr's (2011) model draws attention to the functional nature of anxiety processes, which allow for immediate and fast defensive responses, as well as delayed and slow deliberative processes designed to allow learning to occur that affects the next iteration of defensive behavior. In everyday life, the effects of these processes go largely unnoticed; however, when they are amplified by either external threat and/or heightened sensitivity of the system, then they are labeled problematic and, often, pathological.

CONCLUSION

Although it has long been suspected that anxiety is more than just a symptom of illness (Kierkegaard, 1844/1981), it is only relatively recently that substantial amounts of empirical data have accrued to show that anxiety has a positive, adaptive side, to do with keeping one safe. In this chapter, we have reviewed relevant data on three themes: the occupational value of anxiety, the defensive value of anxiety, and the value of anxiety as part of conscious awareness. All of these themes are unified by a further theme that runs through all of biology, namely evolution by natural selection (Darwin, 1859). By viewing anxiety in the context of natural selection, it can be seen that the subjective unpleasantness of anxiety is no barrier to its preservation, which acts on any attribute, however unpleasant, that aids survival and reproduction.

REFERENCES

Abdel-Khalek, A. M. (1988). The Fear Survey Schedule III and its correlation with personality in Egyptian samples. *Journal of Behavior Therapy and Experimental Psychiatry, 19,* 113–118.

Barlow, D. H. (2000). Unraveling the mysteries of anxiety and its disorders from the perspective of emotion theory. *American Psychologist, 55,* 1247–1263.

Barrick, M. R., & Mount, M. K. (1991). The Big Five personality dimensions and job performance: A meta-analysis. *Personnel Psychology, 44*, 1–26.

Bartram, D. (1995). The predictive validity of the EPI and 16PF for military flying training. *Journal of Occupational and Organizational Psychology, 68*, 229–236.

Bartram, D., & Dale, H. C. A. (1982). The Eysenck Personality Inventory as a selection test for military pilots. *Journal of Occupational Psychology, 55*, 287–296.

Blanchard, D. C., & Blanchard, R. J. (2008). Defensive behaviors, fear and anxiety. In R. J. Blanchard, D. C. Blanchard, G. Griebel, & D. Nutt (Eds.), *Handbook of anxiety and fear* (Vol. 17, pp. 63–79). Amsterdam: Academic Press.

Blanchard, D. C., Blanchard, R. J., & Rodgers, R. J. (1991). Risk assessment and animal models of anxiety. In B. Olivier, J. Mos, & J. L. Slangen (Eds.), *Animal models in psychopharmacology* (pp. 117–134). Basel: Birkhauser.

Blanchard, D. C., Blanchard, R. J., Tom, P., & Rodgers, R. J. (1990). Diazepam changes risk assessment in an anxiety/defense test battery. *Psychopharmacology, 101*, 511–518.

Blanchard, D. C., Griebel, G., & Blanchard, R. J. (2003). The mouse defense test battery: Pharmacological and behavioral assays for anxiety and panic. *European Journal of Pharmacology, 463*, 97–116.

Blanchard, D. C., Hynd, A. L., Minke, K. A., Minemoto, T., & Blanchard, R. J. (2001). Human defensive behaviors to threat scenarios show parallels to fear- and anxiety-related defense patterns of non-human mammals. *Neuroscience and Biobehavioral Reviews, 25*, 761–770.

Bouchard, T. J. (1994). Genes, environment, and personality. *Science, 264*, 1700–1701.

Cattell, R. B., Eber, H. W., & Tatsuoka, M. M. (1970). *Handbook for the Sixteen Personality Factor Questionnaire* (16PF). Champaign, IL: Institute for Personality and Ability Testing.

Cook, E. W., Davis, T. L., Hawk, L. W., Spence, E. L., & Gautier, C. H. (1992). Fearfulness and startle potentiation during aversive visual stimuli. *Psychophysiology, 29*, 633–645.

Corr, P. J. (2010). Automatic and controlled processes in behavioral control: Implications for personality psychology. *European Journal of Personality, 24*, 376–403.

Corr, P. J. (2011). Anxiety: Splitting the phenomenological atom. *Personality and Individual Differences, 50*, 889–897.

Corr, P. J., & Gray, J. A. (1995). Attributional style, socialization and cognitive ability as predictors of sales success: A predictive validity study. *Personality and Individual Differences, 18*, 241–252.

Darwin, C. (1859). *The origin of species by means of natural selection*. London: Murray.

Davis, M., Walker, D. L., Miles, L., & Grillon, C. (2010). Phasic vs. sustained fear in rats and humans: Role of the extended amygdala in fear vs. anxiety. *Neuropsychopharmacology, 35*, 105–135

Deakin, J. F. W., & Graeff, F. G. (1991). 5HT and mechanisms of defense. *Journal of Psychopharmacology, 5*, 305–315.

Eysenck, H. J. (1947). *The dimensions of personality.* London: Kegan Paul, Trench & Trubner.

Fanselow, M. S. (1994). Neural organization of the defensive behavior system responsible for fear. *Psychonomic Bulletin and Review, 1,* 429–438.

Gray, J. A., & McNaughton, N. (2000). *The neuropsychology of anxiety: An enquiry into the functions of the septohippocampal system* (2nd ed.). Oxford, UK: Oxford University Press.

Griebel, G., Blanchard, D. C., Agnes, R., & Blanchard, R. J. (1995). Differential modulation of antipredator defensive behavior in Swiss–Webster mice following acute and chronic treatment with imipramine and fluoxetine. *Psychopharmacology, 120,* 57–66.

Griebel, G., Sanger, D. J., & Perrault, G. (1997). Genetic differences in the mouse defense test battery. *Aggressive Behavior, 23,* 19–31.

Hallam, R. S., & Rachman, S. J. (1980). Courageous acts or courageous actors? *Personality and Individual Differences, 1,* 341–346.

Kierkegaard, S. (1981). *The concept of anxiety.* Princeton, NJ: Princeton University Press. (Original work published 1844)

Leikas, S. S., Mäkinen, S., Lönnqvist, J.-E., & Verkasalo, M. (2009). Cognitive ability × emotional stability interactions on adjustment. *European Journal of Personality, 23,* 329–342.

Matthews, G. (2008). Reinforcement sensitivity theory: A critique from cognitive science. In P. J. Corr (Ed.), *The reinforcement sensitivity theory of personality* (pp. 482–507). Cambridge, UK: Cambridge University Press.

McNaughton, N., & Corr, P. J. (2004). A two-dimensional neuropsychology of defense: Fear/anxiety and defensive distance. *Neuroscience and Biobehavioral Reviews, 28,* 285–305.

Mellanby, J., & Zimdars, A. (2011). Trait anxiety and degree performance. *Higher Education, 61,* 357–370.

Mobbs, D., Petrovic, P., Marchant, J., Hassabis, D., Weiskopf, N., Seymour, B., et al. (2007). When fear is near: Threat imminence elicits prefrontal–periaqueductal gray shifts in humans. *Science, 317,* 1079–1083.

Nikulina, E. M. (1991). Neural control of predatory aggression in wild and domesticated animals. *Neuroscience and Biobehavioral Reviews, 15,* 545–547.

Ormel, J., Bastiaansen, A., Riese, H., Bos, E. H., Servaas, M., Ellenbogen, M., et al. (2013). The biological and psychological basis of neuroticism: Current status and future directions. *Neuroscience and Biobehavioral Reviews, 37,* 59–72.

Perkins, A. M., Cooper, A., Abdelall, M., Smillie, L. D., & Corr, P. J. (2010). Personality and defensive reactions: Fear, trait anxiety and threat magnification. *Journal of Personality, 78,* 1071–1090.

Perkins, A. M., & Corr, P. J. (2005). Can worriers be winners?: The association between worrying and job performance. *Personality and Individual Differences, 38,* 25–31.

Perkins, A. M., & Corr, P. J. (2006). Cognitive ability as a buffer to neuroticism: Churchill's secret weapon? *Personality and Individual Differences, 40,* 39–51.

Perkins, A. M., Ettinger, U., Davis, R., Foster, R., Williams, S. C. R., & Corr, P. J. (2009). Effects of lorazepam and citalopram on human defensive reactions:

Ethopharmacological differentiation of fear and anxiety. *Journal of Neuro-science, 29,* 12617–12624.

Perkins, A. M., Ettinger, U., Weaver, K., Schmechtig, A., Schrantee, A., Morrison, P. D., et al. (2013, April 16). Advancing the defensive explanation for anxiety disorders: Lorazepam effects on human defense are systematically modulated by personality and threat-type. *Translational Psychiatry, 3,* e246 (online).

Perkins, A. M., Ettinger, U., Williams, S. C. R., Reuter, M., Hennig, J., & Corr, P. J. (2011). Flight behavior in humans is intensified by a candidate genetic risk factor for panic disorder: Evidence from a translational model of fear and anxiety. *Molecular Psychiatry, 16,* 242–244.

Perkins, A. M., Inchley-Mort, S. L., Pickering, A. D., Corr, P. J., & Burgess, A. P. (2012). A facial expression for anxiety. *Journal of Personality and Social Psychology, 102,* 910–924.

Perkins, A. M., Kemp, S. E., & Corr, P. J. (2007). Fear and anxiety as separable emotions: An investigation of the revised reinforcement sensitivity theory of personality. *Emotion, 7,* 252–261.

Plomin, R., DeFries, J. C., McClearn, G. E., & McGuffin, P. (2008). *Behavioral genetics* (5th ed.). New York: Worth.

Salgado, J. F. (1997). The five-factor model of personality and job performance in the European community. *Journal of Applied Psychology, 82,* 30–43.

Slater, E. (1943). The neurotic constitution: A statistical study of two thousand neurotic soldiers. *Journal of Neurology and Psychiatry, 6,* 1–16.

Spielberger, C. D. (1966). Theory and research on anxiety. In C. D. Spielberger (Ed.), *Anxiety and behavior* (pp. 3–19). New York: Academic Press.

Stemmelin, J., Cohen, C., Terranova, J. P., Lopez-Grancha, M., Pichat, P., Bergis, O., et al. (2008). Stimulation of the b3–adrenoceptor as a novel treatment strategy for anxiety and depressive disorders. *Neuropsychopharmacology, 33,* 574–587.

Wilson, C. M. (Lord Moran). (1966). *Winston Churchill: The struggle for survival 1940–1965.* London: Constable.

Wittchen H. U., Jacobi, F., Rehm, J., Gustavsson, A., Svensson, M., Jonsson, B., et al (2011). The size and burden of mental disorders and other disorders of the brain in Europe 2010. *European Neuropsychopharmacology, 21,* 655–679.

Wolpe, J., & Lang, P. J. (1977). *Manual for the Fear Survey Schedule.* San Diego, CA: Educational and Industrial Testing Service.

3

Anger Is a Positive Emotion

URSULA HESS

In many ways anger is the prototypical negative emotion. A look into Webster's *Thesaurus* provides a list of related words, which includes *animosity, antagonism, embitterment, enmity, hostility, malevolence,* and *virulence,* all of which refer to strife and destruction. This is also the sense in which Seneca in *De Ira* (*On Anger*) refers to anger: "Certain wise men, therefore, have claimed that anger is temporary madness. For it is equally devoid of self-control, forgetful of decency, unmindful of ties, persistent and diligent in whatever it begins, closed to reason and counsel, excited by trifling causes, unfit to discern the right and true—the very counterpart of a ruin that is shattered in pieces where it overwhelms" (On Anger, n.d., Book 1). And it is with this view in mind that anger is often equated with blind aggression and destruction. In this sense, Berkowitz and Harmon-Jones (2004) define anger as "a syndrome of relatively specific feelings, cognitions, and physiological reactions linked associatively with an urge to injure some target" (p. 108).

However, there is another side to anger as well. A side from which anger can be considered a positive emotion, at least from the perspective of the emoter. The first to remark on this was Aristotle: "since those who do not get angry at things at which it is right to be angry are considered fool-ish, and so are those who do not get angry in the right manner, at the right time, and with the right people. It is thought that they do not feel or resent an injury, and that if a man is never angry he will not stand up for himself;

and it is considered servile to put up with an insult to oneself or suffer one's friends to be insulted" (*Nicomachean Ethics*, n.d., IV.5).

From this perspective anger is a visible sign of strength and a signal that needed action to thwart insult to oneself or close others will be taken.

Obviously this does not imply that Seneca and those who focus on anger as a destructive force have it wrong. Anger can indeed and frequently does wreak great interpersonal havoc and destruction. Yet it is also important in this context to distinguish anger from hostility and aggression, with which it is frequently confused in common parlance. Hostility is a personality trait characterized by negative beliefs about and attitudes toward others, including cynicism and mistrust (cf. Miller, Smith, Turner, Guijarro, & Hallet, 1996). Aggression, in turn, refers to behavior that is intended to cause harm or pain and is often elicited by fear or dominance struggles (e.g., Berkowitz, 1993). And both hostility and aggression contribute to the negative reputation of anger.

This chapter focuses on the important positive side to anger. In what follows, I discuss the two aspects mentioned by Aristotle: anger as a sign of strength and anger as a force that leads to needed action.

In the first part of this chapter I discuss the role of anger as an approach emotion that leads to motivated action and, in the second, the role of anger as a sign of strength. In a third section I discuss the influence of individual differences in regard to these perceptions.

ANGER IS AN APPROACH EMOTION

The notion that anger leads to motivated action is inherent in appraisal theories of emotion (e.g., Frijda, 1986; Scherer, 1987) and finds support in research on anterior cortical asymmetries related to approach and avoidance (Carver & Harmon-Jones, 2009).

According to appraisal theories of emotion (e.g., Frijda, 1986; Scherer, 1987), emotions are elicited and differentiated through a series of appraisals of (internal or external) stimulus events based on the perceived nature of the event. A change in the (internal or external) environment is evaluated according to whether the event is pleasant or unpleasant (pleasantness), as well as whether the change is congruent with the motivational state of the individual or obstructs the individual's goals (goal obstruction). Individuals further evaluate their ability to cope with or adjust to the change (coping potential). A final set of evaluations regards the correspondence with the relevant social and personal norms, that is, how the event is to be judged in terms of ethical, moral, or social considerations (norm incompatibility). According to appraisal theory, each emotion is described by a unique pattern of appraisals. With regard to anger, there is some agreement that

none of these appraisals is necessary or sufficient for a given anger episode (Berkowitz & Harmon-Jones, 2004; Kuppens, Van Mechelen, Smits, & De Boeck, 2003; Parkinson, 1999). However, it is important to note that there is a vast "family" of emotions that all share core appraisals with anger but that differ in details (Frijda, Kuipers, & ter Shure, 1989). Along with anger, Frijda et al. (1989) studied rage, aversion, and annoyance, which also overlap to some degree with disgust and contempt, as all three have implications for moral judgment (Rozin, Lowery, Imada, & Haidt, 1999). Also, as mentioned previously, not all anger episodes can be described as "righteous" anger or as invoked by a clear injustice. Yet even the instances of "unreasonable" anger studied by Parkinson (1999) contain elements of goal obstruction, which seems the common theme for all anger events.

That said, a typical anger event can be characterized by a goal obstruction, blamed on someone else, which is perceived as unjust, combined with strong coping potential, resulting in a desire to act to remove the goal obstruction (Berkowitz & Harmon-Jones, 2004; Frijda et al., 1989). Averill (1997), from a different theoretical perspective, considers power to be an "entrance requirement" for anger. In this manner, anger mobilizes energy and focuses attention on redressing the appraised wrong (Roseman, Wiest, & Swartz, 1994). In this vein, Averill (1982) argues that certain levels of anger can be conceptualized as forms of problem solving, which are generally more beneficial than harmful. In fact, angry individuals tend to feel more energized and active (Frijda et al., 1989; Shaver, Schwartz, Kirson, & O'Connor, 1987) and tend to make more optimistic judgments and choices about themselves. The latter effect is mediated by appraisals of control and of certainty regarding the situation (Lerner, Gonzalez, Small, & Fischhoff, 2003; Lerner & Keltner, 2001). Berkowitz and Harmon-Jones (2004) add that in fact, once aroused, anger may contribute to this feeling of strength and provide the energy for the resulting action. In sum, anger arouses a strong motivation to correct a perceived wrong.

That anger is related to approach is also supported by research on left versus right hemispheric asymmetries related to emotional states. Early research in this domain led to the conclusion that the left frontal cortical region is involved in the experience of positive affect, whereas the right frontal cortical region is involved in the experience of negative affect (see Harmon-Jones, Gable, & Peterson, 2010). Yet more recent research supports the notion that left hemispheric activation is related to approach motivation and right hemispheric activation to withdrawal (Harmon-Jones et al., 2010). Because, by and large, positive emotions are associated with approach and negative emotions with withdrawal, anger proved to be an important element in this argument. Thus Carver and Harmon-Jones (2009) reviewed literature showing that anger is also associated with left frontal activation. This is the case both for trait (Harmon-Jones & Allen,

1998) and state (Harmon-Jones & Sigelman, 2001) anger. In the latter study, only individuals who were insulted showed greater relative left frontal activity, and this activity was correlated with both self-reported anger and a behavioral measure of aggression. In sum, this research supports the notion that anger leads to goal-directed action.

Anger as a Motivational Force for Justice

The role of anger in situations of injustice has also been studied from the perspective of moral emotions, that is, those emotions that are associated with moral transgressions. Haidt (2003) distinguishes between other-condemning emotions (contempt, anger, disgust) and self-conscious emotions. Other-condemning emotions are shown in response to moral violations by others. Their function is to motivate people to change their relationships with moral violators, whereas the function of self-conscious emotions is essentially to enable altruistic behavior and to avoid being the target of other-condemning emotions (e.g., Cosmides & Tooby, 2000; Frank, 1988).

Rozin et al. (1999) link the three other-condemning emotions to specific types of moral violations. Specifically, anger is linked to violations of autonomy, contempt is linked to violations of community, and disgust to violations of divinity. That is, anger is conceived of as an emotion employed to condemn violations linked to notions of justice, freedom, fairness, individualism, individual choice, and liberty.

Evolutionary psychologists posit that moral emotions—in particular, guilt and the other-blaming emotions, including anger—have evolved in the service of the regulation of altruistic behavior and, more specifically, to address the cheater problem in social groups (Trivers, 1971). Cheating is a serious problem because an individual who accepts resources but does not reciprocate adequately harms the group in the long run. Guilt, in turn, motivates individuals either to not cheat at all or to make amends. Conversely, when cheating is detected, it should elicit anger from the cheated. In sum, theories on the role of emotions in moral action converge to see an important role for anger in regulating social relationships in a way that fosters altruistic behavior and the maintenance of positive social relationships.

ANGER AS A SIGN OF STRENGTH

As discussed earlier, Aristotle noted that those who do not show the right anger at the right time are "considered servile to put up with an insult to oneself or suffer one's friends to be insulted." That is, such an individual lacks strength of character and maybe also the competence to show such strength. In this sentence, Aristotle blithely assumed that the expression of

anger in a given situation is indeed indicative of lasting traits of a person. Yet is this the case?

In recent years, the question of whether and how emotions serve as social signals has gained more and more interest (Hareli & Hess, 2012). In fact, when we encounter others, we rapidly and spontaneously make judgments about their personality (see, e.g., Kenny, 2004; Todorov & Uleman, 2002, 2003), and such judgments are often made on the basis of very little information (Ambady, Hallahan, & Rosenthal, 1995; Ambady & Rosenthal, 1992). One relevant source of information about the likely characteristics of others is, as suggested by Aristotle, a person's emotional reactions.

Emotions signal the behavioral intentions, values, and goals, as well as the resources, of a person in a given context. This notion is based on appraisal theory of emotions (Scherer, 1987), and the process of concluding from an expression to a lasting characteristic of the person has been described by Hareli and Hess (2010) as the "reverse engineering of appraisals."

A Model of the Reverse Engineering of Appraisals

As mentioned previously, appraisal theories of emotion posit that emotions are elicited by the spontaneous and intuitive appraisal of (internal or external) relevant stimulus events according to the perceived nature of the event (Arnold, 1960; Scherer, 1987). Importantly, appraisals relate to the subjective perception of the stimulus and not its objective characteristics.

Thus the mere fact that someone reacts with an emotion to an event signals that the event is relevant to that specific person, which in turn provides information about the person's goals and values. For example, the fact that a person reacts with anger to a perceived injustice signals that the person cares about this fact. When such a relevant change in the environment is detected by an organism, it is evaluated according to whether it is pleasant or unpleasant and to what degree it is in line with the motivational state of the individual or obstructs the individual's goals. Thus the second information that is encoded in the resulting emotion is information about preferences (the pleasant–unpleasant evaluation) and motivational goals. The appraisal of coping potential provides information about a person's resources, and the evaluations regarding the correspondence of the event with the relevant social and personal norms provide information about a person's values. All of this information is therefore encoded in the emotional expressions that are generated in this process. In fact, it has been proposed that facial expressions of emotions are a direct readout of appraisals (Scherer, 1992; Smith & Scott, 1997).

Importantly, even though appraisals are typically not the product of reasoning processes, people can and do reconstruct appraisal processes

consciously after the fact (Robinson & Clore, 2002), and they can do so for other people's emotions as well (e.g., Roseman, 1991; Scherer & Grandjean, 2008). As such, emotions can be seen as encapsulated or compacted signals that tell a rather complex story about the emoter (see Figure 3.1).

Thus an angry person experiences a motivation-incongruent (low goal conduciveness) unpleasant state but considers the situation to be potentially under his or her control (high coping potential). An observer who sees a person react with anger to an injustice can hence conclude that the person has values according to which the event in question appears unjust, perceives this injustice as incongruent with his or her own motivational state (which would be to see justice done), and also feels endowed with enough resources to act accordingly. By contrast, the person who does not react with anger to the injustice may be accused—as by Aristotle—of either lacking understanding of the situation or being too weak to defend him- or herself or others against the injustice.

Importantly, the information provided by emotional reactions refers not only to the situation at hand but also to relatively stable characteristics of the person. Specifically, stable traits such as dominance, affiliation, and competence affect the motivational goals, preferences, and resources of a person. Thus a person who is competent may be expected to have more resources for dealing with potential problems than a person who is not. Likewise, an affiliative person can be expected to have affiliative goals. Conversely, seeing a person react with anger in a difficult situation suggests that this person is high in resources in this situation and likely in other situations as well.

In short, emotion displays convey, by their very nature, information regarding not only the senders' emotional states but also their interpersonal intentions (see also Frijda & Mesquita, 1994). However, the attribution of

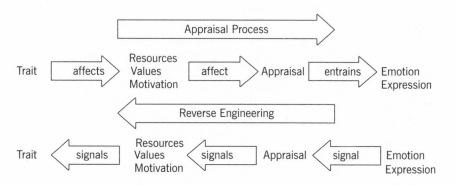

FIGURE 3.1. Reverse engineering of appraisals.

behavioral intentions also depends on the context of the interaction. Such elements as the relative status of the interaction partners, the gender composition of the dyad, and the cultural background of the interaction partners all play important roles. In fact, the social context can be expected to modify the interpretation of a specific expression insofar as context information is used as part of the process of understanding the other; that is, it permits the taking of the other's perspective in a given situation.

What Does Anger Signal?

Research on the social signal function of anger has focused mainly on behavioral intentions—specifically dominance and affiliation—as well as competence, which is related to both status and dominance (Hess, Blairy, & Kleck, 2000; Tiedens, 2001). The impact of anger expressions has also attracted attention in the context of negotiations (Sinaceur & Tiedens, 2006; van Kleef, De Dreu, & Manstead, 2004a, 2004b; see Van Kleef & Côté, Chapter 6, this volume) and with regard to credibility (Hareli et al., 2009).

Dominance and affiliation are of central importance for our interactions with others, as they allow us to judge vital social characteristics of individuals we may interact with. In hierarchical primate societies, for example, highly dominant individuals pose a certain threat insofar as they can claim territory or possessions (food, sexual partners, etc.) from lower status group members (Menzel, 1973, 1974). Hence the presence of a perceived dominant other should lead to increased vigilance and a preparedness for withdrawal (Coussi-Korbel, 1994). In contrast, an affiliation motive is associated with nurturing, supportive behaviors and should lead to approach when the other is perceived to be high on this disposition. When the same person is shown with different facial expressions, observers attribute high levels of dominance and low levels of affiliation to the anger expression (Knutson, 1996). Hess et al. (2000) showed that this effect is moderated by the gender and ethnicity of the expresser, which influence the perceived likelihood that a person of this gender and ethnicity shows anger in everyday life, which in turn—together with the intensity of the expression—influences the level of dominance and affiliation that is attributed to the person as a function of the anger expression (see Figure 3.2).

Specifically, men and European Americans were rated as more likely to display anger than were women and Japanese people. Further, more likely expressions (i.e., those by men and by European American actors) were rated as more dominant; expressions that displayed 80% of maximum intensity led to higher ratings of dominance than did expressions at 40% of maximum intensity.

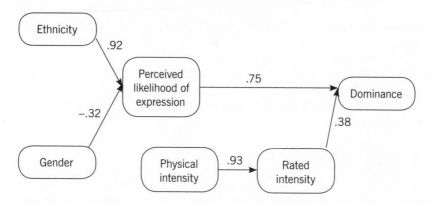

FIGURE 3.2. Moderators of the effect of anger on perceived dominance. Based on Hess, Blairy, and Kleck (2000).

For the affiliation ratings of anger expressions, the likelihood of the expression again predicted the participants' judgments, but intensity did not. Also, in addition to the link mediated by likelihood, a strong direct path between the sex of the actor and affiliation was found indicating that women are generally rated as more affiliative. Thus the degree to which anger expressions signal dominance or affiliation depends importantly on the beliefs that observers hold regarding the likelihood that the expression will be shown by a member of a specific social group. Further, whereas only stronger anger expressions signal dominance, a weak anger expression is already sufficient to signal a lack of affiliation. In short, even though anger per se tends to signal dominance, the strength of this signal depends crucially both on who does the signaling and on the observer's beliefs.

As regards competence, Lerner and Tiedens (2006) provide a review of the literature with regard to the potential positive effects of being angry on decision making. Their review was based on the appraisal-tendency framework (ATF) proposed by Lerner and Keltner (2000, 2001), which assumes that emotions are based on appraisals and serve a coordination role to enable the individual to deal quickly with encountered problems or opportunities. As such, they note the motivating force of anger described herein, as well as its potential to foster optimism (Lerner & Keltner, 2000, 2001). Overall, they conclude that an angry decision maker approaches a situation with the tendency to feel confident, in control, and thinking the worst of others. Such a mind-set can sometimes lead to disaster but at other times can lead to desirable outcomes. They refer in this context to Aristotle's emphasis on being angry at the right time toward the right person.

This finding suits the fact that showing anger positively influences

negotiations in contexts in which the negotiation partner has limited options or low power (Sinaceur & Tiedens, 2006; van Kleef et al., 2004a, 2004b). This positive effect is partially mediated by fear on the side of the recipient (Van Kleef et al., 2004a) but also by a perception of toughness (Sinacoeur & Tiedens, 2006).

Another question is how competent angry people are perceived to be. Tiedens (2001) found that observers attribute higher power to people who express anger rather than sadness. This matches the belief that in failure situations, a high-status person would feel more angry than sad or guilty, as opposed to a person with lower status, who is expected to feel more sad and guilty than angry (Tiedens, Ellsworth, & Mesquita, 2000). Tiedens (2001, Study 4) found that this status conferral is mediated by a perception of competence. Thus individuals who express anger are perceived not only as threatening but also as competent, powerful, and dominant and thus able to assert themselves. This perception is, however, not entirely independent of the expresser and the situation. Thus Lewis (2000) found that male managers who, on receiving bad business news, showed angry or neutral expressions rather than sadness were indeed perceived as more competent. By contrast, female managers who showed anger were rated as equally incompetent as those who showed sadness. Yet, when female managers showed a neutral expression, they were perceived as particularly competent. This finding may be explained by the prevailing workplace norms that tend to emphasize emotional neutrality, objectivity, and professionalism (cf. Ashforth & Humphrey, 1995; Weber, 1968). This and the notion that female emotions may be uncontrolled and hence suspect (Shields, 2005; Warner & Shields, 2007) create an impression of lack of professionalism for the angry woman but not the angry man.

Hareli and colleagues (Hareli et al., 2009; Hareli & Hess, 2010) found that expressing anger can lead to positive assessments by perceivers. Specifically, a complainant who showed anger was perceived as more credible (but only when the complaint was ambiguous). When the anger was appraised as signaling that the protagonist *cared* about the outcome rather than being indifferent, the display of anger can also lead a protagonist to be perceived as more emotional, warm, and gentle (Hareli & Hess, 2010). This latter effect was fully mediated by the observers' perception of the situation as one that the protagonist perceived as both unpleasant and norm incongruent. That is, the person was perceived as warm and gentle because the anger expression signaled concern for the injustice.

In sum, angry individuals are perceived as threatening but at the same time the anger can signal strength and the ability and motivation to address bad situations. However, the above data suggest that there may be

individual differences on the side of the expresser, which may moderate this effect. These are discussed in the following section.

THE ROLE OF BELIEFS
IN EMOTION COMMUNICATION

As stated, the precise effect of an anger expression depends to some degree on who the expresser is. Specifically, for the reverse engineering process to work, an expression must first be classified as anger. However, in a series of studies, Hess, Adams and Kleck (Hess, Adams, & Kleck, 2007, 2008a, 2009b) found that beliefs about the expresser's social group and about the perceived dominance and affiliation of the expresser can influence the perception of anger (as well as of happiness). In particular, as men and women differ in the degree to which they are perceived as dominant, both the perception of their anger (Hess, Blairy, & Kleck, 1997) and the conclusions drawn about the angry man or woman differ as well. In the following I briefly summarize some of these findings. However, first the question needs to be addressed as to why it should matter who shows the emotion to be classified by an observer.

Two Strategies for the Recognition of Emotion

There are two principal strategies for decoding emotion displays (Kirouac & Hess, 1999).The first, *pattern matching*, associates specific features of the expression with specific emotions (Buck, 1984). Thus upturned corners of the mouth or lowered brows are recognized as smiles or frowns, and a perceiver can thus conclude that the individual is happy or angry, respectively. This approach breaks down when the features are either too weak to be classified or lead to contradictory conclusions—such as would be the case when a person both smiles and frowns at the same time. The second decoding strategy, *perspective taking*, depends on the knowledge that the perceiver possesses regarding the sender and/or the social situation in which the interaction is taking place. This information permits the perceiver to take the perspective of the encoder and helps him or her to correctly infer the emotional state that the sender is most likely experiencing. Thus knowing that John encountered an injustice and that John abhors injustice would lead to the conclusion that John is angry. But what happens when we do not know the other person well or at all?

One important aspect of emotion expressions is that the same channels that transmit emotional information—the face, the voice, the body—all tell us a great deal about the social groups to which the emoters belong. These include the sex, age, and race of the other person. This knowledge

can be used by observers to predict the likely emotional reactions of the sender; that is, the beliefs about the likely emotions of others that can then substitute for personalized knowledge and affect the perception and interpretation of emotion expression. Thus Hugenberg and Bodenhausen (2003) found that implicit negative stereotypes toward African Americans were associated with perceivers' sensitivity to anger expressions by African Americans in a change detection task. Also, women are known to cry when angry (Crawford, Clippax, Onyx, Gault, & Benton, 1992; see also Shields, 1987), a behavior very atypical for men. Therefore, when seeing a man cry, we would probably not consider the possibility that he is angry, whereas we might consider this possibility when we see a woman cry.

In addition, as regards facial expressions, the very faces that show the emotions may enhance or obscure some expressive elements and hence bias pattern matching. Thus the facial morphology of women and younger individuals, for example, appears to enhance the cues associated with happiness, whereas those of men and older individuals enhance the cues associated with anger (Becker, Kenrick, Neuberg, Blackwell, & Smith, 2007; Sacco & Hugenberg, 2009). In sum, the same facial expressions shown by two individuals may not be interpreted the same way, either due to the influence of the observers' beliefs about the emoter or because facial features and facial expressions may interact such that pattern-matching errors are made.

This notion of a perceptual overlap between emotion expressions and certain trait markers, which then influences emotion communication, has been more recently proposed by Zebrowitz (see Zebrowitz & Montepare, 2006), as well as by Hess, Adams and Kleck (2007, 2008b, 2009c). Specifically, Hess et al (2007) propose the *functional equivalence hypothesis,* which posits that some aspects of facial expressive behavior and morphological cues to dominance and affiliation are equivalent in their effects on emotional attributions. In what follows I summarize findings on the impact of beliefs on one hand and facial morphology on the other on perceptions of anger in men and women.

Facial Appearance and Beliefs about the Emotionality of Men and Women

In general, men are perceived as more likely than women to express anger (Fischer, 1993). In a number of studies, Hess, Adams, and Kleck (2004, 2005) showed that this belief can be traced in part to beliefs about dominant and affiliative individuals. That is, men's faces were perceived as more dominant in appearance, and men were rated as more likely to show anger, disgust, and contempt. By contrast, women's faces were rated as more affiliative in appearance, and women were expected to be more likely to

show happiness, surprise, sadness, and fear. Mediational analyses showed that the beliefs about men's and women's emotions were partially mediated by their respective perceived affiliation and dominance. Hess, Thibault, Adams, and Kleck (2010) showed that, in fact, the beliefs about men's and women's emotionality are based on facial morphology—the degree to which the faces seem dominant and affiliative—on the one hand and on social roles (nurturing vs. agentic) on the other. When these were taken into account, sex per se did not explain further variance.

Implications for Men's and Women's Anger Expressions

As mentioned earlier, the facial morphological features that make a face appear male or female and in turn dominant or affiliative interact directly with the movement patterns that characterize specific emotional expressions. Thus some of the cues that mark anger expressions, such as lowered eyebrows and tight lips, mimic features also associated with dominance, whereas high eyebrows and smiling in happiness expressions reinforce affiliative features.

Hess, Adams, and Kleck (2009a) showed that these similarities actually lead to perceptual overlap. Specifically, participants had to identify neutral expressions of highly dominant and highly affiliative appearing individuals embedded in either a series of angry, happy, or fear faces. To the degree that anger and dominance look alike, it is harder to identify a dominant neutral face within a series of anger faces. By contrast, the identification of the affiliative neutral faces is comparatively easy. The converse is the case for affiliative faces embedded in a series of happy expressions.

As predicted, participants were slower to identify dominant neutral faces compared with affiliative faces embedded in a series of angry expressions. The converse was the case for affiliative faces embedded in a series of happy faces. These results support the notion that for all intents and purposes a highly dominant face looks angry even when no actual facial movement is present. By contrast, highly affiliative neutral faces look happy. Put another way, the facial configurations that create impressions of dominance and affiliation are the same that make a face appear to show anger and happiness. These perceptual similarities between dominance/anger and affiliation/happiness then can be expected to bias the perception of these emotions, especially when facial expressions are weak and ambiguous.

Importantly, as noted previously, men's faces are generally perceived as more dominant and women's faces as more affiliative. In fact, the high forehead, square jaw, and thicker eyebrows that have been linked to perceptions of dominance (e.g., Keating, Mazur, & Segall, 1981) are also more

typical for men's faces (Brown & Perrett, 1993; Burton, Bruce, & Dench, 1993). On the other hand, a rounded baby face with large eyes is more feminine (Brown & Perrett, 1993; Burton et al., 1993), perceived as more approachable and warm (Berry & Brownlow, 1989) and is more typical for women's faces.

This implies that the preceding findings have implications for the perception of anger in men and women. Thus men who show weak anger are more likely to be perceived as angry than women, and the reverse is true for happiness.

However, this also implies that men's and women's anger will have a different emotional effect on the observer. The reason is that, in addition to the previously described perceptual association between dominance and anger, anger expressions in fact signal dominance on the part of the expresser, whereas happy expressions signal affiliation (Hess et al., 2000; Knutson, 1996). In turn, perceptions of the dominance and affiliation tendencies of others are relevant to the approach–avoidance dimension.

Because anger, dominance, and male sex markers on the one hand and happiness, affiliation, and female sex markers on the other overlap perceptually and are functionally equivalent, anger shown by women and happiness shown by men can be expected to elicit different emotional reactions from observers. Specifically, when anger is shown on a highly dominant face, the threat signal of the expression and the threat signal derived from facial morphology are congruent and reinforce each other. By contrast, when anger is expressed on a highly affiliative face, the two signals contradict each other and hence weaken the overall threat message. The converse is true for happy expressions (Hess, Sabourin, & Kleck, 2007). Following this line of argument, the female anger expression can be viewed as a combination of an appetitive face with a threatening expression. Male anger, on the other hand, represents a less ambiguous example of a threat stimulus. Conversely, female happiness is a clearer appetitive stimulus than male happiness.

Hess, Sabourin, and Kleck (2007) tested this hypothesis using a startle-reflex methodology, which is independent of consciously applied stereotypes. Specifically, the eye-blink reflex to a sudden acoustic probe is modulated by emotional state (e.g., Lang, 1995; Lang, Bradley, & Cuthbert, 1990; Vrana, Spence, & Lang, 1988), such that when an individual is exposed to a threatening or withdrawal-inducing stimulus, the reflex is potentiated. Conversely, a pattern opposite to that of the eye-blink reflex is found for the postauricular reflex, the muscle response that serves to pull the ears back and up (Berzin & Fortinguerra, 1993) such that individuals show an augmented postauricular reaction to an acoustic startle probe when exposed to appetitive stimuli (Benning, Patrick, & Lang, 2004; Johnson, Valle-Inclán, Geary, & Hackley, 2012).

Congruent with the notion that dominance and affiliation signals from the face and facial expressions of anger and happiness interact perceptually, eye-blink startle was potentiated for male anger faces compared with neutral and happy faces, as well as compared with female anger faces. In contrast, the postauricular reflex was potentiated for female happiness faces and attenuated during male anger faces, compared with neutral faces, as well as male happiness faces. Thus anger potentiated eye-blink startle only when shown by a man—that is, shown on a face suggesting social dominance. Conversely, the postauricular reflex was potentiated preferentially for female happy expressions.

In brief, facial features and facial expressions interact when it comes to the perception of anger expressions. The studies reported herein focused on male and female faces because these represent a natural category differing in facial dominance and affiliation. But obviously individuals within each sex differ on these dimensions, and hence we would expect, for example, anger to be more threatening when shown on a highly dominant female face and, conversely, male anger to be less so when shown on a highly affiliative male face. It is important to note that not only do men and women differ with regard to these dimensions but other groups do as well. What this means is that it matters who shows anger and that anger's social signal will vary as a function of its expresser. This is demonstrated in the study reported next.

Whom Do You Trust with Your Money?

The goal of this study was to assess the impact of angry, happy, and neutral facial expressions on trust in an interaction. Smiling is an affiliative signal, and we expect that we can trust smiling people—a logic that salespeople are well aware of. The question in this research was whether anger could stack up to happiness in terms of the trust it inspires, given its association with competence.

In this specific interaction, participants expected to play an economic trust game with a partner but in fact played with the computer. The game required the participants to decide to either cooperate or to make an egoistic decision that favored their own outcome. The payoff matrix was constructed such that cooperative behavior by both participants maximized the payoff for both, with higher payoff when both invested a similar high amount. Egoistic behavior by either game player favored his or her own outcome to the disadvantage of the other player, but the payoff was lower than the one that would be achieved by cooperating. Hence, if participants trusted their partner to cooperate, they could maximize their outcomes. In cases of distrust, an egoistic strategy should be chosen. Thus the fact that

someone invested at all and the amount of investment were both dependent on assuming that the game partner would make similar choices, as the payout was less advantageous when one partner invested much more than the other.

Male and female participants played the game with either a man or a woman. In addition, we varied perceived-expert status by indicating that the game partner was either an economics student (expert) or an arts student (nonexpert). For the manipulation of emotion expression and expert status, participants and the (virtual) partners were introduced to each other prior to the game. They were told to take photos of themselves using the web camera and to provide information on their name, field of study, and age. In turn, each participant received a photo that showed a person with either a slight smile, a slight anger expression, or a perfectly neutral expression, as well as the name, age, and field of study of the partner.

Across all conditions, only 66% ($SD = .48$) of the participants chose the cooperative option. Figure 3.3 shows the average amount invested in a cooperative fashion when playing the game with a man or a woman showing each of the three emotions. Overall, participants invested in a cooperative fashion more when playing with a man rather than a woman, but the gender difference depended on the emotion.

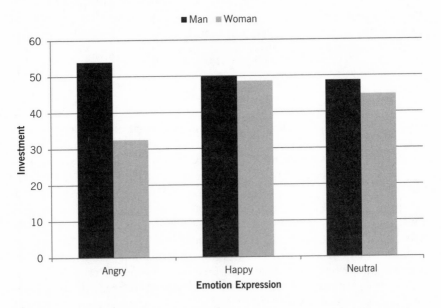

FIGURE 3.3. Mean investment in function of partner sex and facial expressions.

For male game partners, no significant difference between emotion conditions emerged. Thus participants showed the same level of trust in their investments whether the man they played with showed anger, happiness, or a neutral expression. Importantly, showing anger did not lead to any less trust; the pattern, in fact, suggests if anything more trust. For women, however, a different pattern emerged, with a significant drop in trust, when they showed anger compared with either a smiling or a neutral expression. This suggests that anger in women has a notably less positive—in fact, a negative—effect that it does not have for men. Thus anger was indeed a positive emotion—as positive as happiness—when it comes to inspiring trust in a man, but it failed to do this for women, who were trusted more when they smiled or showed a neutral expression. That women are in some way penalized for showing anger resembles the effect found by Lewis (2000) in a business setting. In general, women are not expected to show anger easily, and, as shown by Hess et al. (2000), the degree to which an expression is expected moderates its social signal. Hence, the belief that women—at least nondominant women—do not show anger easily undermines the power of their anger expressions. Hess et al. (2005) found that dominant women are indeed expected to show just as much anger as dominant men but that they pay a price in that they are liked a lot less. Yet this finding suggests, as noted previously, that it is perceived dominance and not gender per se that undermines the power of anger for some women. Hence one could say that anger has positive effects especially for men and for dominant women.

SUMMARY

In sum, there is good evidence that Aristotle was right about anger. Anger both signals that the angry other will act with strength in an adverse situation and provides the motivational force for such actions. However, as was typical for his age, Aristotle thought about men when he formulated this idea; indeed, as regards the signal value of anger, the situation is not quite the same for women as for men. Women are liked less for their anger and women may appear stronger when staying neutral and remote than when "losing control," even in anger. Nevertheless, in most situations anger can be a positive emotion for both men and women. However, one thing must be noted: Anger is a positive emotion for the person who expresses it, but not necessarily for the person it is expressed toward. For the person on the receiving end of righteous anger, the situation may well appear negative.

REFERENCES

Ambady, N., Hallahan, M., & Rosenthal, R. (1995). On judging and being judged accurately in zero-acquaintance situations. *Journal of Personality and Social Psychology, 69,* 518–529.

Ambady, N., & Rosenthal, R. (1992). Thin slices of expressive behavior as predictors of interpersonal consequences: A meta-analysis. *Psychological Bulletin, 111,* 256–274.

Arnold, M. B. (1960). *Emotion and personality.* New York: Columbia University Press.

Ashforth, B. E., & Humphrey, R. H. (1995). Emotion in the workplace: A reappraisal. *Human Relations, 48,* 97–125.

Averill, J. R. (1982). *Anger and aggression.* New York: Springer Verlag.

Averill, J. R. (1997). The emotions: An integrative approach. In R. Hogan, J. A. Johnson, & S. R. Briggs (Eds.), *Handbook of personality psychology* (pp. 513–541). San Diego, CA: Academic Press.

Becker, D. V., Kenrick, D. T., Neuberg, S. L., Blackwell, K. C., & Smith, D. M. (2007). The confounded nature of angry men and happy women. *Journal of Personality and Social Psychology, 92,* 179–190.

Benning, S. D., Patrick, C. J., & Lang, A. R. (2004). Emotional modulation of the post-auricular reflex. *Psychophysiology, 41,* 426–432.

Berkowitz, L. (1993). *Aggression: Its causes, consequences, and control.* New York: McGraw-Hill.

Berkowitz, L., & Harmon-Jones, E. (2004). Toward an understanding of the determinants of anger. *Emotion, 4,* 107–130.

Berry, D. S., & Brownlow, S. (1989). Were the physiognomists right? Personality correlates of facial babyishness. *Personality and Social Psychology Bulletin, 15,* 266–279.

Berzin, F., & Fortinguerra, C. R. (1993). EMG study of the anterior, superior, and posterior auricular muscles in man. *Anatomischer Anzeiger, 175,* 195–197.

Brown, E., & Perrett, D. I. (1993). What gives a face its gender? *Perception, 22,* 829–840.

Buck, R. (1984). Nonverbal receiving ability. In R. Buck (Ed.), *The communication of emotion* (pp. 209–242). New York: Guilford Press.

Burton, A. M., Bruce, V., & Dench, N. (1993). What's the difference between men and women?: Evidence from facial measurement. *Perception, 22,* 153–176.

Carver, C. S., & Harmon-Jones, E. (2009). Anger is an approach-related affect: Evidence and implications. *Psychological Bulletin, 135,* 183–204.

Cosmides, L., & Tooby, J. (2000). Evolutionary psychology and the emotions. In M. Lewis & J. M. Haviland-Jones (Eds.), *Handbook of emotions* (2nd ed., pp. 91–115). New York: Guilford Press.

Coussi-Korbel, S. (1994). Learning to outwit a competitor in mangabeys (*Cercocebus torquatus torquatus*). *Journal of Comparative Psychology, 108,* 164–171.

Crawford, J., Clippax, S., Onyx, J., Gault, U., & Benton, P. (1992). *Emotion and gender: Constructing meaning from memory.* London: Sage.

Fischer, A. H. (1993). Sex differences in emotionality: Fact or stereotype? *Feminism and Psychology, 3,* 303–318.

Frank, R. H. (1988). *Passions within reason: The strategic role of the emotions.* New York: Norton.

Frijda, N. H. (1986). *The emotions.* Cambridge, UK: Cambridge University Press.

Frijda, N. H., Kuipers, P., & ter Shure, E. (1989). Relations among emotion appraisal and emotional action readiness. *Journal of Personality and Social Psychology, 57,* 212–228.

Frijda, N. H., & Mesquita, B. (1994). The social roles and functions of emotions. In S. Kitayama & H. R. Markus (Eds.), *Emotion and culture: Empirical studies of mutual influence* (pp. 51–87). Washington, DC: American Psychological Association.

Haidt, J. (2003). The moral emotions. In R. J. Davidson, K. R. Scherer, & H. H. Goldsmith (Eds.), *Handbook of affective sciences* (pp. 852–870). Oxford, UK: Oxford University Press.

Hareli, S., Harush, R., Suleiman, R., Bergeron, S., Cossette, M., Lavoie, V., et al. (2009). When scowling may be a good thing: The influence of anger expressions on credibility. *European Journal of Experimental Social Psychology, 39,* 631–638.

Hareli, S., & Hess, U. (2010). What emotional reactions can tell us about the nature of others: An appraisal perspective on person perception. *Cognition and Emotion, 24,* 128–140.

Hareli, S., & Hess, U. (2012). The social signal value of emotion. *Cognition and Emotion, 26,* 385–389.

Harmon-Jones, E., & Allen, J. J. B. (1998). Anger and frontal brain activity: EEG asymmetry consistent with approach motivation despite negative affective valence. *Journal of Personality and Social Psychology, 74*(5), 1310–1316.

Harmon-Jones, E., Gable, P. A., & Peterson, C. K. (2010). The role of asymmetric frontal cortical activity in emotion-related phenomena: A review and update. *Biological Psychology, 84,* 451–462.

Harmon-Jones, E., & Sigelman, J. (2001). State anger and prefrontal brain activity: Evidence that insult-related relative left prefrontal activation is associated with experienced anger and aggression. *Journal of Personality and Social Psychology, 80,* 797–803.

Hess, U., Adams, R. B., Jr., & Kleck, R. E. (2004). Facial appearance, gender, and emotion expression. *Emotion, 4,* 378–388.

Hess, U., Adams, R. B., Jr., & Kleck, R. E. (2005). Who may frown and who should smile?: Dominance, affiliation, and the display of happiness and anger. *Cognition and Emotion, 19,* 515–536.

Hess, U., Adams, R. B., Jr., & Kleck, R. E. (2007). When two do the same it might not mean the same: The perception of emotional expressions shown by men and women. In U. Hess & P. Philippot (Eds.), *Group dynamics and emotional expression* (pp. 33–52). New York: Cambridge University Press.

Hess, U., Adams, R. B., Jr., & Kleck, R. E. (2008a). The devil is in the details: The meanings of faces and how they influence the meanings of facial expressions. In J. Or (Ed.), *Affective computing: Focus on emotion expression, synthesis, and recognition* (pp. 45–56). New York: InTech Education.

Hess, U., Adams, R. B., Jr., & Kleck, R. E. (2008b). The role of perceived emotion in first impressions. In N. Ambady & J. J. Skowronski (Eds.), *First impressions* (pp. 234–254). New York: Guilford Press.

Hess, U., Adams, R. B., Jr., & Kleck, R. E. (2009a). The categorical perception of emotions and traits. *Social Cognition, 27,* 319–325.

Hess, U., Adams, R. B., Jr., & Kleck, R. E. (2009b). The face is not an empty canvas: How facial expressions interact with facial appearance. *Philosophical Transactions of the Royal Society London B, 364,* 3497–3504.

Hess, U., Adams, R. B., Jr., & Kleck, R. E. (2009c). Inter-group misunderstandings in emotion communication. In S. Demoulin, J.-P. Leyens, & J. F. Dovidio (Eds.), *Intergroup misunderstandings: Impact of divergent social realities* (pp. 85–100). New York: Psychology Press.

Hess, U., Blairy, S., & Kleck, R. E. (1997). The intensity of emotional facial expressions and decoding accuracy. *Journal of Nonverbal Behavior, 21,* 241–257.

Hess, U., Blairy, S., & Kleck, R. E. (2000). The influence of expression intensity, gender, and ethnicity on judgments of dominance and affiliation. *Journal of Nonverbal Behavior, 24,* 265–283.

Hess, U., Sabourin, G., & Kleck, R. E. (2007). Postauricular and eye-blink startle responses to facial expressions. *Psychophysiology, 44,* 431–435.

Hess, U., Thibault, P., Adams, R. B., Jr., & Kleck, R. E. (2010). The influence of genetics, social roles and social appearance on perceived emotionality. *European Journal of Social Psychology, 40,* 1310–1317.

Hugenberg, K., & Bodenhausen, G. V. (2003). Facing prejudice: Implicit prejudice and the perception of facial threat. *Psychological Science, 14,* 640–643.

Johnson, G. M., Valle-Inclán, F., Geary, D. C., & Hackley, S. A. (2012). The nursing hypothesis: An evolutionary account of emotional modulation of the postauricular reflex. *Psychophysiology, 49*(2), 178–185.

Keating, C. F., Mazur, A., & Segall, M. H. (1981). A cross-cultural exploration of physiognomic traits of dominance and happiness. *Ethology and Sociobiology, 2,* 41–48.

Kenny, D. A. (2004). PERSON: A general model of interpersonal perception. *Personality and Social Psychology Review, 8,* 265–280.

Kirouac, G., & Hess, U. (1999). Group membership and the decoding of nonverbal behavior. In P. Philippot, R. Feldman, & E. Coats (Eds.), *The social context of nonverbal behavior* (pp. 182–210). Cambridge, UK: Cambridge University Press.

Knutson, B. (1996). Facial expressions of emotion influence interpersonal trait inferences. *Journal of Nonverbal Behavior, 20,* 165–182.

Kuppens, P., Van Mechelen, I., Smits, D. J. M., & De Boeck, P. (2003). The appraisal basis of anger: Specificity, necessity and sufficiency of components. *Emotion, 3*(3), 254–269.

Lang, P. J. (1995). The emotion probe: Studies of motivation and attention. *American Psychologist, 50,* 372–385.

Lang, P. J., Bradley, M. M., & Cuthbert, B. N. (1990). Emotion, attention, and the startle reflex. *Psychological Review, 97,* 377–395.

Lerner, J. S., Gonzalez, R. M., Small, D. A., & Fischhoff, B. (2003). Effects of fear and anger on perceived risks of terrorism: A national field experiment. *Psychological Science, 14,* 144–150.

Lerner, J. S., & Keltner, D. (2000). Beyond valence: Toward a model of emotion-specifc influences on judgement and choice. *Cognition and Emotion, 14*, 473–493.

Lerner, J. S., & Keltner, D. (2001). Fear, anger, and risk. *Journal of Personality and Social Psychology, 81*, 146–159.

Lerner, J. S., & Tiedens, L. Z. (2006). Portrait of the angry decision maker: How appraisal tendencies shape anger's influence on cognition. *Journal of Behavioral Decision Making, 19*, 115–137.

Lewis, K. M. (2000). When leaders display emotion: How followers respond to negative emotional expression of male and female leaders. *Journal of Organizational Behavior, 21*, 221–234.

Menzel, E. W., Jr. (1973). Leadership and communication in young chimpanzees. In J. E. W. Menzel (Ed.), *Precultural primate behavior* (pp. 192–225). Basel, Switzerland: Karger.

Menzel, E. W., Jr. (1974). A group of young chimpanzees in a one-acre field. In A. M. Schrier & F. Stollnitz (Eds.), *Behavior of nonhuman primates* (pp. 83–153). San Diego, CA: Academic Press.

Miller, T. Q., Smith, T. W., Turner, C. W., Guijarro, M. L., & Hallet, A. J. (1996). Meta-analytic review of research on hostility and physical health. *Psychological Bulletin, 119*, 322–348.

Parkinson, B. (1999). Relations and dissociations between appraisal and emotion ratings of reasonable and unreasonable anger and guilt. *Cognition and Emotion, 13*(4), 347–385.

Robinson, M., & Clore, G. (2002). Belief and feeling: Evidence for an accessibility model of emotional self-report. *Psychological Bulletin, 128*, 934–960.

Roseman, I. J. (1991). Appraisal determinants of discrete emotions. *Cognition and Emotion, 5*, 161–200.

Roseman, I. J., Wiest, C., & Swartz, T. S. (1994). Phenomenology, behaviors, and goals differentiate discrete emotions. *Journal of Personality and Social Psychology, 67*, 206–221.

Rozin, P., Lowery, L., Imada, S., & Haidt, J. (1999). The CAD triad hypothesis: A mapping between three moral emotions (contempt, anger, disgust) and three moral codes (community, autonomy, divinity). *Journal of Personality and Social Psychology, 76*, 574–586.

Sacco, D. F., & Hugenberg, K. (2009). The look of fear and anger: Facial maturity modulates recognition of fearful and angry expressions. *Emotion, 9*, 39–49.

Scherer, K. R. (1987). Towards a dynamic theory of emotion: The component process model of affective states. *Geneva Studies in Emotion and Communication, 1*, 1–98. Retrieved from *www.unige.ch/fapse/emotion/publications/pdf/tdte_1987.pdf*.

Scherer, K. R. (1992). What does facial expression express? In K. Strongman (Ed.), *International review of studies on emotion* (Vol. 2, pp. 139–165). Chichester, UK: Wiley.

Scherer, K. R., & Grandjean, D. (2008). Facial expressions allow inference of both emotions and their components. *Cognition and Emotion, 22*, 789–801.

Shaver, P., Schwartz, J., Kirson, D., & O'Connor, C. (1987). Emotion knowledge:

Further exploration of a prototype approach. *Journal of Personality and Social Psychology, 52*, 1061–1086.

Shields, S. A. (1987). Women, men, and the dilemma of emotion. In P. Shaver & C. Hendrick (Eds.), *Sex and gender: Review of personality and social psychology* (Vol. 7, pp. 229–250). Thousand Oaks, CA: Sage.

Shields, S. A. (2005). The politics of emotion in everyday life: "Appropriate" emotion and claims on identity. *Review of General Psychology, 9*, 3–15.

Sinaceur, M., & Tiedens, L. Z. (2006). Get mad and get more than even: When and why anger expression is effective in negotiations. *Journal of Experimental Social Psychology, 42*, 314–322.

Smith, C. A., & Scott, H. S. (1997). A componential approach to the meaning of facial expressions. In J. A. Russell & J.-M. Fernández-Dols (Eds.), *The psychology of facial expression* (pp. 229–254). New York: Cambridge University Press.

Tiedens, L. Z. (2001). Anger and advancement versus sadness and subjugation: The effect of negative emotion expressions on social status conferral. *Journal of Personality and Social Psychology, 80*, 86–94.

Tiedens, L. Z., Ellsworth, P. C., & Mesquita, B. (2000). Stereotypes about sentiments and status: Emotional expectations for high- and low-status group members. *Personality and Social Psychology Bulletin, 26*, 500–574.

Todorov, A., & Uleman, J. S. (2002). Spontaneous trait inferences are bound to actors' faces: Evidence from a false recognition paradigm. *Journal of Personality and Social Psychology, 83*, 1051–1065.

Todorov, A., & Uleman, J. S. (2003). The efficiency of binding spontaneous trait inferences to actors' faces. *Journal of Experimental Social Psychology, 39*, 549–562.

Trivers, R. L. (1971). The evolution of reciprocal altruism. *Quarterly Review of Biology, 46*, 35–57.

van Kleef, G. A., De Dreu, C. K. W., & Manstead, A. S. R. (2004a). The interpersonal effects of anger and happiness in negotiations. *Journal of Personality and Social Psychology, 86*, 57–76.

van Kleef, G. A., De Dreu, C. K. W., & Manstead, A. S. R. (2004b). The interpersonal effects of emotions in negotiations: A motivated information processing approach. *Journal of Personality and Social Psychology, 87*, 510–528.

Vrana, S. R., Spence, E. L., & Lang, P. J. (1988). The startle probe response: A new measure of emotion? *Journal of Abnormal Psychology, 97*, 487–491.

Warner, L. A., & Shields, S. A. (2007). The perception of crying in women and men: Angry tears, sad tears, and the "right way" to cry. In U. Hess & P. Philippot (Eds.), *Group dynamics and emotional expression* (pp. 92–117). New York: Cambridge University Press.

Weber, M. (1968). *Economy and society* (G. Roth & C. Wittich, Eds.). New York: Bedminister Press.

Zebrowitz, L. A., & Montepare, J. M. (2006). The ecological approach to person perception: Evolutionary roots and contemporary offshoots. In M. Schaller, J. A. Simpson, & D. T. Kendrick (Eds.), *Evolution and social psychology* (pp. 81–114). New York: Psychology Press.

4

Can Negative Social Emotions Have Positive Consequences?

An Examination of Embarrassment, Shame, Guilt, Jealousy, and Envy

NICOLE E. HENNIGER
CHRISTINE R. HARRIS

One often hears emotions discussed as if some were bad and some were good. Although there is no doubt that some particular emotions feel subjectively positive and others subjectively negative, we argue that emotions do not lend themselves to a simple classification of good versus bad. Asking whether an emotion such as shame or jealousy is bad would be like asking whether a motivational state such as hunger is bad. The answer will be unequivocally "it depends." Although hunger is clearly an evolved state that arose to ensure that an organism does not put off eating for too long, it also can have negative consequences. This is readily evidenced by the growing obesity epidemic in nations such as the United States—the sweet smell of baking cookies in a mall or buttered popcorn in a movie

theatre are often too hard to resist. We suggest that negative emotions, like other motivational states, can serve important functions and need not necessarily be states to avoid at all costs. In particular, we examine five social emotions. The first part of the chapter examines embarrassment, shame, and guilt, three emotions that focus on oneself and arise when one has committed some type of social transgression. We then turn to two emotions that are provoked by the actions, behaviors, or attributes of others, namely, jealousy and envy, both of which have markedly notorious reputations.

We examine the ways in which these subjectively negative emotions can provide potentially beneficial motivations. Much of our discussion of these affective states relies on a *specific emotions* framework. One assumption inherent in many theories that use this framework is that emotions are motivational states that have been shaped by natural selection. Emotions function to prompt an organism to engage in particular types of behaviors that it might otherwise not engage in—behaviors that, over phylogenetic history, have tended to confer some adaptive advantage in a particular class of circumstances (e.g., Ekman, 1992; Frijda, 1986; Haidt & Keltner, 1999). Each specific emotional state is presumed to have its own distinct motivational tendencies (or "urges," to use Fridja's terminology) that are activated by a particular set of appraisals. Fear is perhaps the most straightforward example: The appraisal of threat, which does not need to be conscious, elicits the motivation to avoid or escape a dangerous object or situation. Although one might avoid threat even when not afraid, fear makes it unlikely that one will fail to do so. The five social emotions that we examine here also are proposed to have their own motivational states, although they prove rather more complex and sometimes controversial than does fear.

Thus one way that negative emotions might be considered "positive" is by looking at their proposed evolutionary function. Importantly, the term *function* when used in this way does not refer to psychological well-being in the way that it is often used in common parlance (e.g., a "well-functioning" relationship or a "dysfunctional" person) but rather specifically means that something was likely to produce behaviors that increased an organism's inclusive fitness. In fact, most negative emotions produce psychological discomfort, at least temporarily. Such discomfort often reflects emotions doing exactly what they are designed to do—create an impetus for behavior, which once engaged in helps alleviate the negative psychological state (Kappas, 2011; Nesse, 1990). The emotions discussed in this chapter particularly function by motivating people to respond to problems within their social worlds. (See Baker, McNulty, & Overall, Chapter 5, this volume, for further discussion of some of these emotions in close relationships.)

EMBARRASSMENT

> But that intimacy of mutual embarrassment, in which each feels that the other is
> feeling something, having once existed, its effect is not to be done away with.
> —GEORGE ELIOT

Embarrassment requires the presence of others as an audience, making it a fundamentally social emotion. (When alone, one might recall feeling embarrassed, but even that will entail imagining or recollecting an audience's presence.) At first blush, embarrassment may seem like a rather benign emotion without strong personal or social consequences. However, a closer examination reveals that this emotion can be a powerful motivational force. At its best it can reinforce social bonds and smooth over awkward interactions; at its worst, it can lead people to put their own well-being and that of others at risk.

Theorized Functions

Given its inherent social nature, several theorists have proposed that embarrassment evolved to help overcome and avoid social mistakes and thereby prevent social exclusion from one's group (Harris, 2006; Keltner & Buswell, 1997). Humans have presumably evolved to be group dwellers because doing so provided inclusive fitness benefits to individuals. However, residing among others is not without its difficulties. Social norms are sometimes unintentionally violated, and culprits need a way to readily undo potential damage in such situations. Embarrassment is theorized to help prevent social ostracism through several means. First, it serves as an appeasement gesture to others, communicating that the act was unintentional and not likely to happen again. Second, embarrassment encourages amends making and reparation for the social wrong. Third, it provides a strong warning cue that prompts one to carefully evaluate one's own behavior and others' reaction to it. Finally, the subjective feeling of embarrassment is so dreadful that it motivates people to avoid engaging in similar behaviors in the future. Several findings from the literature are consistent with these proposed functions of embarrassment.

Empirical Studies

A number of experiments have shown that displays of embarrassment produce positive affect in others and appease onlookers. For example, Semin and Manstead (1982) created different video versions of a man knocking over a 5-foot-high display of toilet paper in a grocery market and varied whether the man displayed embarrassment and whether he undid the damage (restacked the display). When participants viewed the videos, they liked

the man more when he showed embarrassment than when he remained calm, and this was the case even if he failed to fix the display. Other work finds that viewing photos of people exhibiting embarrassment elicits positive feelings in viewers (Keltner & Buswell, 1997) and that blushing, a common display during embarrassment, can cause an audience to judge the blusher more favorably (de Jong, 1999). There are, however, limits to the effects of embarrassment displays on others. For example, some work suggests that in order for embarrassment to serve an appeasement function, others must perceive that the transgression was not intentional or that one is truly sorry for the misbehavior (de Jong, Peters, de Cremer, & Vranken, 2002) or that the violation is a minor, temporary one and not suggestive of a deeper personality flaw (Levin & Arluke, 1982).

Research also has found that people tend to behave more prosocially after engaging in embarrassing acts, which is consistent with the proposition that embarrassment motivates one to restore one's self-image and repair potential social damage after a mishap. In an early experiment by Apsler (1975), participants had to engage in either highly embarrassing tasks, such as throwing a temper tantrum, or mildly awkward tasks, such as counting aloud while a confederate watched through a two-way mirror. Afterward, the confederate solicited the participants for help with a school project, which required that the participants complete questionnaires for 30 minutes per day for as many days as they were willing. The control group, who had not engaged in any previous acts, volunteered to help for an average of 5 days. In contrast, participants who had just performed highly embarrassing behaviors offered to help for almost three times as many days (14.9), whereas those who performed the mildly embarrassing acts volunteered an intermediate amount (8.7 days). In an additional study, Apsler (1975) found that embarrassed individuals offered to help more than nonembarrassed individuals even when the person who was asking for help had not been a witness to the embarrassing event. Further evidence that embarrassment produces an urge for remediation can be seen in people's reports of their embarrassing experiences (Miller, 1996); over 30% of the time, they mentioned attempting to repair the event by offering a verbal apology or excuse and trying to redress any harm or damage. In short, embarrassment appears to motivate people to behave in a way that assures others of their prosocial intentions, even when the embarrassing predicament was caused by actions for which they knew they were not truly responsible (i.e., they were following instructions of the experimenter).

Recent work in our lab suggests that this motivation to repair may influence basic cognitive processes such as visual attention. Using an eye tracker, we recorded the gaze patterns of embarrassed people as they looked at still photographs of faces that displayed angry, sad, happy, or neutral expressions (Darby & Harris, 2010). Relative to nonemotional

participants, embarrassed participants focused a larger proportion of their fixations to the eyes and a smaller proportion to the mouths of the faces in the pictures. This pattern was particularly pronounced when the embarrassed participants were viewing angry expressions. These findings suggest that embarrassment may increase attention to the most socially informative area of the face, the eyes, which are critical in recognizing complex emotions, emotional intensity, and direction of attention (Baron-Cohen, Wheelwright, & Jolliffe, 1997; Matsumoto, 2005). Why would embarrassed people be particularly drawn to the information contained in the eyes of others? Darby and Harris (2010) suggest that embarrassed individuals are more motivated to ascertain the emotional response of others because doing so helps determine the best course of action to effectively mitigate a social mistake. For example, if one's audience is laughing at one's transgression, then joining in their laughter might be the best strategy to overcome the situation. However, laughter would likely be a bad strategy when faced with an angry audience. Thus, while embarrassed individuals engage in downward glances and frequent gaze shifts (Harris, 2001; Keltner, 1995), they also appear to be attending to the social and emotional cues of others, perhaps in the service of repairing their social transgressions.

The Dark Side

If displaying and experiencing embarrassment generally has beneficial social consequences, one might wonder why the experience of the emotion is so unpleasant. The subjective unpleasantness provides a strong motivation for people to actively try to avoid future behaviors that might lead them to experience embarrassment—obviously a good goal in many social situations. However, it is this very desire to circumvent embarrassment that produces its most harmful effects, as people will go to great lengths to avoid even the slightest risk of being embarrassed. For example, Sabini and colleagues (Sabini, Siepmann, & Stein, 2001) have argued that a substantial reason that bystanders often fail to intervene during potential emergency situations (known as the *bystander effect* in social psychology) is fear of embarrassment. Bystanders worry about looking silly if they respond as if the situation is a crisis and it turns out not to be. Fear of embarrassment has also been shown to have a variety of detrimental effects in the health domain, including not buying or using condoms, not getting recommended cancer screening exams, and not seeking medical care for potentially serious symptoms such as those that might be indicative of cardiac distress (due to worries of looking silly if it is a false alarm; Harris, 2006; Leary & Dobbins, 1983).

In sum, although embarrassment like any negative emotion can produce unfavorable social and personal consequences, it also has a wide-range of beneficial functions in many day-to-day interactions.

SHAME AND GUILT

The distinction between shame and guilt is very important, since these two emotions may tear a person in opposite directions. The wish to relieve guilt may motivate a confession, but the wish to avoid the humiliation of shame may prevent it.
—PAUL EKMAN (2009, pp. 65–66)

We next turn to two other emotions that arise when one has committed a social transgression, namely, shame and guilt. Some theorists have argued that shame, guilt, and embarrassment are all distinct emotions, although the boundaries between these states are not always clear-cut. Although guilt and embarrassment are rarely confused with one another, shame seems to share elements with both. For example, embarrassment and shame arise over exposure of a flaw and involve the potential negative evaluation of others. Moreover, several languages have just one word to describe both emotions (Haidt & Keltner, 1999; Lutz, 1982). However, people's descriptions of the subjective experience of embarrassment, as well as the antecedent events, suggest some differences from shame. Furthermore, embarrassment is frequently associated with smiling (or smile suppression), whereas smiling is not frequently reported during shameful events and, at least in the United States, people are good at distinguishing between embarrassment and shame displays (Keltner, 1995; Keltner & Buswell, 1996).

In contrast, the distinctions between shame and guilt are less clear-cut. There is a great amount of overlap in participants' descriptions of shame and guilt, and, at least in the United States, participants often do not reliably distinguish between these two emotional states (e.g., Fessler, 2004; Stearns & Parrott, 2012; Tangney & Dearing, 2002). However, among researchers there has been considerable debate about possible differences between these two emotions. For example, it has been proposed that shame and guilt differ according to whether they occur in public versus private, involve a moral violation, motivate approach or avoidance, and focus on feeling bad about the entire self versus feeling bad only about the transgression.

One of the most influential accounts of the difference between shame and guilt has been offered by the clinician Helen Lewis (1971) and championed by June Tangney and colleagues (e.g., Tangney & Dearing, 2002). These theorists argue that shame is a negative emotion with no redeeming qualities, whereas guilt has more constructive social and personal consequences. The differential effects are proposed to be due to shame and guilt being associated with different types of attributions. In both cases, one acknowledges fault for a wrongdoing, but in guilt, one makes attributions about the act itself ("It was a bad thing to do"), whereas in shame, one makes attributions about the entire self ("I'm a bad person"). Thus

shame is argued to arise from condemnation of the whole self, whereas guilt arises from condemnation of the behavior, often referred to as the whole-self-versus-behavior distinction (Lewis, 1971; Tangney & Dearing, 2002). Inherent in this view is the proposition that these differing attributions produce differences in motivations and behaviors (Tangney, Wagner, Hill-Barlow, Marschall, & Gramzow, 1996; Tangney, Stuewig, & Mashek, 2007). Because the core self is the root of the problem in a shame experience, little can be done to resolve the issue (one's core self is presumably hard to change). This difficulty in changing leads to the problematic behaviors that characterize shame, including the motivation to avoid others. In contrast, because a behavior (rather than the whole self) is the root of the problem in a guilt experience, the guilty individual is likely to be able to make amends for the behavior and thus is motivated to engage in more constructive approach behaviors.

Empirical Studies

Most of the evidence for the view that shame leads to destructive outcomes and guilt leads to beneficial outcomes comes from studies of individual differences in the propensity to experience these emotions. Such work has found that a dispositional proneness to feel shame has been correlated with problem behaviors such as drug and alcohol abuse and the willingness to drive drunk and to shoplift, as well as other negative emotional states, such as maladaptive anger and depression (Dearing, Stuewig, & Tangney, 2005; Tangney, Wagner, Fletcher, & Gramzow, 1992; Tangney et al., 1996; Tibbetts, 1997). In contrast, dispositional guilt proneness has been associated with more beneficial states, such as greater empathy and more constructive anger responses (Leith & Baumeister, 1998; Tangney et al., 1996).

However, importantly, not all studies support the hypothesis that the outcomes of shame are exclusively bad and those of guilt good. For example, De Hooge, Zeelenberg, and Breugelmans (2010, 2011) have shown that shame can motivate approach behaviors, which are aimed at restoring the person's self after the damaging transgression, as well as avoidance behaviors, which protect the self from further damage. Research on shame in medical settings also has found that shame can be associated with both constructive and detrimental behaviors (Harris & Darby, 2009). In a survey about interactions with their doctors, over half the respondents acknowledged that they had experienced shame. A fair number of the individuals who reported such experiences attributed undesirable outcomes to the interaction, including enduring distress (32.9%), termination of treatment (20%), and lying to the physician (15.8%). However, similar numbers of participants reported favorable consequences. For example, 33% stated that the shame-provoking interaction led to beneficial behavioral changes,

and 46% said they were appreciative of the physician. Interestingly, men reported better emotional and behavioral consequences than women. Such data clearly suggest that shame need not always lead to exclusively corrosive consequences.

Our lab has been focusing on trying to uncover what factors in shame and guilt are associated with helpful versus harmful effects (Darby & Harris, 2013). As suggested by Lewis (1971), it appears likely that shame is more often associated with negative attributions about the self and guilt with negative attributions about the behavior. However, both types of attributions can occur in either emotion, just as both amends and avoidance motivations can occur with either emotion (e.g., Harris & Darby, 2009; Tangney et al., 1996). Therefore, we suggest that, rather than concentrating on the general emotion labels "shame" or "guilt," a more productive strategy for predicting whether people will engage in amends making versus negative outcomes such as avoidance is to examine the cognitions that occur in a specific instance of shame or guilt. In particular, we propose that amends-making outcomes will be predicted by the extent to which people attribute the transgression to a particular bad act that they performed without indicting themselves in entirety. In contrast, damaging outcomes such as avoidance will result when people attribute the transgression to unchangeable faults within themselves.

Several recent studies conducted in our lab are consistent with this view. For example, participants asked to recall a shame-inducing experience did not report reliably different approach-versus-avoidance motivations compared with participants recalling a guilt-inducing experience (Darby & Harris, 2013). Interestingly, though, regardless of whether participants were recalling shame or guilt, the degree to which they focused on blaming themselves versus blaming their behavior was associated with the types of motivations they experienced. Specifically, greater self-condemnation was correlated with avoiding others, whereas greater behavior condemnation was correlated with making amends (Darby & Harris, 2013). In another study, we also found that specific cognitions predict whether a patient had constructive versus destructive reactions to a shameful medical encounter with a doctor (Darby, Henniger, & Harris, in press). When feeling shame, people reported being motivated to engage in behaviors that were likely to be detrimental to their health (such as avoiding the physician), as well as motivations to engage in health-promoting behaviors (such as working toward solving the medical problem), replicating results of an earlier study by Harris and Darby (2009). However, in the present study, participants also reported on the extent to which they attributed negative aspects of the incident to themselves in entirety or to their behavior. Consistent with our predictions, people who reported greater self-condemnation also reported more health-compromising behavioral outcomes, such as avoiding their

physicians. In contrast, people who reported more behavior condemnation reported engaging in more health-promoting behaviors, such as following the physician's instructions or becoming more careful and knowledgeable about their health. This line of research suggests that understanding the types of attributions that a person makes about his or her shameful encounter is important in predicting subsequent outcomes across a number of situations, including medical settings, which have obvious practical consequences.

JEALOUSY

What makes the pain we feel from shame and jealousy so cutting is that vanity can give us no assistance in bearing them.
—FRANÇOIS DE LA ROCHEFOUCAULD

Jealousy is an emotion that arises when a valued relationship is threatened by a third party (Parrott & Smith, 1993; Salovey, 1991). Societal perceptions of jealousy have varied greatly across time and culture. In the United States, jealousy shifted from being seen as a legitimate motivation for murder in the 19th century to being viewed as a childish personal flaw in the 20th century (Stearns, 2010). As a leading motivation in homicide, spousal abuse, and family breakups (Harris, 2003), jealousy has earned a justly negative reputation for its highly visible destructive consequences. At the same time, at its best, jealousy can lead people to take the actions necessary to protect their most important relationships. This emotion functions to preserve both the rewards of the relationship and the self-esteem that is derived from the relationship (e.g., Harris, 2003; Sabini & Silver, 2005; Salovey & Rothman, 1991).

Jealousy in Nonromantic Relationships

The majority of the research on jealousy has focused on romantic/sexual relationships. However, people also receive many important benefits from nonromantic bonds, such as friendships and parent–child relationships, and therefore, can suffer considerable disadvantages when those relationships are usurped by others. Given this, several theorists have argued that the emotional process that induces jealousy in romantic relationships is also involved in producing jealousy in other types of relationships (Harris, 2003; Parrott, 1991; Salovey & Rodin, 1984). For example, jealousy may play a significant role in the phenomenon of sibling rivalry. Time, affection, and even food can be scarce resources that a parent must divide among offspring. In such situations, jealousy can serve as a means of assuring that

one is not short-changed by a bond between one's parent and a sibling. One intriguing possibility is that jealousy initially may have arisen both ontogenetically and phylogenetically from competition between siblings and only later became an emotion that is integral to romantic relationships.

Developmental studies have found that infants as young as 6 months of age express behaviors that appear to be jealousy (Hart & Carrington, 2002; Legerstee, Ellenbogen, Nienhuis, & Marsh, 2010). For example, babies show more negative affective and attention-seeking behaviors when their mothers interact with what appears to be another baby (but is actually a realistic-appearing doll) but do not show the same behaviors when their mothers attend to a nonsocial item (a book; Hart & Carrington, 2002). This finding suggests that even infants may respond to the potential usurpation of the benefits of the parent–child relationship.

There is also new work emerging with nonhuman species that appears consistent with the hypothesis that jealousy is useful in protecting a range of valuable relationships from potential rivals (Harris & Prouvost, 2013; Morris, Coe, & Godsell, 2008). From a functional standpoint, one might predict that if jealousy is an emotion that evolved to protect social bonds in humans, it might also exist in other social species in which bonds between individuals develop and can be threatened by third parties. Our lab recently examined this issue (Harris & Prouvost, 2012) by testing 36 dogs on a modified version of the infant jealousy paradigm used by Hart and Carrington (2002). The dog owners were instructed to ignore their dogs while engaging in various behaviors. In the jealousy condition, the dog's owner treated a stuffed dog, which wagged its tail and briefly barked, as if it were a real dog (e.g., petting it, speaking in "baby talk" to it). In a second condition, owners engaged in these same behaviors but did so toward a novel object (jack-o'-lantern pail). In the third condition, the owner read a children's book out loud. The dogs exhibited significantly more behaviors that would be consistent with jealousy (e.g., snapping, placing themselves between the owner and the object, pushing/touching the object/owner) when their owners displayed affectionate behaviors toward what appeared to be another dog as compared with their owners' interactions with inanimate objects. These results lend some support to the hypothesis that jealousy may exist in a "primordial" form in at least one other species besides humans.

One interesting implication from the work with infants and dogs is that some form of jealousy can exist without requiring complex interpretations of what the rival relationship means for one's own self-concept or self-esteem. Although cognitive appraisals about the meaning of the betrayal clearly can affect jealousy in adult relationships (White & Mullen, 1989), such cognitions may not be necessary to elicit a more primitive version of jealousy. The simple assessment that a loved one is paying attention to a potential rival may be sufficient to prompt a motivational state aimed

at blocking the liaison. However, as thinking becomes more cognitively sophisticated and self-reflective, what triggers jealousy becomes more complex. For example, developmental work suggests that even by 4 years of age, the specifics of the social triangle (e.g., rival's age) can affect jealous reactions (Masciuch & Kienapple, 1993).

Jealousy in Romantic Relationships

In addition to the parent–child relationship, the type of bond that is likely to have the greatest consequences for a person's own outcomes and those of their offspring is arguably a romantic relationship. Some work finds that people who are more invested in their relationships and whose mates have higher mate values are more likely to experience jealousy (Rydell, McConnell, & Bringle, 2004; Sidelinger & Booth-Butterfield, 2007), suggesting that jealousy is more likely when the cost of the loss of one's partner is higher. In romantic relationships, the experience of jealousy is most often construed as negative, but couples can also view jealousy as being a natural part of being in a relationship and even as a marker of a healthy bond (Staske, 1999). The connection between jealousy and beneficial outcomes finds some support among correlational studies suggesting that jealousy may be related to both the length and the quality of romantic partnerships.

The function of jealousy, to protect relationships, suggests that appropriate jealous reactions should lead to longer lasting relationships. Mathes (1986) conducted a study in which participants completed a questionnaire about jealousy in their current relationships. Seven years later, he followed up with participants on the status of those relationships. Participants who had reported greater jealousy were more likely to still be in committed relationships with those same persons 7 years later. Because this was a correlational study, it is impossible to know whether jealousy directly contributed to protecting and thereby preserving the relationship or whether some third variable (such as valuing the relationship) produced both greater jealousy and greater relationship longevity. Nevertheless, at the very least, this finding suggests that jealousy did not directly harm these relationships, and, in fact, it may have contributed to the persistence of the longer lasting relationships.

Although Mathes (1986) provided evidence that greater jealousy in a relationship was associated with longer relationship duration, he did not investigate whether people were actually happy in their prolonged relationships. There is some other work, however, that suggests that jealousy, despite feeling subjectively unpleasant, can sometimes be associated with other, positive aspects of relationships. Hansen (1983) conducted a survey among men and found that greater marital satisfaction was associated with greater reports of jealousy to hypothetical jealousy-inducing situations.

Other correlational work (Dugosh, 2000) with both men and women found that dispositional jealousy predicted relationship satisfaction (an effect that was particularly strong for participants who were more in love).

However, the positive association between relationship satisfaction and jealousy may be dependent on the type of jealousy being examined. In one study, people who reported higher quality relationships also reported more reactive jealousy to imagining their mate cheating (Barelds & Barelds-Dijkstra, 2007). In contrast, anxious jealousy, measured by people's reports of upset about the possibility of betrayal, was correlated with lower relationship quality. Possessive jealousy (the desire of the person to limit his or her mate's contact with other people) was not consistently related to relationship quality. Thus only jealousy in response to what seemed to be actual betrayal was positively associated with relationship quality.

We do not want to appear to overstate the connection between jealousy and healthy relationship functioning. As discussed in the introduction to this section, jealousy can lead to consequences as dire as death and divorce. Whether jealousy is beneficial in a relationship is clearly a complex matter, and further work on understanding exactly when this emotion serves the best interest of the individual and the relationship is clearly needed. Some factors that are likely to be important in determining the outcomes of jealousy are whether the threat is real and whether there are actions that can be taken to maintain the relationship (Harris & Darby, 2010). The propensity to see threat varies across individuals. The harmful manifestations of jealousy might often occur when the threshold for perceiving threat is set too low and people therefore are responding to their own anxious imaginings rather that to an actual threat. In such cases, jealousy would not be beneficial because the coordinated emotional response is targeted toward solving a problem that does not exist in reality (a threat to the relationship). Jealousy may also be harmful when a relationship is already lost to a rival with no hope for redemption. Indeed, the literature on jealousy and homicide is sprinkled with anecdotal accounts of murderous spouses making remarks such as "if I couldn't have her, then no one would."

Intentionally Inducing Romantic Jealousy

Given the negative perception of jealousy, one might imagine that people try to circumvent jealousy in their lovers as much as possible. Contrary to this expectation, a study of 150 couples found that 31% of women and 17% of males reported attempting to intentionally induce jealousy in their partners (White, 1980). These participants most frequently explained their actions as either a desire to test the relationship or to increase the rewards of the relationship. Participants in another study reported attempting jealousy induction at an even greater rate (Sheets, Fredendall, & Claypool, 1997). In

this work, 73% of participants had tried to induce jealousy at some point in their relationships, most often to gain their partners' attention. Although people may attempt to elicit jealousy in their lovers, it is interesting to note that when people imagine feeling jealous, they predict that they will fight with their partners about the situation more than that they will engage in rewarding behaviors such as paying more attention to their partners (Sheets et al., 1997). This finding suggests that, like the unpleasant subjective feeling of jealousy, the outcomes of this emotion also may not be immediately helpful. However, fighting about a situation may be beneficial in and of itself and may bring about benefits to the relationship in the long term (Brehm, Miller, Perlman, & Campbell, 2002). Further research on the time course of jealousy is necessary in order to understand the complex unfolding of effects for both partners.

ENVY

Envy aims very high.
—OVID

Envy has bred enough hostility and psychological pain to earn the distinction of being considered one of the seven deadly sins in the Western world. This single emotion has been claimed to motivate a wide range of societal phenomena, from the drive toward egalitarianism to the persecution of the Jews in the Holocaust (Glick, 2002; Smith & Kim, 2007). It has even been proposed that the downfall of communism in Russia was partially due to the envy elicited in Russians when they were exposed to American luxuries in a televised debate between the Russian premier and the U.S. president in 1959 (Belk, 2008). Such disparate results display the power of envy to produce both constructive and destructive consequences on a large scale. This section explores some of the factors that underlie the large variation in the outcomes of this emotion.

Envy arises when a person wants what someone else has, whether the envied thing is an object, trait, or circumstance (Parrott & Smith, 1993). This emotion can incorporate both a sense of one's own inferiority and a feeling of hostility toward the comparison target (Smith & Kim, 2007). The comparison target is by definition superior in some way to the person feeling envy. However, people do not envy every better-off person they encounter, nor do they experience the greatest envy toward the person who has the absolute most in any particular domain. Instead, it has been repeatedly observed that people are more likely to envy those who are more similar to them and who excel in a domain that is relevant to the envier (Harris

& Henniger, 2013; Salovey & Rodin, 1984; Schaubroeck & Lam, 2004). For example, people are more likely to envy someone of their own gender and age (Harris & Henniger, 2013).

But why do we envy similar others rather than those who are the absolute best in a domain? This question may be answered by examining the hypothesized function of envy. People's position on a status hierarchy is important for their self-evaluation, as well as their probability of acquiring physical rewards, and envy can motivate people to improve their standing relative to others (D'Arms & Kerr, 2008; Smith & Kim, 2007). Others who are close to an individual on a relevant status hierarchy may be the most appropriate targets for a competitive response because these are the people that the individual has a chance at besting (D'Arms & Kerr, 2008).

In order to achieve the goal of moving one's relative place in a hierarchy, one can either move oneself up in the hierarchy or bring superior people down. Envy, therefore, can motivate people to change themselves in order to acquire the object that they lack (e.g., Crusius & Mussweiler, 2012), or it can motivate people to harm individuals who have already obtained the target object (e.g., Parrott & Smith, 1993). Both of these types of responses contribute toward the overarching goal of eliminating the unfavorable comparison and may ultimately result in beneficial outcomes for the envier, but these ends are achieved through different means. For example, envious anger can motivate hostility toward the other person or provide the motivation to persevere and improve oneself. Of note, some researchers argue that in order for an emotional state to be considered envy it must include an element of hostility (e.g., Smith & Kim, 2007), but this view is challenged by others (e.g., van de Ven, Zeelenberg, & Pieters, 2009).

Hostility and Anger in Envy

The elements of hostility and anger that accompany most envious experiences are largely responsible for the negative reputation of envy. Envious people report feeling hostile toward their rivals (e.g., Parrott & Smith, 1993), and envy has been found to mediate feelings of *schadenfreude* (happiness at the misfortune of others) in response to the downfall of an accomplished person (Brigham, Kelso, Jackson, & Smith, 1997). Hostility can also take the form of an altered appraisal of the rival. For example, bank tellers who had not received a promotion subsequently decreased their liking for the people who had been promoted, and this change was mediated by self-reported feelings of envy (Schaubroeck & Lam, 2004). Presumably, increased disliking would be followed by increased unfriendly behavior as well.

Given its potentially undesirable social consequences, one might assume that the anger component of envy has no redeeming qualities. However, there are intriguing suggestions in the literature that an angry affective state may sometimes have benefits for those who express it (e.g. Smith & Kim, 2007). First, by negatively targeting their rivals, people theoretically can change their standing relative to others. Spite may act as a deterrent and lead to long-term benefits in repeated interactions. Second, apart from the interpersonal effects of anger, this emotion may provide people with the motivation to persevere in order to overcome obstacles.

A number of studies provide insight into the potential benefits of spiteful actions. In economic games, participants who are offered an unfair deal will often reject the offer, even at a cost to themselves (e.g., Zizzo & Oswald, 2001). Such actions may result in long-term benefits, despite the short-term cost, by motivating increased cooperation and fairness in repeated interactions with the same person. In the same way that potentially facing a spiteful reaction may deter people from creating unfair situations, the possibility of encountering a hostile envious reaction might induce people to minimize the difference between themselves and inferior comparison partners in situations in which they could be envied (e.g., Rodriguez Mosquera, Parrott, & de Mendoza, 2010; van de Ven, Zeelenberg, & Pieters, 2010) Indeed, self-reported accounts of being the target of envy include descriptions of worry about the envier's response and the use of various strategies in order to deal with the other person's envy (Rodriguez Mosquera et al., 2010). In an experimental study, participants who unfairly received a reward exhibited increased helping behavior toward people who might envy them, and this increase in helping was mediated by the participant's fear of being maliciously envied (van de Ven et al., 2010). Thus the hostility component in envy sometimes may serve the envier's best interest by inducing the comparison target to act in prosocial ways so as to avoid facing the potential envier's malicious response.

Anger in envious reactions may also help the envier by inducing perseverance in achieving the desired object (see Hess, Chapter 3, this volume). One of the proposed functions of anger is to motivate persistence at a task. Some evidence of this comes from a developmental study by Lewis, Alessandri, and Sullivan (1990). Infants who pulled on a string were rewarded with pleasant music. The string was then detached, and many infants became upset. When the string was subsequently reattached, infants who showed greater expressions of anger relearned the task more quickly relative to those who displayed sad facial expressions. When people experience envious anger, they may be similarly motivated to persevere in their attempts to resolve the comparison situation. In sum, envious people may obtain beneficial outcomes from an increased ability to achieve their goals, as well as from the persuasive effect that their envy can have on others.

Situational Characteristics Influencing Envy

There are hints in the literature that at least two factors might contribute to whether an envious person will be primarily motivated toward interpersonal aggression or toward self-improvement. One important appraisal seems to be whether the situation is perceived as being zero-sum; that is, whether one person's success means that others cannot succeed (e.g., Rodriguez Mosquera et al., 2010; Smith & Kim, 2007; Zizzo, 2008). It has been suggested that hostility may be particularly likely to arise if only one person can obtain the desired object. However, when multiple people can attain the same goal, then envy may have more constructive effects for the individual and even perhaps for the group. Although there is research consistent with this hypothesis (e.g., Rodriguez Mosquera et al., 2010; van de Ven, Zeelenberg, & Pieters, 2011), we are not aware of any experimental studies that directly manipulate the zero-sum characteristic of the situation, and further research is needed in order to evaluate this hypothesis.

A second factor that affects envious responses is perceived control. People who perceive themselves as being able to attain the desired object may be more likely to focus their responses on self-improvement. In contrast, people with low perceived control may react with hostility or depression. This perceived ability to achieve is independent of whether the situation is zero-sum. A student may perceive herself as eventually being capable of being the top student (zero-sum, as there can only be one top student) or capable of getting good grades (not zero-sum, as more than one person can get good grades), or she may believe that either of these results is impossible for some reason, such as poor performance early in a class.

Research directly testing the role of perceived control or efficacy in envious reactions is lacking. However, several findings in the more general literature are consistent with a possible association. In a study of social comparisons that did not directly assess envy, Testa and Major (1990) found that participants in a low-perceived-control condition reported feeling more hostile and depressed and were less persistent at a subsequent task than participants in a high-control condition. Van de Ven and colleagues (2011) found that when participants were led to perceive personal change as easy and then were presented with a vignette about an accomplished person, they were more likely to experience envy without hostility ("benign envy") than malicious envy or admiration and to feel more motivated to improve themselves. In contrast, when participants believed that change was hard, they were more likely to feel admiration and less likely to feel motivated to improve; interestingly, malicious envy was not affected by perceptions of ease of change. However, the main focus of the van de Ven et al. (2011) study was on distinguishing benign envy from malicious envy rather than on fully exploring either emotion. Future research could benefit from

further investigation of the role of perceived control in malicious envy with more comprehensive measures of hostility and its potential ramifications.

CONCLUSION

Each year one of us (C.R.H.) asks the students in her large course on emotions, "If you could choose to never experience unpleasant emotions again, would you?" Inevitably, a large portion answer, "Yes." In this chapter (and subsequently in that course), we argue that the complete elimination of all unpleasant emotional states would likely not be to one's advantage. In an ideal world, we would not find ourselves in situations that elicit feelings such as embarrassment, shame, guilt, envy, or jealousy. However, short of giving up all social contact (which would result in its own tribulations), we will inevitably be faced with social dilemmas that result in negative feelings. These affective states, although undeniably unpleasant, can serve our best interests. In some ways, they are analogous to pain. Few of us would opt to voluntarily experience pain, but its presence warns that something is amiss in our physical world. People who are born with an insensitivity to pain face a host of health consequences, from chewing on their own mouths to major injuries and burns. The negative emotions described here provide signals indicating a problem in our social world and can prompt actions to remedy the situation. This, however, does not mean that the experience of negative emotions is unequivocally good any more than the experience of pain is always good (e.g., as experienced by terminally ill patients).

In this chapter, we have laid out some of the specific situations and cognitions that are associated with personal and social benefits for each of five different emotions. One might wonder whether there are some overarching principles that apply across these emotions to dictate when beneficial effects will emerge. It turns out that generalities are difficult to make. This may speak to just how different these emotions are from one another despite all being subjectively unpleasant emotions arising in social contexts and even often occurring (and co-occurring) in similar situations. Just as hunger and thirst often co-occur and are both key to survival, to state precisely when they are beneficial requires examining each separately, as well as the state of the organism that is experiencing them.

Nonetheless, we do offer some general themes that we see emerging. First, these emotions are likely to motivate constructive behavior when they occur in situations in which the threats are real (or at least highly probable) and in which the person has the ability to modify the situation (or at least senses that she or he does). Some of these emotions' most counterproductive effects result when people are overly concerned with perceived threats

that likely do not exist in reality. The potential harm of such an error can be seen in romantic partners who experience excessive anxious jealousy when no rival actually exists or in patients who avoid doctors for fear of looking silly. (Such a fear likely has little merit in medical contexts, and even when it might, it should not outweigh the benefits of getting needed medical care or screening.)

Second, the perception that one can somehow change the situation or resolve the social dilemma is likely to be associated with more beneficial effects across most of these emotional situations. This proposition is consistent with suggestions in the literature that perceived control influences subsequent motivations in the experience of shame or guilt (e.g., De Hooge et al., 2010; Tracy & Robins, 2006). Global negative attributions about the self after a social transgression likely lead to the perception of a lack of control, as it is difficult to change the core of oneself. This perceived lack of control over the root of the problem may therefore promote less optimal resolution strategies, such as avoiding others. In contrast, attributions that one did a bad thing (but not that one's self is bad) appear more likely to promote amends-making behaviors, perhaps because one perceives greater potential control over one's behavior. Similarly, in experiences of envy, perceptions that a goal is obtainable may be a key factor in motivating people to strive toward the goal themselves rather than focusing efforts on bringing down the envied person who has already obtained the goal (e.g., Smith & Kim, 2007).

In closing, although the social emotions discussed here often have earned their negative reputations, they are states that, at least under some circumstances, serve the interests of those who experience them.

REFERENCES

Apsler, R. (1975). Effects of embarrassment on behavior toward others. *Journal of Personality and Social Psychology, 32,* 145–153.

Barelds, D. P., & Barelds-Dijkstra, P. (2007). Relations between different types of jealousy and self and partner perceptions of relationship quality. *Clinical Psychology and Psychotherapy, 14,* 176–188.

Baron-Cohen, S., Wheelwright, S., & Jolliffe, T. (1997). Is there a "language of the eyes"?: Evidence from normal adults, and adults with autism or Asperger syndrome. *Visual Cognition, 4,* 311–331.

Belk, R. W. (2008). Marketing and envy. In R. H. Smith (Ed.), *Envy: Theory and research* (pp. 211–226). New York: Oxford University Press.

Brehm, S. S., Miller, R. S., Perlman, D., & Campbell, S. M. (2002). Conflict and violence. In S. S. Brehm et al. *Intimate relationships* (pp. 333–366). Boston: McGraw Hill.

Brigham, N. L., Kelso, K. A., Jackson, M. A., & Smith, R. H. (1997). The roles

of invidious comparisons and deservingness in sympathy and *schadenfreude*. *Basic and Applied Social Psychology, 19*, 363–380.

Crusius, J., & Mussweiler, T. (2012). When people want what others have: The impulsive side of envious desire. *Emotion, 12*, 142–153.

Darby, R. S., & Harris, C. R. (2010). Embarrassment's effect on facial processing. *Cognition and Emotion, 24*, 1250–1258.

Darby, R. S., & Harris, C. R. (2013). *The motivations of the self-conscious emotions*. Manuscript in preparation.

Darby, R. S., Henniger, N. E., & Harris, C. R. (in press). Reactions to physician-inspired shame and guilt. *Basic and Applied Social Psychology*.

D'Arms, J., & Kerr, A. D. (2008). Envy in the philosophical tradition. In R. H. Smith (Ed.) *Envy: Theory and research* (pp. 39–59). New York: Oxford University Press.

De Hooge, I. E., Zeelenberg, M., & Breugelmans, S. M. (2010). Restore and protect motivations following shame. *Cognition and Emotion, 24*, 111–127.

De Hooge, I. E., Zeelenberg, M., & Breugelmans, S. M. (2011). A functionalist account of shame-induced behaviour. *Cognition and Emotion, 25*, 939–946.

de Jong, P. J. (1999). Communicative and remedial effects of social blushing. *Journal of Nonverbal Behavior, 23*, 197–217.

de Jong, P. J., Peters, M. L., de Cremer, D., & Vranken, C. (2002). Blushing after a moral transgression in a prisoner's dilemma game: Appeasing or revealing? *European Journal of Social Psychology, 32*, 627–644.

Dearing, R. L., Stuewig, J., & Tangney, J. P. (2005). On the importance of distinguishing shame from guilt: Relations to problematic alcohol and drug use. *Addictive Behaviors, 30*, 1392–1404.

Dugosh, J. W. (2000). On predicting relationship satisfaction from jealousy: The moderating effects of love. *Current Research in Social Psychology, 5*, 254–263.

Ekman, P. (1992). Are there basic emotions? *Psychological Review, 99*, 550–553.

Ekman, P. (2009). *Telling lies: Clues to deceit in the marketplace, politics, and marriage*. New York: Norton.

Fessler, D. M. T. (2004). Shame in two cultures: Implications for evolutionary approaches. *Journal of Cognition and Culture, 4*, 207–262.

Frijda, N. (1986). *The emotions*. Cambridge, UK: Cambridge University Press.

Glick, P. (2002). Sacrificial lambs dressed in wolves' clothing: Envious prejudice, ideology, and the scapegoating of Jews. In L. S. Newman & R. Erber (Eds.), *What social psychology can tell us about the Holocaust* (pp. 113–142). Oxford, UK: Oxford University Press.

Haidt, J., & Keltner, D. (1999). Culture and facial expression: Open-ended methods find more faces and a gradient of recognition. *Cognition and Emotion, 13*, 225–266.

Hansen, G. L. (1983). Marital satisfaction and jealousy among men. *Psychological Reports, 52*, 363–366.

Harris, C. R. (2001). Cardiovascular responses of embarrassment and effects of emotional suppression in a social setting. *Journal of Personality and Social Psychology, 81*, 886–897.

Harris, C. R. (2003). A review of sex differences in sexual jealousy, including

self-report data, psychophysiological responses, interpersonal violence and morbid jealousy. *Personality and Social Psychology Review, 7,* 102–128.

Harris, C. R. (2006). Embarrassment: A form of social pain. *American Scientist, 94,* 524–533.

Harris, C. R., & Darby, R. S. (2009). Shame in physician–patient interactions: Patient perspectives. *Basic and Applied Social Psychology, 31,* 325–334.

Harris, C. R., & Darby, R. S. (2010). Jealousy in adulthood. In S. L. Hart & M. Legerstee (Eds.), *Handbook of jealousy: Theory, research, and multidisciplinary approaches* (pp. 547–571). Oxford, UK: Wiley-Blackwell.

Harris, C. R., & Henniger, N. E. (2013). *Envy in adulthood: Differences across gender and age in the experience of being envied.* Manuscript in preparation.

Harris, C. R., & Prouvost, C. (2013). *Jealousy in dogs: Evidence for a primordial form of jealousy.* Manuscript submitted for publication.

Hart, S. L., & Carrington, H. A. (2002). Jealousy in six-month-old infants. *Infancy, 3,* 395–402.

Kappas, A. (2011). Emotion and regulation are one! *Emotion Review, 3,* 17–25.

Keltner, D. (1995). Signs of appeasement: Evidence for the distinct displays of embarrassment, amusement, and shame. *Journal of Personality and Social Psychology, 68,* 441–454.

Keltner, D., & Buswell, B. N. (1996). Evidence for the distinctness of embarrassment, shame, and guilt: A study of recalled antecedents and facial expressions. *Cognition and Emotion, 10,* 155–171.

Keltner, D., & Buswell, B. N. (1997). Embarrassment: Its distinct form and appeasement functions. *Psychological Bulletin, 122,* 250–270.

Leary, M. R., & Dobbins, S. E. (1983). Social anxiety, sexual behavior, and contraceptive use. *Journal of Personality and Social Psychology, 45,* 1347–1354.

Legerstee, M., Ellenbogen, B., Nienhuis, T., & Marsh, H. (2010). Social bonds, triadic relationships, and goals: Predictions for the emergence of human jealousy. In S. L. Hart & M. Legerstee (Eds.), *Handbook of jealousy: Theory, research, and multidisciplinary approaches* (pp. 163–191). Oxford, UK: Wiley-Blackwell.

Leith, K. P., & Baumeister, R. F. (1998). Empathy, shame, guilt, and narratives of interpersonal conflicts: Guilt-prone people are better at perspective taking. *Journal of Personality, 66,* 1–37.

Levin, J., & Arluke, A. (1982). Embarrassment and helping behavior. *Psychological Report, 51,* 999–1002.

Lewis, H. B. (1971). Shame and guilt in neurosis. *Psychoanalytic Review, 58,* 419–438.

Lewis, M., Alessandri, S. M., & Sullivan, M. W. (1990). Violation of expectancy, loss of control, and anger expressions in young infants. *Developmental Psychology, 26,* 745–751.

Lutz, C. A. (1982). The domain of emotion words in Ifaluk. *American Ethnologist, 9,* 113–128.

Masciuch, S., & Kienapple, K. (1993). The emergence of jealousy in children 4 months to 7 years of age. *Journal of Social and Personal Relationships, 10,* 421–435.

Mathes, E. W. (1986). Jealousy and romantic love: A longitudinal study. *Psychological Reports, 58,* 885–886.

Matsumoto, D. (2005). Face, culture, and judgments of anger and fear: Do the eyes have it? *Journal of Nonverbal Behavior, 13,* 171–188.

Miller, R. S. (1996). *Embarrassment: Poise and peril in everyday life.* New York: Guilford Press.

Morris, P., Coe, C., & Godsell, E. (2008). Secondary emotions in non-primate species?: Behavioral reports and subjective claims by animal owners. *Cognition and Emotion, 22,* 3–20.

Nesse, R. M. (1990). Evolutionary explanations of emotions. *Human Nature, 1,* 263–289.

Parrott, W. G. (1991). The emotional experiences of envy and jealousy. In P. Salovey (Ed.), *The psychology of jealousy and envy* (pp. 3–30). New York: Guilford Press.

Parrott, W. G., & Smith, R. H. (1993). Distinguishing the experiences of envy and jealousy. *Journal of Personality and Social Psychology, 64,* 906–920.

Rodriguez Mosquera, P. M., Parrott, W. G., & Hurtado de Mendoza, A. (2010). I fear your envy, I rejoice in your coveting: On the ambivalent experience of being envied by others. *Journal of Personality and Social Psychology, 99,* 842–854.

Rydell, R. J., McConnell, A. R., & Bringle, R. G. (2004). Jealousy and commitment: Perceived threat and the effect of relationship alternatives. *Personal Relationships, 11,* 451–468.

Sabini, J., Siepmann, M., & Stein, J. (2001). The really fundamental attribution error in social psychological research. *Psychological Inquiry, 12,* 1–15.

Sabini, J., & Silver, M. (2005). Ekman's basic emotions: Why not love and jealousy? *Cognition and Emotion, 19,* 693–712.

Salovey, P. (Ed.). (1991). *The psychology of jealousy and envy.* New York: Guilford Press.

Salovey, P., & Rodin, J. (1984). Some antecedents and consequences of social-comparison jealousy. *Journal of Personality and Social Psychology, 47,* 780–792.

Salovey, P., & Rothman, A. (1991). Envy and jealousy: Self and society. In P. Salovey (Ed.), *The psychology of jealousy and envy* (pp. 271–286). New York: Guilford Press.

Schaubroeck, J., & Lam, S. S. K. (2004). Comparing lots before and after: Promotion rejectees' invidious reactions to promotees. *Organizational Behavior and Human Decision Processes, 94,* 33–47.

Semin, G. R., & Manstead, A. S. R. (1982). The social implications of embarrassment displays and restitution behaviour. *European Journal of Social Psychology, 12,* 367–377.

Sheets, V. L., Fredendall, L. L., & Claypool, H. M. (1997). Jealousy evocation, partner reassurance, and relationship stability: An exploration of the potential benefits of jealousy. *Evolution and Human Behavior, 18,* 387–402.

Sidelinger, R. J., & Booth-Butterfield, M. (2007). Mate value discrepancy as predictor of forgiveness and jealousy in romantic relationships. *Communication Quarterly, 55,* 207–223.

Smith, R. H., & Kim, S. H. (2007). Comprehending envy. *Psychological Bulletin, 133,* 46–64.

Staske, S. A. (1999). Creating relational ties in talk: The collaborative construction of relational jealousy. *Symbolic Interaction, 22,* 213–246.

Stearns, D. C., & Parrott, W. G. (2012). When feeling bad makes you look good: Guilt, shame, and person perception. *Cognition and Emotion, 26,* 407–430.

Stearns, P. N. (2010). Jealousy in adulthood. In S. L. Hart & M. Legerstee (Eds.), *Handbook of jealousy: Theory, research, and multidisciplinary approaches* (pp. 7–26). Oxford, UK: Wiley-Blackwell.

Tangney, J. P., & Dearing, R. L. (2002). *Shame and guilt.* New York: Guilford Press.

Tangney, J. P., Stuewig, J., & Mashek, D. J. (2007). Moral emotions and moral behavior. *Annual Review of Psychology, 58,* 345–372.

Tangney, J. P., Wagner, P., Fletcher, C., & Gramzow, R. (1992). Shamed into anger?: The relation of shame and guilt to anger and self-reported aggression. *Journal of Personality and Social Psychology, 62,* 669–675.

Tangney, J. P., Wagner, P. E., Hill-Barlow, D., Marschall, D. E., & Gramzow, R. (1996). Relation of shame and guilt to constructive versus destructive responses to anger across the lifespan. *Journal of Personality and Social Psychology, 70,* 797–809.

Testa, M., & Major, B. (1990). The impact of social comparison after failure: The moderating effects of perceived control. *Basic and Applied Social Psychology, 11,* 205–218.

Tibbetts, S. G. (1997). Shame and rational choice in offending decisions. *Criminal Justice and Behavior, 24,* 234–255.

Tracy, J. L., & Robins, R. W. (2006). Appraisal antecedents of shame and guilt: Support for a theoretical model. *Personality and Social Psychology Bulletin, 32,* 1339–1351.

van de Ven, N., Zeelenberg, M., & Pieters, R. (2009). Leveling up and down: The experiences of benign and malicious envy. *Emotion, 9,* 419–429.

van de Ven, N., Zeelenberg, M., & Pieters, R. (2010). Warding off the evil eye: When the fear of envy increases prosocial behavior. *Psychological Science, 21,* 1671–1677.

van de Ven, N., Zeelenberg, M., & Pieters, R. (2011). Why envy outperforms admiration. *Personality and Social Psychology Bulletin, 37,* 784–795.

White, G. L. (1980). Inducing jealousy: A power perspective. *Personality and Social Psychology Bulletin, 6,* 222–227.

White, G., & Mullen, P. E. (1989). *Jealousy: Theory, research, and clinical strategies.* New York: Guilford Press.

Zizzo, D. (2008). The cognitive and behavioral economics of envy. In R. H. Smith (Ed.), *Envy: Theory and research* (pp. 190–210). New York: Oxford University Press.

Zizzo, D. J., & Oswald, A. (2001). Are people willing to pay to reduce others' incomes? *Annales d'Economie et de Statistique, 63–64,* 39–62.

PART II

SOCIAL AND CULTURAL ASPECTS OF NEGATIVE EMOTIONS

5

When Negative Emotions Benefit Close Relationships

LEVI R. BAKER
JAMES K. McNULTY
NICKOLA C. OVERALL

People frequently enter close relationships expecting them to be a fountain of positive emotions. Although close relationships do provide people with some of their most positive emotions (Wallbott & Scherer, 1986), even in the best close relationships people will still experience problems (McGonagle, Kessler, & Schilling, 1992) and thus experience negative emotions (Averill, 1983; Schwartz & Shaver, 1987). For example, people commonly experience anger due to a partner's transgressions, fear due to concerns that a partner will abandon them, jealousy due to concerns about a partner's fidelity, and/or loneliness due to a lack of support from the partner (Leary, 2000; Tangney & Salovey, 1999).

Although these and other negative emotions may be unpleasant, they are not inherently harmful and may serve important functions in relationships. One function of negative emotions is to signal that something is wrong (e.g., Klinger, 1996; Nesse & Ellsworth, 2009). In the context of a close relationship, negative emotions may thus signal that something is wrong with the relationship (Davila, Karney, Hall, & Bradbury, 2003; Fisher & McNulty, 2008; Karney & Bradbury, 1997; Karney, Bradbury, Fincham, & Sullivan, 1994; McNulty, 2008). Another function of negative

emotions is to motivate people to address their problems (Frijda, Kuipers, & ter Schure, 1989; Hiller et al., 2009; McCaul, Branstetter, O'Donnell, Jacobson, & Quinlan, 1998). In the context of a close relationship, negative emotions may thus motivate people to improve the relationship (Baker & McNulty, 2011, 2013; Gonzales, Pederson, Manning, & Wetter, 1990). In other words, although negative emotions may be unpleasant, they can benefit relationships by making individuals aware of their relationship problems and by motivating resolutions of those problems.

Of course, just as negative emotions are not inherently harmful, they are not inherently beneficial, either. The goal of this chapter is to clarify when negative emotions may benefit close relationships. In pursuit of this goal, the first section describes the ways in which *experiencing* negative emotions can benefit relationships—it can increase individuals' understanding of and motivation to resolve their relationship problems. The second section describes the ways in which *expressing* negative emotions can benefit relationships—it can increase partners' intimacy, elicit support, and regulate partner's behavior to better resolve relationship problems. The third section provides a more in-depth analysis of how three specific negative emotions—anger, romantic jealousy, and guilt—lead to distinct behaviors that help resolve unique relationship problems (see Roseman, Wiest, & Swartz, 1994). The last section concludes with a cautionary note about the circumstances in which the benefits of negative emotions for close relationships may not outweigh their negative implications.

EXPERIENCING EMOTIONS

Experiencing negative emotions in the face of a problem can benefit individuals by helping them to recognize and understand, and thus be more likely to address and resolve, that problem (Frijda, 1986; Levenson, 1999; Tooby & Cosmides, 2008). Although the amount and severity of problems can vary across relationships, nearly all people acknowledge experiencing problems that have negatively affected their relationship at some point (e.g., McGonagle et al., 1992). Frequently, these problems emerge when partners have incompatible goals or interests (e.g., Kelley & Thibaut, 1978) or when they encounter external stressors (e.g., Karney & Bradbury, 1995). For example, some of the most common problems that romantic partners experience relate to finances, sex, children, communication, emotional intimacy, household management, decision making, and jealousy (Henry & Miller, 2004; Levenson, Carstensen, & Gottman, 1993; Miller, Yorgason, Sandberg, & White, 2003). Experiencing negative emotions as a result of a problem should help individuals (1) become more aware of the problem and (2) be more motivated to resolve it.

Problem Awareness

Several theoretical accounts of emotions suggest that people are more aware of problems that elicit greater negative emotional responses than they are of problems that are less distressing. For example, evolutionary theories of emotion (e.g., Nesse & Ellsworth, 2009; Plutchik, 2003; Tooby & Cosmides, 2008) suggest that one function of negative emotions is to shift perception and attention toward potential threats and problems to ensure that they are recognized. Similarly, Leary, Tambor, Terdal, and Downs's (1995) sociometer model proposes that the negative emotions that result from decreases in self-esteem function to warn us that others may regard us poorly—a relational problem. Finally, several clinical models, such as Prochaska and DiClemente's (1983) transtheoretical model, Mechanic's (1975) sociopsychological model of help seeking, and Zwaanswijk, Verhaak, Bensing, van der Ende, and Verhulst's (2003) model of help seeking emphasize that individuals must encounter the negative implications of their problems, such as negative emotions, before recognizing that such problems exist.

Existing research provides support for these ideas. At a perceptual level, humans recognize distressing objects faster and pay greater attention to them than they do to objects that are not distressing (e.g., Eastwood, Smilek, & Merikle, 2001; Öhman, Flykt, & Esteves, 2001). For example, Öhman and colleagues (2001) found that people participating in a picture recognition task identified pictures that elicited fear responses (e.g., snakes, spiders) faster than pictures that did not elicit a fear response (e.g., flowers, mushrooms). Similarly, clinical research provides considerable evidence that greater distress predicts better problem recognition (e.g., Angold et al., 1998; Farmer & Ferraro, 1997; Farmer, Stangl, Burns, Costello, & Angold, 1999; Wu et al., 1999, 2001; Yokopenic, Clark, & Aneshensel, 1983). For example, Yokopenic and colleagues (1983) found that the severity of the negative emotions that people experienced predicted better recognition of their psychological problems. Similarly, Wu and colleagues (1999) demonstrated that children who experienced greater depressive affect were more likely to report needing mental health services, suggesting a greater awareness of their psychological problems, than were children who experienced lower depressive affect.

Given that people appear to be more aware of their problems when they are in greater distress, they should be more aware of their *relationship* problems when such problems cause greater distress. For example, if Lindsay has a greater negative emotional reaction upon finding out that her husband, Tobias, has bounced a check, she should be more aware that Tobias's handling of finances is a problem than if she were not distressed by the news. A few studies provide indirect support for this idea by demonstrating that individuals who tend to experience greater negative emotions within

close relationships tend to report recognizing more relationship problems than do individuals who tend to experience less negative emotions (e.g., Baker & McNulty, 2010; McNulty, 2008; Mattson, Frame, & Johnson, 2011; Murray, Holmes, & Griffin, 2000; Murray, Holmes, MacDonald, & Ellsworth, 1998). For example, McNulty (2008) demonstrated that intimates high in neuroticism, who tend to experience more negative emotions, viewed their partner's behaviors during a conflict discussion more negatively than did intimates low in neuroticism. Similarly, Mattson et al. (2011) demonstrated that intimates' negative affect was positively associated with the severity of their relationship problems. Of course, it is unclear from this research whether negative emotions lead to a better understanding of relationship problems or to an exaggerated view of problems or are simply a result of more severe problems. Future research may benefit from directly addressing this issue.

Motivation to Resolve Problems

In addition to helping individuals to be more aware of their interpersonal problems, there is reason to believe that negative emotions should help motivate individuals to directly address those problems. In particular, several theoretical accounts of emotions posit that people are more motivated to resolve problems that cause more negative emotions than problems that cause less negative emotions. For example, Hull (1943) argued that negative emotions lead to aversive drives, which motivate people to avoid or reduce unpleasant situations that cause negative emotions, such as bodily injury or a lack of food. Similarly, Maslow (1955) proposed that people are broadly motivated to diminish negative emotional states. More recent evolutionary explanations of emotion (e.g., Nesse & Ellsworth, 2009; Plutchik, 2003; Tooby & Cosmides, 2008) argue that emotions evolved because they motivate behavior and that negative emotions in particular aid in motivating people to prevent or resolve problems. Finally, Leary and colleagues' (1995) sociometer model also posits that the negative emotions that result from low self-esteem motivate people to resolve their interpersonal problems.

Empirical evidence supports these ideas as well (e.g., Frijda et al., 1989; Hiller et al., 2009; McCaul et al., 1998; Roseman et al., 1994; Wohl & Thompson, 2011). For example, Frijda and colleagues (1989) found that many negative emotions, such as fear, sadness, and anger, were associated with greater intentions to improve one's emotional state. Anger, for example, was associated with a greater desire to overcome difficulties. Similarly, Hiller and colleagues (2009) found that drug-addicted inmates who reported greater distress were more motivated to be treated for their addiction than were inmates who reported less distress. Finally, McCaul and colleagues (1998) found that women who were more worried about

breast cancer were more likely to take preventative measures against developing cancer, such as requesting screening procedures, than were women who were less worried.

Given that people should be more motivated to resolve their problems when they are more distressed, people should be more motivated to resolve their *relationship* problems when such problems cause greater distress. For example, the more upset Tobias is about bouncing the check, the more likely he is to monitor the balance of his checking account in the future. Empirical evidence supports this idea as well (e.g., Baker & McNulty, 2011, 2013; Gonzales et al., 1990). For example, Baker and McNulty (2011) demonstrated that self-criticism, which frequently causes negative emotions (e.g., Leary, Tate, Adams, Batts, Allen, & Hancock, 2007), was associated with greater motivation to resolve relationship problems among men who lacked other dispositional sources of motivation—conscientiousness. Similarly, Baker and McNulty (2013) demonstrated that intimates with low self-esteem, who tend to experience greater negative emotions (e.g., Leary et al., 1995), are more likely to engage in interdependence-promoting behaviors that can repair relationships when such relationships are an important aspect of their self-concept. Finally, Gonzales and colleagues (1990) led people to believe that they had committed either small or large interpersonal offenses and found that those who believed they had committed large offenses felt more negatively about the offenses and, in turn, made more reparative efforts (e.g., apologies, attempts to resolve the problem) than did those who committed smaller offenses.

EXPRESSING EMOTIONS

Negative emotions do not affect only the person experiencing them. That is, negative emotions are routinely expressed to others, especially in the context of close relationships (e.g., Clark & Finkel, 2004; Pennebaker, Zech, Rimé, 2001), and the expression of negative emotions frequently affects partners' thoughts and behaviors (Altman & Taylor, 1973; Graham, Huang, Clark, & Helgeson, 2008). One of the most common ways that people communicate emotions is through nonverbal behaviors (e.g., Coulson, 2004; de Meijer, 1989; Matsumoto, Keltner, Shiota, Frank, & O'Sullivan, 2008). For example, facial expressions effectively communicate negative emotions; people across most cultures, and nonhuman primates, easily recognize the facial expressions of basic emotions such as anger, fear, and sadness (for a review, see Matsumoto et al., 2008). Other nonverbal cues, such as postures, hand gestures, and touch, also communicate emotions (Coulson, 2004; de Meijer, 1989). Of course, verbal communication conveys emotions as well. Content-free features of vocal communication,

such as pitch, volume, and rate of speech, express emotion (Bachorowski & Owren, 2008; Frick, 1985). For example, faster speech signals anxiety and louder speech signals anger. And the content of verbal communication can certainly signal a communicator's emotional state (Johnson-Laird & Oatley, 1989). For example, blaming a romantic partner for a problem or demanding that he or she change can signal anger. Through these different modes of expression, negative emotions may benefit relationships by (1) leading to a better understanding by the partner, (2) eliciting support from the partner, and (3) regulating the partner's behavior.

Understanding

Honesty and open communication are central to any quality close relationship (Noller & Ruzzene, 1991). Indeed, people value being able to accurately recognize their partner's thoughts, emotions, motivations, and behavioral intentions (Collins & Miller, 1994; Ickes, 1993; Regan, Levin, Sprecher, Christopher, & Cate, 2000; Wieselquist, Rusbult, Foster, & Agnew, 1999). Several theories account for why expressing even negative emotions may be beneficial. For example, theories of emotional self-disclosure (e.g., Altman & Taylor, 1973; Collins & Miller, 1994) suggest that emotional self-disclosures tend to increase intimacy for both the person expressing the emotion and the person receiving the disclosure. Similarly, Ickes's (1993) theoretical descriptions of empathic accuracy suggest that people are motivated to understand other's emotional states because such understanding leads to greater insight about them and the issues that they face. Furthermore, such emotional understanding often results in greater trust and closeness, assuming that such emotions are not threatening to the relationship (Simpson, Oriña, & Ickes, 2003). Of course, expressing even relationship-threatening negative emotions may have long-term positive implications if they motivate resolution behaviors (see the section on partner regulation later in this chapter). Finally, theories of emotional suppression (e.g., John & Gross, 2004) and associated research (Butler et al., 2003; Impett et al., 2012) suggest that inhibiting emotional expressions hinders the development of intimacy because people who inhibit their emotional expressions (1) are not disclosing important information and (2) appear avoidant to their partners. In sum, these theories suggest that although expressing negative emotions can be unpleasant, it can increase understanding and intimacy between partners.

Empirical evidence supports these ideas (Graham et al., 2008; Larzelere & Huston, 1980; Laurenceau, Barrett, & Pietromonaco, 1998; Noller & Venardos, 1986). For example, Graham and colleagues (2008) found that people who were more willing to express their negative emotions developed more intimate friendships than did people who were less

willing to express their negative emotions. Similarly, Laurenceau and colleagues (1998) found that emotional self-disclosures led to greater intimacy between romantic partners and that intimates experienced greater intimacy to the extent that their partners disclosed negative emotions. Finally, Noller and Venardos (1986) demonstrated that people who were more accurate at reading their spouses' emotions were more satisfied with their marriages than were people who were less accurate.

Eliciting Support

Expressing distress may also serve the valuable function of signaling to a relationship partner that one's needs are not being met (Levenson, 1994). For example, Mike might express to his friend the sadness he is experiencing over the death of a relative because he needs to be consoled, Tiara might express to her husband her fear that she will not be successful in her new job because she needs to be reassured of her competence, and Andre might express to his boyfriend his anxiety about being unable to afford his rent and thus be more likely to receive financial assistance. Although it can be disconcerting for individuals to realize that their partners' needs are not being met, expressing distress may benefit close relationships by increasing provisions of support. Indeed, according to Clark and Mills' (1979) notion of communal relationships, partners genuinely care about fulfilling each other's needs. Accordingly, expressing negative emotions should be beneficial within close relationships because it likely motivates partners to provide support (see Clark & Finkel, 2004).

Extensive research demonstrates that expressions of distress do indeed elicit support from close others (Clark, Oullette, Powell, & Milberg, 1987; Graham et al., 2008; Shimanoff, 1987; for a review, see Batson & Shaw, 1991). For example, Shimanoff (1987) found that the extent to which people express negative emotions to their partners is positively associated with the quality of emotional support their partners provide. Similarly, Clark and colleagues (1987) demonstrated that people who were primed by a communal orientation were more likely to help individuals who expressed sadness than people who were not. Finally, Graham and colleagues (2008) demonstrated that people provided more help to others who appeared nervous while preparing to give a speech than to others who appeared calm.

Such provisions of support can benefit both recipients' and their partners' relationship well-being (Laurenceau, Barrett, & Rovine, 2005; Pasch & Bradbury, 1998; Sullivan, Pasch, Johnson, & Bradbury, 2010). For example, Sullivan and colleagues (2010) demonstrated that better quality partner support predicted less subsequent distress in the recipient and, consequently, less steep declines in marital satisfaction over time. Similarly,

Laurenceau and colleagues (2005) found that the partners' responsiveness was positively associated with subsequent intimacy.

Partner Regulation

Beyond promoting understanding and eliciting support, expressing negative emotions can also provide another benefit for close relationships—helping people resolve their relationship problems. Specifically, many relationship problems require change in one or both partners (Caughlin & Vangelisti, 1999; Margolin, Talovic, & Weinstein, 1983), and partners often attempt to regulate one another's behavior to resolve such problems (Oriña, Wood, & Simpson, 2002; Overall, Fletcher, & Simpson, 2006; Overall, Fletcher, Simpson, & Sibley, 2009; Tucker & Mueller, 2000). One way that individuals try to regulate one another is by expressing their negative emotions (Cohen & Lichtenstein, 1990; Overall et al., 2009). For example, Melissa might angrily demand that Joan take out the trash before she leaves for work, and Mike might blame his wife for spending too much time writing academic manuscripts in an attempt to increase the amount of time they spend together.

Expressions of negative emotions, although unpleasant, may benefit relationships by helping with several aspects of the problem-resolution process. First, expressing negative emotions to a partner should make that partner more aware of the problem. This idea is consistent with evolutionary perspectives of emotional expression (e.g., Levenson, 1994), which suggest that expressions of negative emotions developed as a way to communicate to others that one's needs are not being met. An infant's cry, for example, signals to her parents that she is facing a problem. Likewise, if Eduardo expresses anger over Chantel's excessive alcohol use, Chantel may be more likely to recognize that her alcohol use is a problem. Overall and colleagues (2006) illustrated the benefits of expressing negative emotions in romantic relationships by demonstrating that the partners of intimates who expressed more negative emotions were more aware that they did not match those intimates' ideals and viewed their relationships as more problematic compared with the partners of intimates who expressed less negative emotions.

Second, expressions of negative emotions can also communicate a solution to the problem. For example, if Angela is upset that her husband, Justin, is gambling too much, she might communicate her frustration by demanding that he stop gambling. Although her commands might bother Justin, she is effectively communicating the solution to the problem—that Justin stop gambling. Ample research demonstrates that partners can influence each other's behavioral intentions in order to resolve problems (Oriña et al., 2002; Overall et al., 2006; Tucker & Mueller, 2000). For example,

Tucker and Mueller (2000) demonstrated that requesting that partners change their health-related behaviors is an effective way to get them to do so.

Third, expressing negative emotions to a partner might increase that partner's motivation to resolve the problem. Expressing negative emotions to a partner tends to increase that partner's negative emotions (Eisenberger, Lieberman, & Williams, 2003; Gottman, Markman, & Notarius, 1977), and, as noted in the first section of this chapter, experiencing negative emotions can increase motivation to resolve relationship problems (Baker & McNulty, 2010, 2013; Frijda, 1986; Hiller et al., 2009; McCaul et al., 1998; Roseman et al., 1994). This idea is consistent with partner regulation theory (Overall et al., 2006, 2009), which posits that "negative communication behavior motivates partners to bring about desired change" (Overall et al., 2009, p. 621). For example, if Lindsay expresses her anger at Tobias for bouncing the check, Tobias should be more likely to feel guilty about his mistake and should be more motivated to make sure it does not happen again than if Lindsay appeared unbothered by Tobias's behavior.

Empirical evidence supports the idea that, although expressing negative emotions may be immediately distressing, it can help individuals resolve their relationship problems and strengthen the relationship in the long term (e.g., Cohan & Bradbury, 1997; Heavey, Layne, & Christensen, 1993; Karney & Bradbury, 1997; McNulty & Russell, 2010; Overall et al., 2009). For example, Overall and colleagues (2009) demonstrated that although expressions of negative emotions, such as anger, derogation, and blaming, were perceived to be less successful and were associated with greater distress immediately after the behaviors took place, they were also associated with a greater reduction of problems over the course of a year. Similarly, Heavey and colleagues (1993) demonstrated that although the extent to which husbands demanded changes from their wives was initially negatively associated with lower marital satisfaction, it was associated with increases in marital satisfaction over time. Recent research demonstrates that expressing negative emotions can even help partners accomplish their personal goals. Meltzer, McNulty, and Karney (2012) demonstrated that husbands who displayed a lack of motivation while discussing a personal goal, such as personal health, gained less weight over time to the extent that their wives directly expressed negative emotions.

SPECIFIC NEGATIVE EMOTIONS

Until now, we have discussed the general implications of experiencing and expressing negative emotions for close relationships. Nevertheless, humans likely evolved to experience specific negative emotions that uniquely affect

attention, perception, goal choice, motivation, communication, and behavioral intentions (Tooby & Cosmides, 2008) to meet the specific challenges that humans faced in the evolutionary environment (Nesse & Ellsworth, 2009; Plutchik, 2003). For example, fear is often experienced in response to physical threats and prevents physical harm by causing adaptive responses, including increased perceptual alertness and behavioral responses that prevent harm, such as hiding, fleeing, or defending (Tooby & Cosmides, 2008). In contrast, disgust is often experienced in response to offensive objects, such as spoiled food, corpses, or insects, and triggers adaptive responses, such as nausea and distancing from disgust-inducing objects (Rozin, Haidt, & McCauley, 2008). Accordingly, specific negative emotions should have unique implications for close relationships. The remainder of this section discusses how three of these specific negative emotions—anger, romantic jealousy, and guilt—should uniquely affect close relationships.

Anger

People experience anger when they believe that others are neglecting their well-being (Sell, Tooby, & Cosmides, 2009). One function of experiencing anger is that it can motivate individuals to attempt to regulate a partner to behave in a way that is more beneficial for the angry individual (e.g., Fischer & Roseman, 2007; Lemay, Overall, & Clark, 2012; for reviews, see Canary, Spitzberg, & Semic, 1998; Hess, Chapter 3, this volume). For example, Lemay and colleagues (2012) demonstrated that experiencing anger in response to a transgression was associated with greater motivation to change the perpetrator's behavior and with engaging in greater regulation behaviors, such as blaming, criticizing, and yelling. Similarly, Fischer and Roseman (2007) had participants recall a time when they felt angry toward another person and found that the extent of their anger was associated with greater regulatory goals (i.e., wanting the partner to understand the extent of the transgression, apologize, avoid future transgressions) and regulatory behaviors (i.e., criticizing and confronting the partner). As noted in the previous section, such partner regulation behaviors can effectively motivate the partner to change.

Furthermore, *expressing* anger signals to the partner that the expresser is unhappy with the partner's behavior and gives the partner the opportunity to rectify the situation, and this can be an effective form of partner regulation itself (Fischer & Roseman, 2007). Empirical evidence is consistent with this idea (Averill, 1983; Cohan & Bradbury, 1997; Tiedens, 2001; Van Kleef, De Dreu, & Manstead, 2004). For example, Averill (1983) had people recall a time when they expressed anger and found that most people reported that such expressions led to a change in another's behavior. Similarly, Van Kleef and colleagues (2004) found that people made larger

concessions to an angry opponent than to a happy opponent during a negotiation task (see Van Kleef & Côté, Chapter 6, this volume).

Romantic Jealousy

Most people in close relationships are motivated to secure their partner's romantic and sexual fidelity (Greeley, 1991), and doing so can have benefits (see Henniger & Harris, Chapter 4, this volume). From an evolutionary perspective, men who could secure a partner's fidelity could be certain that they would not commit resources to an offspring that was not theirs (Buss & Schmitt, 1993). For women, securing a partner's fidelity decreased the likelihood that their partner diverted resources to an alternative mate, increasing their offspring's chance of survival (Buss, 1988; Trivers, 1972). Indeed, infidelity is associated with decreased relationship satisfaction (Spanier & Margolis, 1983) and stability (Amato & Rogers, 1997), decreased self-esteem (Shackelford, 2001), and increased risk of mental health problems (e.g., Cano & O'Leary, 2000).

Romantic jealousy is a negative social emotion that frequently arises from the belief that a romantic partner has engaged in or might engage in romantic infidelity (Buunk & Dijkstra, 2000). Emotionally, romantic jealousy often involves a combination of fear over a relational loss and anger over betrayal (Parrott & Smith, 1993). Although unpleasant, romantic jealousy serves an adaptive function: It motivates behaviors that reduce the likelihood that a partner will engage in infidelity (Buss, Larsen, Westen, & Semmelroth, 1992). For example, jealous intimates often attempt to prove their commitment to romantic partners, confront potential rivals, prevent their partners from seeing potential rivals, and closely monitor and demand explanations for their partners' behavior (Guerrero, Andersen, Jorgensen, Spitzberg, & Eloy, 1995; Kasian & Painter, 1992). Furthermore, there is evidence that the behaviors that arise from romantic jealousy assist with mate retention (Buss, 1988; Buss & Shackelford, 1997; Sheets, Fredendall, & Claypool, 1997). For example, Sheets and colleagues (1997) found that although expressing romantic jealousy led to more initial relationship conflict, it led to greater relationship stability over time. In short, although romantic jealousy may be distressing, it can be beneficial to the extent that it reduces infidelity, a behavior that harms relationship well-being.

Guilt

Guilt arises from the recognition that one has behaved in an unacceptable manner (Guerrero & Andersen, 2000). Within close relationships, people can feel guilty for various transgressions, such as neglecting household duties, insulting a partner, or engaging in an extra-dyadic relationship.

Like other negative emotions, experiencing guilt can be distressing; however, it can also serve a beneficial function by motivating behaviors that correct transgressions, such as expressing apologies or remorse, making amends, and avoiding future transgressions (Baumeister, Stillwell, & Heatherton, 1995; for a review, see Baumeister, Stillwell, & Heatherton, 1994). For example, Baumeister and colleagues (1995) found that participants responded to their guilt by engaging in behaviors that compensated for transgressions, including apologizing and changing their subsequent behavior. Similarly, when people feel guilty, they demonstrate greater perspective taking, generate higher quality solutions to relationship problems, and report more constructive intentions (Covert, Tangney, Maddux, & Heleno, 2003; Leith & Baumeister, 1998; Tangney, Wagner, Hill-Barlow, Marschall, & Gramzow, 1996). Such tendencies also produce lower aggressive responses, more constructive problem solving, and greater efforts to make amends (Covert et al., 2003; Lopez, et al., 1997; Tangney et al., 1996). Consistent with extensive research demonstrating that these types of reparative efforts improve relationship well-being (Hannon, Rusbult, Finkel, & Kamashiro, 2010; Silk, 1998), people who experience greater guilt in response to specific transgressions or conflict episodes also report better long-term outcomes, such as problem resolution and relationship improvement (Baumeister et al., 1994; Leith & Baumeister, 1998).

THE IMPORTANCE OF CONTEXT

The evidence presented here indicates that negative emotions help individuals resolve their relationship problems. Why, then, are negative emotions frequently considered harmful for close relationships (e.g., Bell, 1978; Sommers, 1984)? As previously noted, negative emotions do have costs, including immediate negative evaluations of the relationship (Jacobson & Margolin, 1979; for a review, see Heyman, 2001). Although these short-term costs may be offset by the potential benefits of negative emotions described throughout this chapter, there are situations in which negative emotions may not produce benefits or in which the benefits are inconsequential compared with the costs incurred. In the remainder of this section, we describe several contexts in which negative emotions may be more costly to relationships than they are beneficial.

Infrequent or Mild Relationship Problems

For negative emotions to benefit close relationships, they need to help individuals resolve relationship problems that negatively affect their relationships. Experiencing and expressing negative emotions that result from

minor problems may help to resolve such problems, but the benefits from resolving inconsequential problems may not outweigh the immediate relationship distress such negative emotions can cause. For example, if Margaret frequently yells at Latoya for minor transgressions, such as chewing too loudly, Latoya is likely to change her behavior (i.e., chew less loudly), but the resulting improvement of such minor problems is unlikely to counterbalance the costs of Latoya's feelings of rejection and anger.

Research is consistent with this idea (Baker & McNulty, 2010; Cohan & Bradbury, 1997; Fisher, Benson, & Tessler, 1990; McNulty & Russell, 2010; Rusbult, Verette, Whitney, Slovik, & Lipkus, 1991). For example, people appear to be less responsive to negative emotions that they perceive as unjustified (Fisher et al., 1990; Rusbult et al., 1991). Similarly, McNulty and Russell (2010) demonstrated that reacting too negatively to minor relationship problems can decrease relationship satisfaction and increase the severity of those problems. Specifically, they found that although expressions of negative emotions, such as blaming one's partner for a problem and commanding one's partner to change his or her behavior, were associated with more stable marital satisfaction and decreases in marital problems among newlyweds facing more severe problems, those same behaviors were associated with sharper decreases in satisfaction and increases in marital problems among newlyweds facing less severe problems.

Unsolvable Relationship Problems

Likewise, given that the ultimate benefit of negative emotions is that they help individuals resolve their relationship problems, they may not benefit close relationships if they are in response to problems that cannot be resolved. For example, although a husband may experience frustration and express anger at his wife if the couple finds out that she is unable to have children for medical reasons, such negative emotions can do nothing to resolve this problem and thus are likely to lead to costs that are not offset by any benefits. Consistent with this idea, Ickes and Simpson (1997) argue that an accurate understanding of a partner's emotions may not be beneficial when those emotions involve disputes that cannot be resolved. Further, the assumption that confrontational attempts to change irreconcilable differences is ultimately damaging to the relationship is central to Jacobson and Christensen's (1998) integrative behavioral couples therapy. They argue that improving relationships involves promoting accepting and tolerance of differences in personalities, views, values, and communication styles that cannot be altered. Nevertheless, we are unaware of research that has directly examined how the solvability of relationship problems affects the implications of negative emotions for close relationships. Future research examining this possibility may prove fruitful.

Indirect Expression of Negative Emotions

Although we noted that expressing negative emotions can help resolve relationship problems by signaling to a partner that something is wrong, by suggesting a solution, and by motivating behavior that helps resolve the problem, not all expressions of negative emotions effectively communicate the problem or solution. Specifically, indirect expressions, which are passive or covert means for resolving problems (Overall et al., 2009), are a less effective strategy for resolving relationship problems. For example, sulking, refusing to talk to a partner, reminding a partner of unrelated previous transgressions, and making fun of a partner does not help that partner to understand what he or she is doing wrong or how to fix it. Similarly, indirect expressions of distress, such as whining and sighing, do not effectively communicate one's needs to a partner. For example, McNulty and Russell (2010) demonstrated that indirect emotional expressions such as sarcasm, asking hostile questions, and exaggeration were associated with greater increases in relationship problems, regardless of the severity of the problems couples faced in their relationships. Similarly, Overall and colleagues (2009) demonstrated that direct emotional expressions such as criticizing partners' behavior, demanding they change their behavior, and suggesting negative consequences for noncompliance, were more successful at changing partners' problematic behavior than were indirect strategies such as sulking, making partners feel guilty, and debasing oneself. Finally, a similar pattern also emerges within contexts of supportive discussions. Indirect emotional expressions when seeking support, such as sighing, sulking, or whining, are less effective at gaining responsive partner support than direct expressions of sadness and anger (Barbee & Cunningham, 1995).

Interpersonal Violence

Although experiencing and expressing negative emotions such as anger and jealousy may sometimes have the advantage of motivating people to resolve their problems in a constructive manner, at times such negative emotions may cause people to behave aggressively toward their partners. In particular, theoretical models of interpersonal violence, such as I³ theory (Finkel, 2007; Slotter & Finkel, 2011) and supporting research (e.g., Finkel et al., 2012; Finkel, DeWall, Slotter, Oaten, & Foshee, 2009), posit that impelling forces are most likely to lead people to behave violently when those people (1) experience an instigating force (e.g., being the recipient of expressed negative emotions) and (2) are unable to inhibit their resultant aggressive impulses (e.g., experience self-regulatory depletion). For example, Finkel and colleagues (2012, Study 4) demonstrated that intimates who experienced more anger across the course of a week, an impeller, were more likely

to behave aggressively when they also experienced the depleting forces of stress and had partners who tended to express negative emotions. Consequently, experiencing negative emotions and being the target of expressions of negative emotions may be dangerous when individuals possess a tendency to behave in an aggressive manner and are in situations in which they are unable to inhibit such impulses.

Sustained Depressive Mood

Although negative emotions typically motivate people to resolve their problems, there is reason to expect that sustained depressive mood may have an opposite effect. Evolutionary theories of depression (e.g., Carver & Scheier, 1990; Nesse, 2000; Nesse & Ellsworth, 2009; Tooby & Cosmides, 2008), for example, argue that although negative emotions, such as sadness, should initially increase motivation because individuals who invested time and effort into resolving distressing problems should have had a distinct advantage over those who did not attempt to resolve them, prolonged depressive affect should eventually decrease motivation because it is costly to continue investing time and effort into a problem that is unsolvable. Similarly, theories of learned helplessness argue that people experience depressive affect if they believe that their problems are unsolvable, which leads them to disengage effort (see Abramson, Seligman, & Teasdale, 1978).

Research is consistent with the idea that prolonged depressive mood may inhibit motivation (Layne, Merry, Christian, & Ginn, 1982; Miller & Markman, 2007; Reinecke, DuBois, & Schultz, 2001; for reviews, see Nestler & Carlezon, 2006; Trew, 2011). For example, Reinecke and colleagues (2001) demonstrated that dysphoria was positively associated with an avoidant problem-solving style. Similarly, Miller and Markman (2007) found that people with more severe depressive mood focused less on promotion goals and were consequently less motivated to improve their academic performance than were people with less severe depressive mood. Finally, Layne and colleagues (1982) found that people high in depressive mood were less motivated to avoid punishing stimuli, such as criticism, than were people low in depressive mood. Consistent with these lines of research, clinical depression is strongly negatively related to relationship satisfaction in both partners (e.g., Coyne, Thompson, & Palmer, 2002; Davila et al., 2003).

CONCLUSIONS

Although experiencing and expressing negative emotions may be unpleasant, negative emotions serve a valuable function by making people more

aware of their problems and motivating behaviors that help them resolve such problems. Indeed, people who underreact to serious relationship problems are unlikely to notice their problems and thus be unmotivated to resolve them. Nevertheless, emotional responses that are not justified by the severity of relationship problems should do more harm than good. Indeed, when people overreact to minor relationship problems, the benefit of resolving minor issues is likely to be overshadowed by the harmful effects of those negative emotions for both oneself and one's partner. The research covered in this chapter, therefore, suggests that for negative emotions to be beneficial, people need to accurately assess the severity of their problems, experience emotions that match the severity of such problems, and directly communicate those emotions to ensure that problems are effectively resolved.

REFERENCES

Abramson, L. Y., Seligman, M. E., & Teasdale, J. D. (1978). Learned helplessness in humans: Critique and reformulation. *Journal of Abnormal Psychology, 87,* 49–74.

Altman, I., & Taylor, D. A. (1973). *Social penetration: The development of interpersonal relationships.* Oxford, UK: Holt, Rinehart & Winston.

Amato, P. R., & Rogers, S. J. (1997). A longitudinal study of marital problems and subsequent divorce. *Journal of Marriage and the Family, 59,* 612–624.

Angold, A., Messer, S. C., Stangl, D., Farmer, E. M. Z., Costello, E. J., & Burns, B. J. (1998). Perceived parental burden and service use for child and adolescent psychiatric disorders. *American Journal of Public Health, 88,* 75–80.

Averill, J. R. (1983). Studies on anger and aggression: Implications for theories of emotion. *American Psychologist, 38,* 1145–1160.

Bachorowski, J.-A., & Owren, M. J. (2008). Vocal expressions of emotion. In M. Lewis, J. M. Haviland-Jones, & L. F. Barrett (Eds.), *Handbook of emotions* (3rd ed., pp. 196–210). New York: Guilford Press.

Baker, L. R., & McNulty, J. K. (2010). Shyness and marriage: Does shyness shape even established relationships? *Personality and Social Psychology Bulletin, 36,* 665–676.

Baker, L. R., & McNulty, J. K. (2011). Self-compassion and relationship maintenance: The moderating roles of conscientiousness and gender. *Journal of Personality and Social Psychology, 100,* 853–873.

Baker, L. R., & McNulty, J. K. (2013). When low self-esteem encourages behaviors that risk rejection to increase interdependence: The role of relational self-construal. *Journal of Personality and Social Psychology, 104,* 995–1018.

Barbee, A. P., & Cunningham, M. R. (1995). An experimental approach to social support communications: Interactive coping in close relationships. *Communication Yearbook, 18,* 381–413.

Batson, C. D., & Shaw, L. L. (1991). Evidence for altruism: Toward a pluralism of prosocial motives. *Psychological Inquiry, 2,* 107–122.

Baumeister, R. F., Stillwell, A. M., & Heatherton, T. F. (1994). Guilt: An interpersonal approach. *Psychological Bulletin, 115*, 243–267.

Baumeister, R. F., Stillwell, A. M., & Heatherton, T. F. (1995). Personal narratives about guilt: Role in action control and interpersonal relationships. *Basic and Applied Social Psychology, 17*, 173–198.

Bell, P. A. (1978). Affective state, attraction and affiliation: Misery loves happy company too. *Personality and Social Psychology Bulletin, 4*, 616–619.

Buss, D. M. (1988). From vigilance to violence: Tactics of mate retention in American undergraduates. *Ethology and Sociobiology, 9*, 291–317.

Buss, D. M., Larsen, R. J., Westen, D., & Semmelroth, J. (1992). Sex differences in jealousy: Evolution, physiology, and psychology. *Psychological Science, 3*, 251–255.

Buss, D. M., & Schmitt, D. P. (1993). Sexual strategies theory: An evolutionary perspective on human mating. *Psychological Review, 100*, 204–232.

Buss, D. M., & Shackelford, T. K. (1997). From vigilance to violence: Mate retention tactics in married couples. *Journal of Personality and Social Psychology, 72*, 346–361.

Butler, E. A., Egloff, B., Wilhelm, F. H., Smith, N. C., Erickson, E. A., & Gross, J. J. (2003). The social consequences of expressive suppression. *Emotion, 3*, 48–67.

Buunk, A. P., & Dijkstra, P. (2000). Extradyadic relationships and jealousy. In C. Hendrick & S. S. Hendrick (Eds.), *Close relationships: A sourcebook* (pp. 317–330). Thousand Oaks, CA: Sage.

Canary, D. J., Spitzberg, B. H., & Semic, B. A. (1998). The experience and expression of anger in interpersonal settings. In P. A. Andersen & L. K. Guerrero (Eds.), *Handbook of communication and emotion: Research, theory, applications, and contexts* (pp. 189–213). San Diego, CA: Academic Press.

Cano, A., & O'Leary, K. D. (2000). Infidelity and separations precipitate major depressive episodes and symptoms of nonspecific depression and anxiety. *Journal of Consulting and Clinical Psychology, 68*, 774–781.

Carver, C. S., & Scheier, M. F. (1990). Origins and functions of positive and negative affect: A control-process view. *Psychological Review, 97*, 19–35.

Caughlin, J. P., & Vangelisti, A. L. (1999). Desire for change in one's partner as a predictor of the demand/withdraw pattern of marital communication. *Communication Monographs, 66*, 66–89.

Clark, M. S., & Finkel, E. J. (2004). Does expressing emotion promote well-being? It depends on relationship context. In L. Z. Tiedens & C. W. Leach (Eds.), *The social life of emotions* (pp. 105–126). New York: Cambridge University Press.

Clark, M. S., & Mills, J. (1979). Interpersonal attraction in exchange and communal relationships. *Journal of Personality and Social Psychology, 37*, 12–24.

Clark, M. S., Oullette, R., Powell, M. C., & Milberg, S. (1987). Recipient's mood, relationship type, and helping. *Journal of Personality and Social Psychology, 53*, 94–103.

Cohan, C. L., & Bradbury, T. N. (1997). Negative life events, marital interaction, and the longitudinal course of newlywed marriage. *Journal of Personality and Social Psychology, 73*, 114–128.

Cohen, S., & Lichtenstein, E. (1990). Partner behaviors that support quitting smoking. *Journal of Consulting and Clinical Psychology, 58*, 304–309.

Collins, N. L., & Miller, L. C. (1994). Self-disclosure and liking: A meta-analytic review. *Psychological Bulletin, 116*, 457–475.

Coulson, M. (2004). Attributing emotion to static body postures: Recognition accuracy, confusions, and viewpoint dependence. *Journal of Nonverbal Behavior, 28*, 117–139.

Covert, M. V., Tangney, J. P., Maddux, J. E., & Heleno, N. M. (2003). Shame-proneness, guilt-proneness, and interpersonal problem solving: A social cognitive analysis. *Journal of Social and Clinical Psychology, 22*, 1–12.

Coyne, J. C., Thompson, R., & Palmer, S. C. (2002). Marital quality, coping with conflict, marital complaints, and affection in couples with a depressed wife. *Journal of Family Psychology, 16*, 26–37.

Davila, J., Karney, B. R., Hall, T. W., & Bradbury, T. N. (2003). Depressive symptoms and marital satisfaction: Within-subject associations and the moderating effects of gender and neuroticism. *Journal of Family Psychology, 17*, 557–570.

de Meijer, M. (1989). The contribution of general features of body movement to the attribution of emotions. *Journal of Nonverbal Behavior, 13*, 247–268.

Eastwood, J. D., Smilek, D., & Merikle, P. M. (2001). Differential attentional guidance by unattended faces expressing positive and negative emotion. *Perception and Psychophysics, 63*, 1004–1013.

Eisenberger, N. I., Lieberman, M. D., & Williams, K. D. (2003). Does rejection hurt?: An fMRI study of social exclusion. *Science, 302*, 290–292.

Farmer, E. M. Z., Stangl, D. K., Burns, B. J., Costello, E. J., & Angold, A. (1999). Use, persistence, and intensity: Patterns of care for children's mental health across one year. *Community Mental Health Journal, 35*, 31–46.

Farmer, M. M., & Ferraro, K. F. (1997). Distress and perceived health: Mechanisms of health decline. *Journal of Health and Social Behavior, 38*, 298–311.

Finkel, E. J. (2007). Impelling and inhibiting forces in the perpetration of intimate partner violence. *Review of General Psychology, 11*, 193–207.

Finkel, E. J., DeWall, C. N., Slotter, E. B., McNulty, J. K., Pond, R. S., Jr., & Atkins, D. C. (2012). Using I³ theory to clarify when dispositional aggressiveness predicts intimate partner violence perpetration. *Journal of Personality and Social Psychology, 102*, 533–549.

Finkel, E. J., DeWall, C. N., Slotter, E. B., Oaten, M., & Foshee, V. A. (2009). Self-regulatory failure and intimate partner violence perpetration. *Journal of Personality and Social Psychology, 97*, 483–499.

Fischer, A. H., & Roseman, I. J. (2007). Beat them or ban them: The characteristics and social functions of anger and contempt. *Journal of Personality and Social Psychology, 93*, 103–115.

Fisher, G., Benson, P., & Tessler, R. (1990). Family response to mental illness: Developments since deinstitutionalization. In J. Greenly (Ed.), *Research in community and mental health* (pp. 203–236). Greenwich, CT: JAI Press.

Fisher, T. D., & McNulty, J. K. (2008). Neuroticism and marital satisfaction: The mediating role played by the sexual relationship. *Journal of Family Psychology, 22*, 112–122.

Frick, R. W. (1985). Communicating emotion: The role of prosodic features. *Psychological Bulletin, 97,* 412–429.

Frijda, N. H. (1986). *The emotions.* London: Cambridge University Press.

Frijda, N. H., Kuipers, P., & ter Schure, E. (1989). Relations among emotion, appraisal, and emotional action readiness. *Journal of Personality and Social Psychology, 57,* 212–228.

Gonzales, M. H., Pederson, J. H., Manning, D. J., & Wetter, D. W. (1990). Pardon my gaffe: Effects of sex, status, and consequence severity on accounts. *Journal of Personality and Social Psychology, 58,* 610–621.

Gottman, J., Markman, H., & Notarius, C. (1977). The topography of marital conflict: A sequential analysis of verbal and nonverbal behavior. *Journal of Marriage and the Family, 39,* 461–477.

Graham, S. M., Huang, J. Y., Clark, M. S., & Helgeson, V. S. (2008). The positives of negative emotions: Willingness to express negative emotions promotes relationships. *Personality and Social Psychology Bulletin, 34,* 394–406.

Greeley, A. T. (1991). Patterns of college women's development: A cluster analysis approach. *Journal of College Student Development, 32,* 516–524.

Guerrero, L. K., & Andersen, P. A. (2000). Emotion in close relationships. In C. Hendrick & S. S. Hendrick (Eds.), *Close relationships: A sourcebook* (pp. 171–183). Thousand Oaks, CA: Sage.

Guerrero, L. K., Andersen, P. A., Jorgensen, P. F., Spitzberg, B. H., & Eloy, S. V. (1995). Coping with the green-eyed monster: Conceptualizing and measuring communicative responses to romantic jealousy. *Western Journal of Communication, 59,* 270–304.

Hannon, P. A., Rusbult, C. E., Finkel, E. J., & Kamashiro, M. (2010). In the wake of betrayal: Amends, forgiveness, and the resolution of betrayal. *Personal Relationships, 17,* 253–278.

Heavey, C. L., Layne, C., & Christensen, A. (1993). Gender and conflict structure in marital interaction: A replication and extension. *Journal of Consulting and Clinical Psychology, 61,* 16–27.

Henry, R. G., & Miller, R. B. (2004). Marital problems occurring in midlife: Implications for couples therapists. *American Journal of Family Therapy, 32,* 405–417.

Heyman, R. E. (2001). Observation of couple conflicts: Clinical assessment applications, stubborn truths, and shaky foundations. *Psychological Assessment, 13,* 5–35.

Hiller, M. L., Narevic, E., Webster, J. M., Rosen, P., Staton, M., Leukefeld, C., et al. (2009). Problem severity and motivation for treatment in incarcerated substance abusers. *Substance Use and Misuse, 44,* 28–41.

Hull, C. L. (1943). *Principles of behavior: An introduction to behavior theory.* Oxford, UK: Appleton–Century.

Ickes, W. (1993). Empathic accuracy. *Journal of Personality, 61,* 587–610.

Ickes, W., & Simpson, J. (1997). Managing empathic accuracy in close relationships. In W. Ickes (Ed.), *Empathic accuracy* (pp. 218–250). New York: Guilford Press.

Impett, E. A., Kogan, A., English, T., John, O., Oveis, C., Gordon, A. M., et al. (2012). Suppression sours sacrifice: Emotional and relational costs of

suppressing emotions in romantic relationships. *Personality and Social Psychology Bulletin, 38,* 707–720.

Jacobson, N. S., & Christensen, A. (1998). *Acceptance and change in couple therapy: A therapist's guide to transforming relationships.* New York: Norton.

Jacobson, N. S., & Margolin, G. (1979). *Marital therapy: Strategies based on social learning and behavior exchange principles.* New York: Brunner/Mazel.

John, O. P., & Gross, J. J. (2004). Healthy and unhealthy emotion regulation: Personality processes, individual differences, and life span development. *Journal of Personality, 72,* 1301–1333.

Johnson-Laird, P., & Oatley, K. (1989). The language of emotions: An analysis of a semantic field. *Cognition and Emotion, 3,* 81–123.

Karney, B. R., & Bradbury, T. N. (1995). The longitudinal course of marital quality and stability: A review of theory, methods, and research. *Psychological Bulletin, 118,* 3–34.

Karney, B. R., & Bradbury, T. N. (1997). Neuroticism, marital interaction, and the trajectory of marital satisfaction. *Journal of Personality and Social Psychology, 72,* 1075–1092.

Karney, B. R., Bradbury, T. N., Fincham, F. D., & Sullivan, K. T. (1994). The role of negative affectivity in the association between attributions and marital satisfaction. *Journal of Personality and Social Psychology, 66,* 413–424.

Kasian, M., & Painter, S. L. (1992). Frequency and severity of psychological abuse in a dating population. *Journal of Interpersonal Violence, 7,* 350–364.

Kelley, H. H., & Thibaut, J. (1978). *Interpersonal relations: A theory of interdependence.* New York: Wiley.

Klinger, E. (1996). The contents of thoughts: Interference as the downside of adaptive normal mechanisms in thought flow. In I. G. Sarason, B. R. Sarason, & G. R. Pierce (Eds.), *Cognitive interference: Theories, methods, and findings* (pp. 3–23). Hillsdale, NJ: Erlbaum.

Larzelere, R. E., & Huston, T. L. (1980). The dyadic trust scale: Toward understanding interpersonal trust in close relationships. *Journal of Marriage and the Family, 42,* 595–604.

Laurenceau, J., Barrett, L. F., & Pietromonaco, P. R. (1998). Intimacy as an interpersonal process: The importance of self-disclosure, partner disclosure, and perceived partner responsiveness in interpersonal exchanges. *Journal of Personality and Social Psychology, 74,* 1238–1251.

Laurenceau, J., Barrett, L. F., & Rovine, M. J. (2005). The interpersonal process model of intimacy in marriage: A daily-diary and multilevel-modeling approach. *Journal of Family Psychology, 19,* 314–323.

Layne, C. C., Merry, J., Christian, J., & Ginn, P. (1982). Motivational deficit in depression. *Cognitive Therapy and Research, 6,* 259–274.

Leary, M. R. (2000). Affect, cognition, and the social emotions. In J. P. Forgas (Ed.), *Feeling and thinking: The role of affect in social cognition* (pp. 331–356). New York: Cambridge University Press.

Leary, M. R., Tambor, E. S., Terdal, S. K., & Downs, D. L. (1995). Self-esteem as an interpersonal monitor: The sociometer hypothesis. *Journal of Personality and Social Psychology, 68,* 518–530.

Leary, M. R., Tate, E. B., Adams, C. E., Batts Allen, A., & Hancock, J. (2007). Self-compassion and reactions to unpleasant self-relevant events: The implications of treating oneself kindly. *Journal of Personality and Social Psychology, 92*, 887–904.

Leith, K. P., & Baumeister, R. F. (1998). Empathy, shame, guilt, and narratives of interpersonal conflicts: Guilt-prone people are better at perspective taking. *Journal of Personality, 66*, 1–37.

Lemay, E. P., Overall, N. C., & Clark, M. S. (2012). Experiences and interpersonal consequences of hurt feelings and anger. *Journal of Personality and Social Psychology, 103*, 982–1006.

Levenson, R. W. (1994). Human emotion: A functional view. In P. Ekman & R. J. Davidson (Eds.), *The nature of emotion: Fundamental questions* (pp. 123–126). New York: Oxford University Press.

Levenson, R. W. (1999). The intrapersonal functions of emotion. *Cognition and Emotion, 13*, 481–504.

Levenson, R. W., Carstensen, L. L., & Gottman, J. M. (1993). Long-term marriage: Age, gender, and satisfaction. *Psychology and Aging, 8*, 301–313.

Lopez, F. G., Gover, M. R., Leskela, J., Sauer, E. M., Schirmer, L., & Wyssmann, J. (1997). Attachment styles, shame, guilt, and collaborative problem-solving orientations. *Personal Relationships, 4*, 187–199.

Margolin, G., Talovic, S., & Weinstein, C. D. (1983). Areas of change questionnaire: A practical approach to marital assessment. *Journal of Consulting and Clinical Psychology, 51*, 920–931.

Maslow, A. (1955). Deficiency motivation and growth motivation. In M. R. Jones (Ed.), *Nebraska Symposium on Motivation* (pp. 1–30). Lincoln: University of Nebraska Press.

Matsumoto, D., Keltner, D., Shiota, M. N., Frank, M. C., & O'Sullivan, M. (2008). What's in a face?: Facial expressions as signals of discrete emotions. In M. Lewis, J. M. Haviland-Jones, & L. F. Barrett (Eds.), *Handook of emotions* (3rd ed., pp. 211–234). New York: Guilford Press.

Mattson, R. E., Frame, L. E., & Johnson, M. D. (2011). Premarital affect as a predictor of postnuptial marital satisfaction. *Personal Relationships, 18*, 532–546.

McCaul, K. D., Branstetter, A. D., O'Donnell, S. M., Jacobson, K., & Quinlan, K. B. (1998). A descriptive study of breast cancer worry. *Journal of Behavioral Medicine, 21*, 565–579.

McGonagle, K. A., Kessler, R. C., & Schilling, E. A. (1992). The frequency and determinants of marital disagreements in a community sample. *Journal of Social and Personal Relationships, 9*, 507–524.

McNulty, J. K. (2008). Neuroticism and interpersonal negativity: The independent contributions of behavior and perceptions. *Personality and Social Psychology Bulletin, 34*, 1439–1450.

McNulty, J. K., & Russell, V. M. (2010). When "negative" behaviors are positive: A contextual analysis of the long-term effects of problem-solving behaviors on changes in relationship satisfaction. *Journal of Personality and Social Psychology, 98*, 587–604.

Mechanic, D. (1975). Sociocultural and social-psychological factors affecting personal responses to psychological disorder. *Journal of Health and Social Behavior, 16,* 393–404.

Meltzer, A. L., McNulty, J. K., & Karney, B. R. (2012). Social support and weight maintenance in marriage: The interactive effects of support seeking, support provision, and gender. *Journal of Family Psychology, 26,* 678–687.

Miller, A. K., & Markman, K. D. (2007). Depression, regulatory focus, and motivation. *Personality and Individual Differences, 43,* 427–436.

Miller, R. B., Yorgason, J. B., Sandberg, J. G., & White, M. B. (2003). Problems that couples bring to therapy: A view across the family life cycle. *American Journal of Family Therapy, 31,* 395–407.

Murray, S. L., Holmes, J. G., & Griffin, D. W. (2000). Self-esteem and the quest for felt security: How perceived regard regulates attachment processes. *Journal of Personality and Social Psychology, 78,* 478–498.

Murray, S. L., Holmes, J. G., MacDonald, G., & Ellsworth, P. C. (1998). Through the looking glass darkly?: When self-doubts turn into relationship insecurities. *Journal of Personality and Social Psychology, 75,* 1459–1480.

Nesse, R. M. (2000). Is depression an adaptation? *Archives of General Psychiatry, 57,* 14–20.

Nesse, R. M., & Ellsworth, P. C. (2009). Evolution, emotions, and emotional disorders. *American Psychologist, 64,* 129–139.

Nestler, E. J., & Carlezon, W. A. (2006). The mesolimbic dopamine reward circuit in depression. *Biological Psychiatry, 59,* 1151–1159.

Noller, P., & Ruzzene, M. (1991). Communication in marriage: The influence of affect and cognition. In G. J. O. Fletcher & F. D. Fincham (Eds.), *Cognition in close relationships* (pp. 203–233). Hillsdale, NJ: Erlbaum.

Noller, P., & Venardos, C. (1986). Communication awareness in married couples. *Journal of Social and Personal Relationships, 3,* 31–42.

Öhman, A., Flykt, A., & Esteves, F. (2001). Emotion drives attention: Detecting the snake in the grass. *Journal of Experimental Psychology, 130,* 466–478.

Oriña, M. M., Wood, W., & Simpson, J. A. (2002). Strategies of influence in close relationships. *Journal of Experimental Social Psychology, 38,* 459–472.

Overall, N. C., Fletcher, G. J. O., & Simpson, J. A. (2006). Regulation processes in intimate relationships: The role of ideal standards. *Journal of Personality and Social Psychology, 91,* 662–685.

Overall, N. C., Fletcher, G. J. O., Simpson, J. A., & Sibley, C. G. (2009). Regulating partners in intimate relationships: The costs and benefits of different communication strategies. *Journal of Personality and Social Psychology, 96,* 620–639.

Parrott, W. G., & Smith, R. H. (1993). Distinguishing the experiences of envy and jealousy. *Journal of Personality and Social Psychology, 64,* 906–920.

Pasch, L. A., & Bradbury, T. N. (1998). Social support, conflict, and the development of marital dysfunction. *Journal of Consulting and Clinical Psychology, 66,* 219–230.

Pennebaker, J. W., Zech, E., & Rimé, B. (2001). Disclosing and sharing emotion: Psychological, social, and health consequences. In M. S. Stroebe, R. O. Hansson, W. Stroebe, & H. Schut (Eds.), *Handbook of bereavement research:*

Consequences, coping, and care (pp. 517–544). Washington, DC: American Psychological Association.

Plutchik, R. (2003). *Emotions and life: Perspectives from psychology, biology, and evolution.* Washington, DC: American Psychological Association.

Prochaska, J. O., & DiClemente, C. C. (1983). Stages and processes of self-change of smoking: Toward an integrative model of change. *Journal of Consulting and Clinical Psychology, 51,* 390–395.

Regan, P. C., Levin, L., Sprecher, S., Christopher, F. S., & Cate, R. (2000). Partner preferences: What characteristics do men and women desire in their short-term sexual and long-term romantic partners? *Journal of Psychology and Human Sexuality, 12,* 1–21.

Reinecke, M. A., DuBois, D. L., & Schultz, T. M. (2001). Social problem solving, mood, and suicidality among inpatient adolescents. *Cognitive Therapy and Research, 25,* 743–756.

Roseman, I. J., Wiest, C., & Swartz, T. S. (1994). Phenomenology, behaviors, and goals differentiate discrete emotions. *Journal of Personality and Social Psychology, 67,* 206–221.

Rozin, P., Haidt, J., & McCauley, C. R. (2008). Disgust. In M. Lewis, J. M. Haviland-Jones, & L. F. Barrett (Eds.), *Handbook of emotions* (3rd ed., pp. 757–776). New York: Guilford Press.

Rusbult, C. E., Verette, J., Whitney, G. A., Slovik, L. F., & Lipkus, I. (1991). Accommodation processes in close relationships: Theory and preliminary empirical evidence. *Journal of Personality and Social Psychology, 60,* 53–78.

Schwartz, J., & Shaver, P. R. (1987). Emotions and emotion knowledge in interpersonal relations. In W. Jones & D. Perlman (Eds.), *Advances in personal relationships* (Vol. 1, pp. 197–241). Greenwich, CT: JAI Press.

Sell, A., Tooby, J., & Cosmides, L. (2009). Formidability and the logic of human anger. *Proceedings of the National Academy of Sciences, 106,* 15073–15078.

Shackelford, T. K. (2001). Self-esteem in marriage. *Personality and Individual Differences, 30,* 371–390.

Sheets, V. L., Fredendall, L. L., & Claypool, H. M. (1997). Jealousy evocation, partner reassurance and relationship stability: An exploration of the potential benefits of jealousy. *Evolution and Human Behavior, 18,* 387–402.

Shimanoff, S. B. (1987). Types of emotional disclosures and request compliance between spouses. *Communication Monographs, 54,* 85–100.

Silk, J. B. (1998). Making amends: Adaptive perspectives on conflict remediation in monkeys, apes, and humans. *Human Nature, 9,* 341–368.

Simpson, J. A., Oriña, M. M., & Ickes, W. (2003). When accuracy hurts, and when it helps: A test of the empathic accuracy model in marital interactions. *Journal of Personality and Social Psychology, 85,* 881–893.

Slotter, E. B., & Finkel, E. J. (2011). I[3] theory: Instigating, impelling, and inhibiting factors in aggression. In P. R. Shaver & M. Mikulincer (Eds.), *Human aggression and violence: Causes, manifestations, and consequences* (pp. 35–52). Washington, DC: American Psychological Association.

Sommers, S. (1984). Reported emotions and conventions of emotionality among college students. *Journal of Personality and Social Psychology, 46,* 207–215.

Spanier, G. B., & Margolis, R. L. (1983). Marital separation and extramarital sexual behavior. *Journal of Sex Research, 19*, 23–48.

Sullivan, K. T., Pasch, L. A., Johnson, M. D., & Bradbury, T. N. (2010). Social support, problem solving, and the longitudinal course of newlywed marriage. *Journal of Personality and Social Psychology, 98*, 631–644.

Tangney, J. P., & Salovey, P. (1999). Problematic social emotions: Shame, guilt, jealousy, and envy. In R. M. Kowalski & M. R. Leary (Eds.), *The social psychology of emotional and behavioral problems: Interfaces of social and clinical psychology* (pp. 167–195). Washington, DC: American Psychological Association.

Tangney, J. P., Wagner, P., Hill-Barlow, D., Marschall, D. E., & Gramzow, R. (1996). Relation of shame and guilt to constructive versus destructive responses to anger across the life-span. *Journal of Personality and Social Psychology, 70*, 797–809.

Tiedens, L. Z. (2001). Anger and advancement versus sadness and subjugation: The effect of negative emotion expressions on social status conferral. *Journal of Personality and Social Psychology, 80*, 86–94.

Tooby, J., & Cosmides, L. (2008). The evolutionary psychology of the emotions and their relationship to internal regulatory variables. In M. Lewis, J. M. Haviland-Jones, & L. F. Barrett (Eds.), *Handbook of emotions* (3rd ed., pp. 114–137). New York: Guilford Press.

Trew, J. L. (2011). Exploring the roles of approach and avoidance in depression: An integrative model. *Clinical Psychology Review, 31*, 1156–1168.

Trivers, R. L. (1972). Parental investment and sexual selection. In B. Campbell (Ed.), *Sexual selection and the descent of man: 1871–1971* (pp. 136–179). Chicago: Aldine.

Tucker, J. S., & Mueller, J. S. (2000). Spouses' social control of health behaviors: Use and effectiveness of specific strategies. *Personality and Social Psychology Bulletin, 26*, 1120–1130.

Van Kleef, G. A., De Dreu, C. K., & Manstead, A. S. (2004). The interpersonal effects of anger and happiness in negotiations. *Journal of Personality and Social Psychology, 86*, 57–76.

Wallbott, H. G., & Scherer, K. R. (1986). The antecedents of emotional experiences. In K. R. Scherer, H. G. Wallbott, & A. B. Summerfield (Eds.), *Experiencing emotion: A crosscultural study* (pp. 69–83). Cambridge, UK: Cambridge University Press.

Wieselquist, J., Rusbult, C. E., Foster, C. A., & Agnew, C. R. (1999). Commitment, pro-relationship behavior, and trust in close relationships. *Journal of Personality and Social Psychology, 77*, 942–966.

Wohl, M. J. A., & Thompson, A. (2011). A dark side to self-forgiveness: Forgiving the self and its association with chronic unhealthy behaviour. *British Journal of Social Psychology, 50*, 354–364.

Wu, P., Hoven, C. W., Bird, H. R., Moore, R. E., Cohen, P., Alegria, M., et al. (1999). Depressive and disruptive disorders and mental health service utilization in children and adolescents. *Journal of the American Academy of Child and Adolescent Psychiatry, 38*, 1081–1090.

Wu, P., Hoven, C. W., Cohen, P., Liu, X., Moore, R. E., Tiet, Q., et al. (2001). Factors associated with use of mental health services for depression by children and adolescents. *Psychiatric Services, 52,* 189–195.

Yokopenic, P. A., Clark, V. A., & Aneshensel, C. S. (1983). Depression, problem recognition, and professional consultation. *Journal of Nervous and Mental Disease, 171,* 15–23.

Zwaanswijk, M., Verhaak, P. F. M., Bensing, J. M., van der Ende, J., & Verhulst, F. C. (2003). Help seeking for emotional and behavioural problems in children and adolescents: A review of recent literature. *European Child and Adolescent Psychiatry, 12,* 153–161.

6

On the Social Influence of Negative Emotional Expressions

GERBEN A. VAN KLEEF
STÉPHANE CÔTÉ

Social influence is a defining feature of life. Wherever people interact, they influence each other's opinions, judgments, and behaviors— or they attempt to do so. This is often an emotional endeavor. Consider how easily a conversation about politics can turn into a heated debate. Despite the inherently emotional nature of social influence processes, scientific understanding of the role of emotion in such processes is still embryonic. Scattered evidence suggests, however, that emotional expressions may be used deliberately to influence others. For instance, anecdotal reports indicate that people may strategically use displays of sadness to solicit help (Clark, Pataki, & Carver, 1996). Furthermore, people have been observed to express anger in an attempt to intimidate and control others (Fitness, 2000; Frank, 1988). Emotional expressions, it seems, are a potential source of social influence (Côté & Hideg, 2011; Van Kleef, Van Doorn, Heerdink, & Koning, 2011).

This chapter is concerned with the ways in which people engender social influence by means of negative emotional expressions. We begin with a brief discussion of recent theoretical developments that are pertinent to our analysis of emotion in social influence. Next we review emerging empirical evidence, highlighting four illustrative domains of research in

which negative emotional expressions have been shown to engender social influence. First, we consider how negative emotional expressions influence the provision of social support to those who are in need. Second, we discuss research on the effects of emotional expressions on concessions in negotiation. Third, we consider how leaders' emotional expressions shape effort expenditure and task performance of followers. Fourth, we address the effects of emotional expressions on conformity versus deviance in groups. This review informs our subsequent discussion of emotions as agents of social influence. We conclude the chapter with a discussion of theoretical implications and avenues for future research.

CONCEPTUALIZING THE ROLE OF EMOTION IN SOCIAL INFLUENCE

In conceptualizing the role of emotion in social influence, it is useful to distinguish between intrapersonal and interpersonal effects of emotions. At the intrapersonal level of analysis, scholars seek to understand how people's attitudes, cognitions, and behaviors are influenced by their own emotional states. For instance, researchers explore whether certain emotional states render people more susceptible to influence attempts (e.g., are happy people more likely than sad people to provide help when asked?). At the interpersonal level of analysis, studies are aimed at uncovering how people are influenced by the emotional expressions of *others*. In other words, research at the interpersonal level of analysis investigates how the emotional expressions of a source shape the attitudes, cognitions, and behaviors of a target (e.g., are people more likely to extend help to a person who smiles than to a person who frowns?).

The focus of this chapter is on the interpersonal level of analysis, because this is where emotional influence takes place. People continuously influence one another through their emotional expressions, whether deliberately or unconsciously, in their private lives or at work. When a shopper refuses to donate to a charity collector, the collector's disappointment may lead the shopper to reconsider and offer some change. When a negotiator gets angry upon receiving his counterpart's demands, the counterpart may feel pressured to make a concession. When a manager expresses dissatisfaction about the performance of a work team, the team may become motivated to work harder. When a group of scientists at a conference attempts to decide where to go for dinner, their annoyance with one person's deviating preferences may lead that person to conform to the group's position. Although the idea that we influence other people through our emotional expressions may sound plausible, this notion has only recently started to find its way into psychological theorizing.

A nice example of the emergence of this thinking is a recent theoretical argument by Côté and Hideg (2011). These authors proposed a new dimension of emotional intelligence: using emotional expressions to influence others. Emotional intelligence consists of a set of abilities to process emotions and emotional information (Mayer & Salovey, 1997; Salovey & Mayer, 1990). The dominant model of emotional intelligence includes four sets of abilities concerned with perceiving emotions, using emotions to facilitate thinking, understanding the sources of emotions, and regulating emotions (Mayer & Salovey, 1997). These abilities have an interpersonal aspect. For instance, in addition to aptly perceiving their own emotions, individuals can also aptly perceive the emotions that others display. In addition to effectively regulating their own emotions, individuals can also effectively regulate the emotions that other people feel.

The emerging research on the social effects of emotions suggests that individuals can also exhibit emotional intelligence in interpersonal contexts by strategically displaying emotions to influence the attitudes and behaviors of other people. Through this process, individuals display certain emotions so as to elicit specific attitudes and behaviors in others. For instance, leaders may strategically display enthusiasm to boost the motivation of their followers, and negotiators may strategically display anger to claim more value in a distributive negotiation. As such, individuals high on this dimension of emotional intelligence leverage the several social effects of emotions described in this chapter for their benefit.

Another manifestation of the emerging conceptualization of emotions as agents of social influence is a recent theory paper by Van Kleef and colleagues (2011). These authors applied emotion as social information (EASI) theory (Van Kleef, 2009, 2010; Van Kleef, De Dreu, & Manstead, 2010; Van Kleef, Homan, & Cheshin, 2012) to the domain of social influence. EASI theory provides a social account of emotion by focusing on the interpersonal consequences of emotional expressions. As such, it complements existing models that attempt to explain the *intra*personal effects of emotions on cognition, judgment, and behavior (e.g., Forgas, 1995; Schwarz & Clore, 1983). EASI theory moves beyond the valence approach that characterizes many other models and posits that each discrete emotion conveys specific social information (for a detailed account, see Van Kleef, De Dreu, & Manstead, 2010). The theory specifies two processes through which emotional expressions exert social influence (inferences vs. affective reactions), and it identifies two classes of moderators (information processing and the appropriateness of the emotional expression) that determine which of these processes takes precedence. The predictive strength of the inferential pathway increases to the extent to which the target is motivated and able to engage in thorough information processing and to which he or she

perceives the emotional expression as appropriate; the predictive strength of the affective-reactions pathway increases to the extent to which the target's information processing is reduced and he or she perceives the emotional expression as inappropriate.

Inspired by the early writings of Darwin (1872), many emotion theorists have embraced the notion that emotions are functional in that they help the individual to adapt to the (social) environment (e.g., Frijda, 1986; Lazarus, 1991). In fact, many have argued that these intrapersonal consequences of emotional experience are the cornerstone of emotion's functionality: Consider the classic example of a person who sees a snake, feels afraid, and runs away, thereby increasing his or her chances of surviving and contributing to the gene pool. Although EASI theory does not deny such individual-level functionality, it does question whether intrapersonal effects capture the whole story about emotion. After all, if emotions were functional only at the individual level, why would they show on our faces? Why would they be audible in our voices? And why would they become manifest in our postures? The very fact that emotions are *expressed* implies that they may serve social functions. Building on EASI theory, Van Kleef et al. (2011) proposed that a primary function of emotions—and perhaps the reason that they have survived over the course of evolution (cf. Fridlund, 1994)—is to engender social influence.

EMPIRICAL SUPPORT FOR THE VIEW OF EMOTIONS AS AGENTS OF SOCIAL INFLUENCE

The theoretical perspectives just outlined have surfaced hand in hand with a growing body of research on various aspects of emotional influence. In this section we provide an overview of emerging empirical support for the conceptualization of emotions as agents of social influence. We discuss evidence from four different domains in turn: social support, negotiation, leadership, and conformity.

Negative Emotional Expressions Can Elicit Social Support

Several pieces of evidence converge to support the idea that sadness and related "supplication" emotions (e.g., disappointment, worry) trigger a tendency to "move toward" the expresser (Van Kleef, De Dreu, & Manstead, 2010), resulting in increased cooperation and support. Expressions of sadness (e.g., crying) and worry increase perceptions of neediness and dependency (Clark & Taraban, 1991) and evoke helping behavior in both

children (Barnett, Howard, Melton, & Dino, 1982) and adults (Clark, Ouellette, Powell, & Milberg, 1987; Labott, Martin, Eason, & Berkey, 1991; Yee & Greenberg, 1998).

Van Kleef and colleagues (2008) prompted same-sex dyads of unacquainted individuals to talk about instances in their lives that had caused them a great deal of suffering and distress. Participants who were motivated to get to know and collaborate with their counterparts responded more compassionately and supportively to their partners' distress than did those who were less motivated to befriend their partners. Interestingly, individuals who relayed a story of suffering to conversation partners who were motivated to invest emotionally in the conversation experienced more trust and understanding than did those whose partners were not so motivated, indicating that supportive responses to another's suffering contribute to the quality of cooperative interpersonal relationships.

Tendencies to support those who express sadness can also become manifested in helping behavior. In an illustrative study described by Clark and colleagues (1996), participants were invited to the lab supposedly to participate in a text-proofing experiment. Participants were led to believe that they would work in a group of three and that one participant could leave early while the other two would proofread each other's work. The experimenter explained to the target participant that the other two participants were hoping to be allowed to leave early and that the target participant could choose who would be dismissed and who would have to stay. Target participants then received the work of the other participants, which included ratings of how they were supposedly feeling at the time. The results showed that fellow students who were described as sad were more likely to be selected by target participants to leave the experiment early than those who were described as nonemotional or angry.

Other studies have investigated the interpersonal effects of emotional expressions on compliance with explicit requests for help (Van Doorn, Van Kleef, & Van der Pligt, 2013). In one experiment, participants were asked to imagine that while out shopping they encountered a charity collector. After the participant had donated a 50-cent coin, the charity collector paused in front of them, as if he expected an additional donation. Participants were shown a picture of the collector's face, which expressed either anger, disappointment, or no emotion. Participants in the disappointment condition were willing to more than double their initial donation, whereas those in the neutral and angry conditions did not intend to make an additional donation. In fact, several participants in the anger condition indicated that they wanted to *take back* their initial donation. The difference between the disappointment and anger conditions was mediated by the perceived appropriateness of the charity collector's emotional expression, which was higher in the case of disappointment than in the case of anger.

In another experiment by Van Doorn and colleagues (2013), participants played a computer-simulated donation game. They first made a donation in a practice round, upon which they were informed that previous players had on average made either low or high allocations (i.e., a descriptive norm). Then they received a message from their "partners," who asked them to be more generous in the real game than they had been in the trial round. This request was paired with anger or disappointment about the participant's allocation in the trial round or with no emotional expression. In the absence of an emotional expression, participants conformed to the descriptive norm, giving more or less generously according to what others had given in the past. When the partner had expressed disappointment, participants donated substantially more regardless of the norm; when the partner had expressed anger, participants donated substantially less regardless of the norm. The difference between the anger and disappointment conditions was again mediated by perceived appropriateness.

These studies demonstrate that expressing emotions as part of a request can affect targets' willingness to comply with the request. Interestingly, the predictive value of emotional expressions outweighed that of an explicit descriptive norm, indicating that emotional expressions can be a powerful source of social influence. The studies also corroborate EASI theory's proposition that the effectiveness of emotional expressions in engendering social influence depends on their perceived appropriateness within the social context. In the context of a request for help, expressions of disappointment are perceived as more appropriate than expressions of anger, which explains why the former are effective whereas the latter are not.

Negative Emotional Expressions Can Elicit Concessions in Negotiation

Negotiation is defined as a discussion between two or more parties aimed at solving a (perceived) divergence of interests (Pruitt & Carnevale, 1993). Social influence is central to this process. Typically, parties in negotiation attempt to persuade each other to make concessions using a variety of strategies. In that sense, negotiation can be seen as a sequence of reciprocal requests (akin to compliance). The main difference between negotiation and a request is that the former situation is typically characterized by competitive incentives, whereas the latter is not (Van Kleef, De Dreu, & Manstead, 2010).

In a first study of the interpersonal effects of emotions in negotiation, Van Kleef, De Dreu, and Manstead (2004a) investigated the interpersonal effects of anger and happiness using a computer-mediated negotiation task. In the course of the negotiation, participants received emotional messages from their (simulated) opponents (e.g., "This negotiation pisses me off").

Negotiators who received angry messages estimated the opponents' limits to be high, and to avoid costly impasse they made relatively large concessions. Conversely, negotiators who received happy messages judged the opponents' limits to be low, felt no need to concede to avoid impasse, and therefore made smaller concessions. A recent study further showed that the inferences that negotiators draw from their counterparts' emotions continue to influence behavior in later encounters with the same people. In second encounters with opponents who had previously expressed anger, negotiators conceded again because they believed that the others had ambitious limits, even when the opponents expressed no emotion during the second encounter (Van Kleef & De Dreu, 2010).

In line with the idea that emotions provide relevant information, research has shown that the tendency of negotiators to concede more to angry opponents than to happy ones is moderated by the extent to which individuals are motivated and able to systematically and deliberately process information during the negotiation. Thus negotiators with a low dispositional need for cognitive closure, those who were under low time pressure, and those who depended strongly on their counterparts were influenced by their counterparts' expressions of anger versus happiness. In contrast, those with a high need for closure, those who were under high time pressure, and those who did not depend on their counterparts were uninfluenced by the counterparts' emotional expressions (Van Kleef, De Dreu, & Manstead, 2004b). Other studies showed that the interpersonal effects of anger and happiness are similarly moderated by power, with low-power negotiators being more strongly affected by their counterparts' emotions than high-power negotiators (Sinaceur & Tiedens, 2006; Van Dijk, Van Kleef, Steinel, & Van Beest, 2008; Van Kleef, De Dreu, Pietroni, & Manstead, 2006).

Several other moderators of the interpersonal effects of anger and happiness in negotiations have been identified. Inspired by the classic advice to "separate the people from the problem" (Fisher & Ury, 1981), Steinel, Van Kleef, and Harinck (2008) differentiated between emotions that are directed toward a negotiator's *offer* and emotions that are directed toward the negotiator *as a person*. When emotional statements were directed at the participants' offers, participants used the opponents' emotions to assess their limits, and consequently they conceded more to angry opponents than to happy ones. However, when the emotions were directed at the negotiator as a person, negotiators conceded *less* to an angry opponent than to a happy one. In this case, participants did not find useful information in their opponents' emotions, but instead felt affronted by the angry remarks (see also Lelieveld, Van Dijk, Van Beest, Steinel, & Van Kleef, 2011). Other work has demonstrated that expressions of anger may be effective when they are perceived as appropriate but elicit negative affective reactions and

retaliation when they are deemed inappropriate, for instance because they violate a display rule (Van Kleef & Côté, 2007).

Another recent study also illustrates how the social context shapes the perceived appropriateness of emotional expressions and subsequent behavioral responses to those expressions. Adam, Shirako, and Maddux (2010) examined the interpersonal effects of verbal expressions of anger across cultures. They found that European American participants conceded more to angry than to neutral opponents, whereas Asian American participants conceded *less* to angry than to neutral opponents. This reversal could be explained in terms of different cultural norms about the appropriateness of anger expressions in negotiations. Asian American participants deemed expressions of anger inappropriate, and therefore they responded negatively to such expressions. (See Chentsova-Dutton, Senft, & Ryder, Chapter 7, this volume, for a review of how cultural norms moderate the effects of negative emotions.)

Relatively few studies have addressed the effects of emotions other than anger and happiness. In one such study, Van Kleef, De Dreu, and Manstead (2006) found that participants whose opponents expressed guilt or regret developed a positive impression of their opponents but were nonconciliatory in their demands. By contrast, participants whose opponents expressed disappointment or worry rated their opponents less positively, but they made larger concessions. Additional experiments revealed that another's expressions of guilt are interpreted as a sign that the other has claimed too much, whereas disappointment is taken as a signal that the other has received too little. Furthermore, the effects of guilt and disappointment were eliminated when the target had low trust, because lack of trust undermined thorough processing of the implications of the opponent's emotional expressions.

In sum, these studies show that expressing emotions can be a powerful influence strategy in negotiation but that success depends on which emotion is expressed under which circumstances. In line with EASI theory (e.g., Van Kleef, 2009), expressions of anger help to elicit concessions when targets are motivated to engage in thorough information processing, because this increases the relative predictive strength of inferential processes compared with affective reactions. Conversely, expressions of anger evoke retaliation when targets deem the anger inappropriate, because this increases the relative predictive strength of affective reactions.

Negative Emotional Expressions of Leaders Can Stimulate Effort and Performance

Leadership refers to the process of influencing others to accomplish a goal (Yukl, 2010). Following a leader shares resemblances with obedience—a

special type of compliance that occurs in response to orders by an authority figure (Cialdini & Goldstein, 2004). In the past 15 years, researchers have begun to explore the effects of leaders' emotional expressions on followers. Early studies focused on the effects of leader emotional displays on follower ratings of leadership quality (e.g., Glomb & Hulin, 1997) and charisma (Bono & Ilies, 2006), showing that positive emotional expressions of leaders generally elicit more favorable ratings from followers than do negative expressions.

More recently, researchers started to focus on actual follower behavior as a function of leaders' emotional expressions. Sy, Côté, and Saavedra (2005) studied the effects of leader moods on the moods of their followers and team functioning. They invited groups of participants to the lab and randomly selected one of them to play the role of leader. This person then saw a film clip that induced either a positive or a negative mood. The leader then joined the rest of the group and coached them as they built up a tent together while blindfolded. Teams that were exposed to a leader in a positive mood developed a positive mood themselves and, as a result, exhibited better coordination than teams with a leader in a negative mood. Teams with a leader in a negative mood expended more effort, presumably because they interpreted the leader's negative mood as a signal that performance was unsatisfactory. Teams with a leader in a positive mood expended less effort, presumably because they interpreted the leader's positive mood as a signal that performance was adequate and did not need to be improved.

Van Kleef and colleagues examined the effects of expressions of anger versus happiness by a leader on team performance as a function of followers' information-processing motivation (Van Kleef et al., 2009). Four-person teams collaborated on a task, during which they were supposedly observed by their leader via a video camera setup. After a while, the leader (a trained actor) appeared on a video screen and provided standardized feedback and tips to the team, expressing either anger or happiness by means of facial expressions, vocal intonation, and bodily postures. Teams consisting of members with low information-processing motivation (measured in terms of need for structure; Neuberg & Newsom, 1993) performed better when the leader expressed happiness because they experienced positive emotions themselves and developed favorable impressions of the leader. Teams consisting of members with high information-processing motivation, in contrast, performed better when the leader expressed anger because they inferred from the leader's anger that their performance was suboptimal and that they needed to expend more effort.

Another recent study addressed the moderating role of followers' desire for social harmony, operationalized in terms of individual differences in agreeableness (Van Kleef, Homan, Beersma, & van Knippenberg,

2010). In a first experiment, participants read a scenario about a leader who expressed either anger or no emotion about his or her performance, with emotion being manipulated via pictures of emotional expressions. Participants high on agreeableness reported lower motivation in the anger condition compared with the neutral condition, whereas those low on agreeableness reported higher motivation in the anger condition than in the neutral condition. In a second experiment, participants performed a task in four-person teams, and they received angry or happy feedback from their leader, as described previously. Teams consisting of followers with high levels of agreeableness performed better when the leader expressed happiness, whereas teams consisting of followers with low agreeableness performed better when the leader expressed anger. Additional analyses revealed that agreeable followers experienced high levels of stress when confronted with an angry leader, which undermined their performance on the task.

These studies indicate that the emotional expressions of leaders are an important source of influence. Although leaders who express negative emotions such as anger tend to receive poorer evaluations than leaders who express positive emotions, in some cases expressing anger appears to be an effective way to motivate followers and to get them to perform—at least in the short run. In line with the predictions of EASI theory (e.g., Van Kleef, 2009), the effects of leaders' emotional displays on followers' performance are mediated by both affective reactions (emotional contagion and impressions of the leader) and inferential processes (inferences about performance quality), and the relative predictive strength of both processes depends on followers' information-processing motivation and their desire for social harmony, which may be seen as a proxy of the perceived appropriateness of expressions of anger versus happiness.

Negative Emotional Expressions Can Enforce Conformity in Groups

A final line of research that has recently emerged aims to understand how emotional expressions shape conformity processes in groups. Conformity refers to the act of changing one's behavior to match the responses of others (Cialdini & Goldstein, 2004). Heerdink, Van Kleef, Homan, and Fischer (2013) performed a first exploration of the interpersonal effects of anger and happiness on conformity in groups. They reasoned that expressions of anger may signal that certain behavior is not tolerated by the group and may be sanctioned. Groups fulfill individuals' need to belong (Baumeister & Leary, 1995), and, as research on ostracism has shown, threatened belongingness is highly aversive and motivates behavior aimed at improving acceptance (Williams, 2007). By conforming to the group norm, the deviant can show that he or she is a "good" group member and thus increase

chances of acceptance (Steinel et al., 2010). Happiness, on the other hand, is usually construed as a signal of affiliation (Clark et al., 1996) and acceptance (Cacioppo & Gardner, 1999). Targets of happy expressions can therefore be expected to feel safe in the group and to feel free to be unique and to deviate from the group's position, as their behavior is unlikely to compromise their group membership.

In a first study testing these ideas, Heerdink and colleagues (2013) asked participants to recall incidents in which their opinions had differed from that of the majority of the group. After describing the situation, they reported which emotions the majority had shown and how this had made them feel. The more anger the majority had expressed, the more the participant had felt excluded; the more happiness the majority had expressed, the more the participant had felt accepted. These feelings of inclusion versus exclusion in turn predicted the extent to which participants felt pressure to conform to the majority position.

In a second study the majority emotion was manipulated using a scenario. Participants read about a situation in which they were attempting to decide on a vacation destination with three of their friends. It turned out that the three friends all had the same destination in mind, but the participant preferred a different destination. The majority did not agree with the participant's proposal. Depending on the condition, the majority expressed anger, enthusiasm, or no emotion about the situation. Heerdink and colleagues also manipulated the availability of an alternative group with whom participants could go on vacation, reasoning that expressions of anger might prompt conformity in the absence of an alternative but not in the presence of an alternative. Expressions of anger led to greater feelings of exclusion than expressions of enthusiasm, with neutral expressions falling in between. Feelings of exclusion in turn motivated participants to conform when no alternative group was available, whereas they motivated participants to leave the group when such an alternative was available.

In a third study, Heerdink et al. (2013) explored these mechanisms in the context of a computer-simulated group discussion (see Homan, Greer, Jehn, & Koning, 2010) on aesthetic preferences. In one condition, participants learned that their responses on several questionnaires indicated that they were very prototypical members of the group, meaning that their personalities overlapped strongly with the personalities of the other group members. In the other condition they learned that they were rather peripheral members of the group, because their personality structures were different from those of the other group members (see Van Kleef, Steinel, van Knippenberg, Hogg, & Svensson, 2007). Participants then privately rated a number of abstract paintings. To generate discussion, their ratings were supposedly sent to the "other group members," who were preprogrammed to express different preferences than the participant. All group members

then sent a few messages to the rest of the group to initiate the discussion. Depending on the condition, participants received messages expressing anger or happiness about their deviating opinions. Then participants rated the paintings for a second time, and this time their ratings could supposedly be seen by the rest of the group. Participants who occupied peripheral positions in their groups exhibited conformity after receiving angry reactions, but not after receiving happy reactions. Participants with prototypical positions in the groups were not influenced by their group members' emotional expressions, because they experienced little fear of social exclusion and, consequently, little pressure to change their opinions.

These studies indicate that the emotional expressions of group members may be interpreted as signals of future acceptance or exclusion, which in turn influence conformity depending on the security of the target's position in the group and on the extent to which the target depends on the group. As such, these studies present initial evidence that emotional expressions can provide a means to engender conformity in groups, lending further support to the conceptualization of emotions as agents of social influence.

IMPLICATIONS AND SUGGESTIONS FOR FUTURE RESEARCH

We have seen that emotional expressions can engender social influence by triggering inferential processes and/or affective reactions in targets. We have also seen that the consequences of emotional expressions differ widely. In line with EASI theory (e.g., Van Kleef, 2009), the effects of emotional expressions depend heavily on the target's information-processing depth and on the perceived appropriateness of the emotional expression. In this section we consider a number of implications of the present theory and review and outline some avenues for future inquiry.

The Emerging View of Emotions as Agents of Social Influence

Research on social influence aims to uncover the processes through which and the circumstances under which individuals come to adapt their attitudes, cognitions, and/or behavior to other individuals. Besides an interest in fundamental processes, the social influence literature reveals a strong interest in tactics that can be used deliberately to influence other people. Classic examples are the foot-in-the-door technique (making a small request that is almost certainly granted and then following up with a larger, related request; Freedman & Fraser, 1966) and the door-in-the-face technique

(making an extreme request that is likely to get rejected so that a subsequent smaller request for a truly desired action is more likely to be granted; Cialdini et al., 1975). These strategies rely on individuals' desires for consistency and for reciprocity, respectively. Other strategies capitalize more on emotional processes. For instance, "fear appeals" can be used to frighten targets (e.g., by showing pictures of tarred lungs to smokers), which may in some circumstances help to establish behavioral change (Rogers, 1983). The theory and findings reviewed here suggest that interpersonal emotional strategies should be added to the social influence toolbox.

Our review also indicates, however, that the use of emotional expressions as a strategy of social influence is a delicate enterprise. A particular emotional expression may work in one situation but not in the next. The effectiveness of emotional expressions depends on which emotion is expressed to whom and under which circumstances. The many contingencies of the effects of emotional expressions in social influence are perhaps best illustrated by research on anger, which is by far the most studied emotion in this context. For instance, expressions of anger elicit concessions in negotiation when they are deemed appropriate and the target is motivated to consider the implications of the anger, but they backfire when they are perceived as inappropriate and/or the target is not motivated to process the information that the anger conveys (e.g., Steinel et al., 2008; Van Kleef & Côté, 2007; Van Kleef et al., 2004a, 2004b; Van Kleef, De Dreu, Pietroni, & Manstead, 2006). Furthermore, expressions of anger by a leader may stimulate effort but at the same time undermine coordination (Sy et al., 2005). In addition, expressions of anger may increase motivation and performance among followers who are high on epistemic motivation and among those who are low on agreeableness, whereas anger undermines motivation and performance of followers low on epistemic motivation and high on agreeableness (Van Kleef et al., 2009; Van Kleef, Homan, et al., 2010). Finally, expressions of anger may engender conformity in groups when targets depend on the group and/or occupy a peripheral position in it, whereas anger undermines conformity when targets do not depend on the group and/or occupy a central position in the group (Heerdink et al., 2013).

It is clear, then, that anger can be a powerful instrument of social influence, but it should be used with care. Expressing anger is likely to have desired effects on targets only when a number of conditions are met, as specified in EASI theory (see Van Kleef et al., 2011, for details). Future research is needed to illuminate whether the effects of other negative emotional expressions (e.g., sadness, disappointment, worry, fear, guilt, regret) are subject to the same moderating influences as are expressions of anger. When we learn more about the contingencies of the effectiveness of emotional expressions, we can start to consider, for instance, how emotional

expressions can be used in marketing or incorporated in governmental campaigns to promote desired behavior and discourage undesired behavior.

This chapter also suggests that successful emotion-based social influence requires adequate emotion regulation. Individuals who understand which emotional expressions work under which circumstances are likely to be more successful at exerting social influence than those who lack such knowledge (Côté & Hideg, 2011). Importantly, successful emotion regulation requires not just showing the right emotion at the right time but also showing the right emotion in the right way. In an illustrative study, participants felt more trust toward and cooperated more with a person who showed an authentic rather than an inauthentic smile (Krumhuber et al., 2007). In another study, "deep acted" displays of anger (which appear authentic) elicited concessions in negotiation, whereas "surface acted" displays of anger (which appear inauthentic) had the opposite effect (Côté, Hideg, & Van Kleef, 2013). This difference could be explained in terms of lower levels of trust in the latter condition, which may have fueled reactance.

Valence, Discrete Emotions, and Emotion Blends

There is a pervasive tendency in the literature to conceptualize emotions mainly in terms of their positive or negative valence. This chapter challenges this practice. Together with a growing body of research outside the domain of emotion-based social influence (e.g., Bodenhausen, Sheppard, & Kramer, 1994; DeSteno, Petty, Wegener, & Rucker, 2000; Fischer & Roseman, 2007; Keltner, Ellsworth, & Edwards, 1993; Lerner & Keltner, 2001; Tiedens & Linton, 2001), the theory and research reviewed here suggest that there is more promise in conceptualizing emotions in terms of their unique appraisal patterns and action tendencies than in terms of their valence. For instance, the "core relational themes" of anger and guilt are other-blame and self-blame, respectively (Smith, Haynes, Lazarus, & Pope, 1993), which helps to explain why they have opposite effects in negotiations even though both have a negative valence (Van Kleef et al., 2004a; Van Kleef, De Dreu, & Manstead, 2006). Further, the fact that disappointment does not involve assigning blame to another person whereas anger does helps to explain why expressing disappointment is more effective in securing compliance with a request (Van Doorn et al., 2013). Accordingly, future research would do well to measure or manipulate discrete emotions rather than focusing solely on positive or negative valence.

Without exception, the studies reviewed here have examined the effects of single emotional states and expressions (e.g., "pure" anger, sadness, disappointment, or guilt). However, in everyday life individuals often experience "blends" of emotions (Scherer & Tannenbaum, 1986). These

blends may even comprise emotions with different valences. For instance, individuals reported that they simultaneously experienced happiness and sadness on graduation day (Larsen, McGraw, & Cacioppo, 2001). Little is known about the interpersonal effects of mixed emotional displays. One series of studies found that negotiators who express emotional ambivalence claim little value in negotiations, because their opponents perceive them to be submissive and, in turn, are particularly intransigent in their interactions with them (Rothman, 2011). Other evidence, however, suggests that the alternating or simultaneous expression of positive and negative emotions can be an effective instrument of social influence.

In a classic study, Rafaeli and Sutton (1991) investigated the use of "emotional contrast strategies" as a social influence tactic. They discovered that criminal interrogators and bill collectors often use combinations of expressed positive and negative emotions to elicit compliance in others, a strategy that may be regarded as a variation of the "good cop, bad cop" technique. Such emotional contrast strategies can be effective in exerting social influence, although it is not clear exactly why. Further exploration of the mechanisms and contingencies of emotional contrast strategies and other forms of mixed emotional expressions is needed to develop a more complete understanding of emotion-based social influence.

Another investigation examined the social effects of transitions between happy and angry displays (Filipowicz, Barsade, & Melwani, 2011). Individuals who "became angry" (by transitioning from happiness to anger) claimed more value than individuals who displayed only anger. This effect was driven by two mechanisms. First, partners inferred that negotiators who "became angry" were more intransigent than negotiators who were always angry, because they were thought to react to something that occurred during the negotiation. Second, the partners of negotiators who "became angry" caught some of the happiness that was initially shown by their partners, and this caught happiness led them to be more accepting of suboptimal offers. This research shows that changing one's display from happy to angry can be an even more powerful influence strategy than constantly showing anger.

CONCLUSION

Our goal in this chapter has been to demonstrate that negative emotional expressions are powerful tools of social influence. Consistent with EASI theory (Van Kleef, 2009), we have seen that emotional expressions may exert social influence by triggering affective reactions and/or inferential processes in targets, depending on the target's information-processing depth and the perceived appropriateness of the emotional expression. We

have applied this framework to several domains of social influence, including requests for social support, negotiation, leadership, and conformity in groups. Although emerging evidence from these domains supports our analysis, more work is needed to establish the generalizability of the theory to other areas of social influence. We expect that such research will further underline the emerging conceptualization of emotions as agents of social influence.

ACKNOWLEDGMENTS

Preparation of this chapter was supported by a grant from the Netherlands Organisation for Scientific Research (No. NWO 452-09-010) awarded to Gerben A. Van Kleef.

REFERENCES

Adam, H., Shirako, A., & Maddux, W. W. (2010). Cultural variance in the interpersonal effects of anger in negotiations. *Psychological Science, 21*, 882–889

Barnett, M. A., Howard, J. A., Melton, E. M., & Dino, G. A. (1982). Effect of inducing sadness about self or other on helping behavior in high- and low-empathic children. *Child Development, 53*, 920–923.

Baumeister, R. F., & Leary, M. R. (1995). The need to belong: Desire for interpersonal attachments as a fundamental human motivation. *Psychological Bulletin, 117*, 497–529.

Bodenhausen, G. V., Sheppard, L. A., & Kramer, G. P. (1994). Negative affect and social judgment: The differential impact of anger and sadness. *European Journal of Social Psychology, 24*, 45–62.

Bono, J. E., & Ilies, R. (2006). Charisma, positive emotions, and mood contagion. *Leadership Quarterly, 17*, 317–334.

Cacioppo, J. T., & Gardner, W. L. (1999). Emotion. *Annual Review of Psychology, 50*, 191–214.

Cialdini, R. B., & Goldstein, N. J. (2004). Social influence: Compliance and conformity. *Annual Review of Psychology, 55*, 591–621.

Cialdini, R. B., Vincent, J. E., Lewis, S. K., Catalan, J., Wheeler, D., & Darby, B. L. (1975). Reciprocal concessions procedure for inducing compliance: The door-in-the-face technique. *Journal of Personality and Social Psychology, 31*, 206–215.

Clark, M. S., Ouellette, R., Powell, M. C., & Milberg, S. (1987). Recipient's mood, relationship type, and helping. *Journal of Personality and Social Psychology, 53*, 94–103.

Clark, M. S., Pataki, S. P., & Carver, V. H. (1996). Some thoughts and findings on self-presentation of emotions in relationships. In G. J. O. Fletcher & J. Fitness (Eds.), *Knowledge structures in close relationships: A social psychological approach* (pp. 247–274). Mahwah, NJ: Erlbaum.

Clark, M. S., & Taraban, C. B. (1991). Reactions to and willingness to express emotion in two types of relationships. *Journal of Experimental Social Psychology, 27,* 324–336.

Côté, S., & Hideg, I. (2011). The ability to influence others via emotion displays: A new dimension of emotional intelligence. *Organizational Psychology Review, 1,* 53–71.

Côté, S., Hideg, I., & Van Kleef, G. A. (2013). The consequences of faking anger in negotiations. *Journal of Experimental Social Psychology, 49,* 453–463.

Darwin, C. (1872). *The expression of the emotions in man and animals* (3rd ed.). London: HarperCollins.

DeSteno, D., Petty, R., Wegener, D. T., & Rucker, D. D. (2000). Beyond valence in the perception of likelihood: The role of emotion specificity. *Journal of Personality and Social Psychology, 78,* 397–416.

Filipowicz, A., Barsade, S., & Melwani, S. (2011). Understanding emotional transitions: The interpersonal consequences of changing emotions in negotiations. *Journal of Personality and Social Psychology, 101,* 541–556.

Fischer, A. H., & Roseman, I. J. (2007). Beat them or ban them: The characteristics and social functions of anger and contempt. *Journal of Personality and Social Psychology, 93,* 103–115.

Fisher, R., & Ury, W. (1981). *Getting to yes.* New York: Penguin Books.

Fitness, J. (2000). Anger in the workplace: An emotion script approach to anger episodes between workers and their superiors, co-workers, and subordinates. *Journal of Organizational Behavior, 21,* 147–162.

Forgas, J. P. (1995). Mood and judgment: The affect infusion model (AIM). *Psychological Bulletin, 117,* 39–66.

Frank, R. H. (1988). *Passions within reason: The strategic role of the emotions.* New York: Norton.

Freedman, J. L., & Fraser, S. C. (1966). Compliance without pressure: The foot-in-the-door technique. *Journal of Personality and Social Psychology, 4,* 195–202.

Fridlund, A. J. (1994). *Human facial expression: An evolutionary view.* San Diego, CA: Academic Press.

Frijda, N. H. (1986). *The emotions.* Cambridge, UK: Cambridge University Press.

Glomb, T. M., & Hulin, C. L. (1997). Anger and gender effects in observed supervisor–subordinate dyadic interactions. *Organizational Behavior and Human Decision Processes, 72,* 281–307.

Heerdink, M. W., Van Kleef, G. A., Homan, A. C., & Fischer, A. H. (2013). On the social influence of emotions in groups: Interpersonal effects of anger and happiness on conformity versus deviance. *Journal of Personality and Social Psychology, 105,* 262–284.

Homan, A. C., Greer, L. L., Jehn, K. A., & Koning, L. (2010). Believing shapes seeing: The impact of diversity beliefs on the construal of group composition. *Group Processes and Intergroup Relations, 13,* 477–493.

Keltner, D., Ellsworth, P. C., & Edwards, K. (1993). Beyond simple pessimism: Effects of sadness and anger on social perception. *Journal of Personality and Social Psychology, 64,* 740–752.

Krumhuber, E., Manstead, A. S. R., Cosker, D., Marshall, D., Rosin, P. L., & Kappas, A. (2007). Facial dynamics as indicators of trustworthiness and cooperative behavior. *Emotion, 7,* 730–735.

Labott, S. M., Martin, R. B., Eason, P. S., & Berkey, E. Y. (1991). Social reactions to the expression of emotion. *Cognition and Emotion, 5,* 397–417.

Larsen, J. T., McGraw, A. P., & Cacioppo, J. (2001). Can people feel happy and sad at the same time? *Journal of Personality and Social Psychology, 81,* 684–696.

Lazarus, R. S. (1991). *Emotion and adaptation.* New York: Oxford University Press.

Lelieveld, G.-J., Van Dijk, E., Van Beest, I., Steinel, W., & Van Kleef, G. A. (2011). Disappointed in you, angry about your offer: Distinct negative emotions induce concessions via different mechanisms. *Journal of Experimental Social Psychology, 47,* 635–641.

Lerner, J. S., & Keltner, D. (2001). Fear, anger, and risk. *Journal of Personality and Social Psychology, 81,* 146–159.

Mayer, J. D., & Salovey, P. (1997). What is emotional intelligence? In P. Salovey & D. J. Sluyter (Eds.), *Emotional development and emotional intelligence* (pp. 3–31). New York: Basic Books.

Neuberg, S. L., & Newsom, J. T. (1993). Personal need for structure: Individual differences in the desire for simpler structure. *Journal of Personality and Social Psychology, 65,* 113–131.

Pruitt, D. G., & Carnevale, P. J. (1993). *Negotiation in social conflict.* Buckingham, UK: Open University Press.

Rafaeli, A., & Sutton, R. I. (1991). Emotional contrast strategies as means of social influence: Lessons from criminal interrogators and bill collectors. *Academy of Management Journal, 34,* 749–775.

Rogers, R. W. (1983). Cognitive and physiological processes in fear appeals and attitude change: A revised theory of protection motivation. In J. T. Cacioppo & R. E. Petty (Eds.), *Social psychophysiology: A sourcebook* (pp. 153–176). New York: Guilford Press.

Rothman, N. B. (2011). Steering sheep: How expressed emotional ambivalence elicits dominance in interdependent decision-making contexts. *Organizational Behavior and Human Decision Processes, 116,* 66–82.

Salovey, P., & Mayer, J. D. (1990). Emotional intelligence. *Imagination, Cognition, and Personality, 9,* 185–211.

Scherer, K. R., & Tannenbaum, P. H. (1986). Emotional experiences in everyday life: A survey approach. *Motivation and Emotion, 10,* 295–314.

Schwarz, N., & Clore, G. L. (1983). Mood, misattribution, and judgments of well-being: Informative and directive functions of affective states. *Journal of Personality and Social Psychology, 45,* 513–523.

Sinaceur, M., & Tiedens, L. Z. (2006). Get mad and get more than even: When and why anger expression is effective in negotiations. *Journal of Experimental Social Psychology, 42,* 314–322.

Smith, C. A., Haynes, K. N., Lazarus, R. S., & Pope, L. K. (1993). In search of the "hot" cognitions: Attributions, appraisals, and their relation to emotion. *Journal of Personality and Social Psychology, 65,* 916–929.

Steinel, W., Van Kleef, G. A., & Harinck, F. (2008). Are you talking to me?!: Separating the people from the problem when expressing emotions in negotiation. *Journal of Experimental Social Psychology, 44*, 362–369.

Steinel, W., Van Kleef, G. A., Van Knippenberg, D., Hogg, M. A., Homan, A. C., & Moffit, G. (2010). How intragroup dynamics affect behavior in intergroup conflict: The role of group norms, prototypicality, and need to belong. *Group Processes and Intergroup Relations, 13*, 779–794.

Sy, T., Côté, S., & Saavedra, R. (2005). The contagious leader: Impact of the leader's mood on the mood of group members, group affective tone, and group processes. *Journal of Applied Psychology, 90*, 295–305.

Tiedens, L. Z., & Linton, S. (2001). Judgment under emotional certainty and uncertainty: The effects of specific emotions on information processing. *Journal of Personality and Social Psychology, 81*, 973–988.

Van Dijk, E., Van Kleef, G. A., Steinel, W., & Van Beest, I. (2008). A social functional approach to emotions in bargaining: When communicating anger pays and when it backfires. *Journal of Personality and Social Psychology, 94*, 600–614.

Van Doorn, E. A., Van Kleef, G. A., & Van der Pligt, J. (2013). *Emotional expressions shape prosocial behavior: Interpersonal effects of anger and disappointment on compliance with requests.* Manuscript submitted for publication.

Van Kleef, G. A. (2009). How emotions regulate social life: The emotions as social information (EASI) model. *Current Directions in Psychological Science, 18*, 184–188.

Van Kleef, G. A. (2010). The emerging view of emotion as social information. *Social and Personality Psychology Compass, 4/5*, 331–343.

Van Kleef, G. A., & Côté, S. (2007). Expressing anger in conflict: When it helps and when it hurts. *Journal of Applied Psychology, 92*, 1557–1569.

Van Kleef, G. A., & De Dreu, C. K. W. (2010). Longer-term consequences of anger expression in negotiation: Retaliation or spill-over? *Journal of Experimental Social Psychology, 46*, 753–760.

Van Kleef, G. A., De Dreu, C. K. W., & Manstead, A. S. R. (2004a). The interpersonal effects of anger and happiness in negotiations. *Journal of Personality and Social Psychology, 86*, 57–76.

Van Kleef, G. A., De Dreu, C. K. W., & Manstead, A. S. R. (2004b). The interpersonal effects of emotions in negotiations: A motivated information processing approach. *Journal of Personality and Social Psychology, 87*, 510–528.

Van Kleef, G. A., De Dreu, C. K. W., & Manstead, A. S. R. (2006). Supplication and appeasement in conflict and negotiation: The interpersonal effects of disappointment, worry, guilt, and regret. *Journal of Personality and Social Psychology, 91*, 124–142.

Van Kleef, G. A., De Dreu, C. K. W., & Manstead, A. S. R. (2010). An interpersonal approach to emotion in social decision making: The emotions as social information model. *Advances in Experimental Social Psychology, 42*, 45–96.

Van Kleef, G. A., De Dreu, C. K. W., Pietroni, D., & Manstead, A. S. R. (2006). Power and emotion in negotiation: Power moderates the interpersonal effects of anger and happiness on concession making. *European Journal of Social Psychology, 36*, 557–581.

Van Kleef, G. A., Homan, A. C., Beersma, B., & van Knippenberg, D. (2010). On angry leaders and agreeable followers: How leaders' emotions and followers' personalities shape motivation and team performance. *Psychological Science, 21,* 1827–1834.

Van Kleef, G. A., Homan, A. C., Beersma, B., van Knippenberg, D., van Knippenberg, B., & Damen, F. (2009). Searing sentiment or cold calculation? The effects of leader emotional displays on team performance depend on follower epistemic motivation. *Academy of Management Journal, 52,* 562–580.

Van Kleef, G. A., Homan, A. C., & Cheshin, A. (2012). Emotional influence at work: Take it EASI. *Organizational Psychology Review, 2,* 311–339.

Van Kleef, G. A., Oveis, C., Van der Löwe, I., LuoKogan, A., Goetz, J., & Keltner, D. (2008). Power, distress, and compassion: Turning a blind eye to the suffering of others. *Psychological Science, 19,* 1315–1322.

Van Kleef, G. A., Steinel, W., van Knippenberg, D., Hogg, M., & Svensson, A. (2007). Group member prototypicality and intergroup negotiation: How one's standing in the group affects negotiation behaviour. *British Journal of Social Psychology, 46,* 129–154.

Van Kleef, G. A., Van Doorn, E. A., Heerdink, M. W., & Koning, L. F. (2011). Emotion is for influence. *European Review of Social Psychology, 22,* 114–163.

Williams, K. D. (2007). Ostracism. *Annual Review of Psychology, 58,* 425–452.

Yee, J. L., & Greenberg, M. S. (1998). Reactions to crime victims: Effects of victims' emotional state and type of relationship. *Journal of Social and Clinical Psychology, 17,* 209–226.

Yukl, G. A. (2010). *Leadership in organizations* (7th ed.). Upper Saddle River, NJ: Pearson.

7

Listening to Negative Emotions
How Culture Constrains What We Hear

YULIA E. CHENTSOVA-DUTTON
NICOLE SENFT
ANDREW G. RYDER

I knew there'd be a lot of sorrow but I'd rather know bittersweet
happiness than a grey, uneventful life. . . . There was a lot of grief,
and fear, and pain, but I've never regretted it, nor envied anyone.
It's just fate. It's life.
—"STALKER'S WIFE" in Andrey Tarkovsky's film *Stalker*
(Demidova & Tarkovsky, 1979)

Negative emotions, such as anger, sadness, disgust, fear, or guilt,
signal threats and losses and are generally experienced as unpleasant. Yet
people in different cultural contexts hear different things when listening
to their own negative emotions and those of others. European American
cultural contexts foster the idea that these emotions are not just unpleasant but problematic, even pathological. Over the course of the last century,
shared cultural ideas of what it means to function well in these contexts
have increasingly emphasized the ability to avoid or down-regulate negative emotions and cultivate positivity (Davies, 2011; Kotchemidova, 2005;
Stearns & Stearns, 1989). Americans sign up for anger management and
grief-resolution workshops and purchase best-selling books guiding them
to "cool the flames" of anger (Hanh, 2002), imagine "life without fear"

(Lucado, 2009), and "let go of rage, frustration, and irritation" (Childre, Rozman & McKay, 2003). Parents can avail themselves of books promising to help them "take the *grrrr* out of anger" (Verdick & Lisovskis, 2002), and "free your child from anxiety" (Chansky, 2004).

These self-help books illustrate a particular cultural model of negative emotions—a set of cultural beliefs, values, and scripts organizing knowledge about these emotions and ways of enacting them and responding to them. The core assumption of this particular model is that feeling bad is bad for you and should be avoided. There is some legitimacy to this emphasis. Recent psychological research conducted in European American cultural contexts provides ample evidence that negative emotions carry significant costs for relationships, health, and well-being (Dickerson, Gruenewald, & Kemeny, 2004; Gottman & Levenson, 1992; Kubzansky & Kawachi, 2000). Other studies promote the cultivation of positive emotions (Folkman & Moskowitz, 2000; Fredrickson, 2000; Fredrickson & Levenson, 1998; Moskowitz & Epel, 2006; Xu & Roberts, 2010), although there is also emerging work on the costs of positive emotions (Graham, Huang, Clark & Helgeson, 2008; Gruber, Mauss, & Tamir, 2011; Hershfield, Scheibe, Sims, & Carstensen, 2012). Negative emotions are discouraged by parents during socialization of children, starting early in infancy (Malatesta, Grigoryev, Lamb, Albin, & Culver, 1986; Miller & Sperry, 1987). Experience and expression of negative emotions have increasingly become linked to psychopathology (Horwitz & Wakefield, 2007). A shared understanding in European American cultural contexts is that negative emotions signal significant concerns; hence, when they are expressed, they grab attention and demand a response.

These assumptions about negative emotions are not universal. Cultural contexts differ in their basic assumptions regarding the desirability of feeling bad. Low hedonic value is paramount in the European American milieu, but many other cultural contexts incorporate the understanding that there are many aspects to negative emotions—for example, their perceived effects on attention, cognition, motivation, and interpersonal relationships. East Asian contexts, for example, are less likely than European American contexts to foster the belief that negative emotions are undesirable and inappropriate (Eid & Diener, 2001). Although the perceived unpleasantness of negative emotions is acknowledged across a wide range of cultural contexts (Church, Katigbak, Reyes, & Jensen, 1999; Russell, Lewicka, & Niit, 1989; Thompson, 2007), the avoidance of unpleasantness does not universally dominate beliefs about these emotions. Consider our opening quotation, illustrating a commonly held Russian belief (Rancour-Laferriere, 1995, 2003; Wierzbicka, 1998, 1999) that positive and negative emotions are intimately connected and that a well-lived life includes both. Similarly, East Asian cultural contexts foster the idea that positive

and negative emotions can coexist (Miyamoto, Uchida, & Ellsworth, 2010; Schimmack, Oishi, & Diener, 2002).

Anthropological research has demonstrated that these beliefs are far from unusual (Gaines & Farmer, 1986; Lock, 1995; Lutz, 1988; Obeyesekere, 1985). For example, Gaines and Farmer (1986) observed that in Catholic Mediterranean cultural contexts, women who experience and express negative emotions are likely to gain attention, empathy, and public prestige. A widely shared belief in these contexts is that although suffering and negative emotions may not feel good, they are ennobling, making one a better, more respectable, and saintly person. In some cultural contexts, negative emotions, particularly those that promote socialization, are so valued that adults encourage children to feel bad. Feelings of loneliness are emphasized in Japanese preschools (Hayashi, Karasawa, & Tobin, 2009), and shame is fostered in Taiwanese (Fung, 1999) and Tamang families (the Tamang are indigenous people of the Himalayas; Cole, Bruschi, & Tamang, 2002). Despite their unpleasantness, experience and expression of these emotions are sanctioned and even admired in these contexts. Cross-cultural studies demonstrate that cultural models of emotions affect the actual experience of these emotions (Eid & Diener, 2001; Kitayama, Markus, & Kurokawa, 2000; Mesquita & Karasawa, 2002; Scollon, Diener, Oishi, & Biswas-Diener, 2004). For example, European American and Japanese people differ in the balance between experienced positive and negative emotions, with European Americans experiencing more positive emotions for each negative emotion than do Japanese (Kitayama et al., 2000). Thus culture affects not only what we believe but also what we feel and communicate to others.

HOW SHOULD WE THINK ABOUT THE INTERRELATION OF CULTURE AND EMOTION?

When speaking of culture, we refer to intersubjectively held meanings (beliefs, values, norms), combined with consensually understood meaningful practices, that both constitute and are constituted by the evolved brain and the social mind (Ryder, Ban, & Chentsova-Dutton, 2011). These meaningful practices shape our models of how to respond to environmental challenges and how to balance individual versus group needs. Cultural contexts affect how emotions are represented "in the head" (e.g., beliefs about emotions) as well as "in the world" (e.g., events that trigger negative emotions; cultural products, such as children's books or popular songs). Because emotions are expressed to others and encoded in cultural products, such as songs and memorials, cultural models of emotions shape not only what we attend to, feel, and think but also what is objectively present in our

cultural worlds. For example, the portrayal of emotions in East versus West German newspapers was shown to correspond with emotions displayed by people in East and West Berlin bars (Oettingen & Seligman, 1990). People are profoundly shaped by the cultural models available to them, regardless of whether they respond to them with uncritical acceptance, vehement rejection, or something in between.

Human emotions are inherently cultural. William James famously stated that stripping emotions of their bodily symptoms leaves nothing behind but a "cold and neutral state of intellectual perception," which no longer resembles a fully realized human emotion (James, 1890/2007, p. 451). He saw human emotions as phenomena that are rooted in the realities of the human body. We agree that emotions are emergent phenomena that depend on physiological activation but add that human emotions evolved to aid us in the contexts of cultural meanings and shared ways of feeling (Laland, Odling-Smee, & Myles, 2010). Cultural influences interact with situational demands and biological predispositions to shape the way negative emotions are experienced, expressed, conceptualized, and regulated. Stripping emotions of their cultural values and meanings leaves us with "hot" responses in a social vacuum not shaped by consensual models of how to think about them, feel them, and respond to them. As such, they fall far short of the full complexity of human emotions, which are rooted in the realities of cultural worlds. As such, the cultural shaping of negative emotions is best seen as a built-in adaptation to complex and varied cultural environments rather than a mere overlay on evolved responses to universally encountered threats. The role of culture is important and pervasive.

Cultural models and natural selection pressures jointly constrain experience and expression of negative emotions. Natural selection places limits on many aspects of emotions, including the ways our bodies and brains respond to elicitors of these emotions, types of elicitors themselves, and typical duration of emotional response (LeDoux, 2000; Levenson, 2003; Panksepp, 2004). A parent has to work hard to train a curious baby to fear electric plugs and cars, yet the task is much easier in case of heights or dogs, a pattern of emotional responses that is constrained by our evolutionary past. Cultural models of negative emotions further constrain their meanings and behavioral consequences. By encouraging attention to culturally salient aspects of emotional elicitors and responses, cultural models shape the ways in which emotions are detected, construed, experienced, and enacted.

For example, although the face communicates important emotional information across cultural contexts, different contexts encourage attention to different facial features. Compared with European Americans, Japanese are more likely to focus on information conveyed by the eyes and less likely to attend to the mouth when interpreting expressions of emotions

(Yuki, Maddux, & Masuda, 2007). Moreover, Japanese are more likely than Americans to take the larger social context into account when evaluating emotional facial expressions (Masuda, Ellsworth, Mesquita, Leu, Tanida, & Veerdonk, 2008). These variations in attention constrain the effectiveness of different emotional cues in signaling negative emotions.

Cultural models can also extend meanings, expressions, and functions of negative emotions (Fessler, 2007; Keltner, Haidt, & Shiota, 2006; Simon, 1990). As cultural creatures, we are able to experience uniquely human emotions, such as moral disgust and outrage, sweet sadness, shame, guilt, and embarrassment. Cultural functions of emotions can "hitchhike" on previously evolved characteristics (Boyd & Richerson, 1992; Simon, 1990). Consider the ways in which moral disgust builds upon evolutionarily older mechanisms that help the organism avoid ingestion of dangerous substances. Negative emotions may also function differently in cultural contexts that tolerate or encourage negativity. Unlike their European American counterparts, when Asian Americans are highly pessimistic they perform better, not worse, at problem solving (Chang, 1996). Russians who ruminate on negative life events are less likely than European Americans to blame other people for their misfortunes (Grossmann & Kross, 2010).

Such variation raises the possibility that psychological theories of negative emotions need to make more room for culture as an important constituent of these emotions. By constraining and extending negative emotions as they are represented in the head and in the world, cultures shape the ability of these emotions to effectively signal threats and coordinate behavioral responses to these threats. In the remainder of this chapter, we review research on culture and functions of negative emotions conducted by anthropologists and psychologists. To ensure that we consider the full spectrum of negative emotions, we include basic research on culture and negative emotions and also clinical studies on culture and emotional distress.

WHAT ARE THE FUNCTIONS
OF NEGATIVE EMOTIONS?

Within the field of affective science, an overemphasis on the hedonic value of negative emotions is a relatively recent phenomenon. Much of the early theoretical and empirical work in the field emphasized functions of negative emotions to the relative exclusion of positive emotions. By the time the importance of positive emotions was acknowledged (Fredrickson, 1998), the field had developed a shared understanding that negative emotions evolved to maximize our chances of survival. They do so by signaling threats and coordinating physiological changes, attention, thoughts, and behavior to

allow us to rapidly respond to these threats and spread the threat signal across social groups (Cosmides & Tooby, 2000; Ekman, Friesen, & Ellsworth, 1972; Tooby & Cosmides, 1990; Frijda, 1989; Izard, 1992). Negative emotions are particularly adaptive when they are executed with some degree of context specificity and when the intensity of response is neither too weak (failing to signal important threats) nor too strong (overwhelming one's ability to act in response to threats). Constrained by features of our ancestral environments, negative emotions do not always fit the demands of the worlds that we live in today (Tooby & Cosmides, 1990).

This perspective on negative emotions emphasizes their capacity to prepare people for threats in the natural world—the bear in the woods, the snake in the grass. Relatively less attention is allocated to the role of these emotions in guiding our responses to the social world and its interpersonal and culturally shaped challenges. Yet emotional responses show a considerable degree of heterogeneity, suggesting that they are far more sensitive to contextual inputs than the traditional conceptualization of emotions as evolved programs of responses to threats allows (see Feldman Barrett, 2006). It appears that human emotions evolved to be input-dependent, showing considerable responsiveness to cultural shaping. Emotions are fundamentally interpersonal phenomena that unfold in and take their meanings from the social context (Keltner & Haidt, 2001; Turner, 2000). In comparison with our closest animal relatives, our emotions can be described as ultrasocial (Keltner et al., 2006). We experience them in response to interpersonal threats and losses, enact them in the interpersonal sphere, and share them with others (Rimé, Mesquita, Boca, & Philippot, 1991; Berger, 2011). Emotions reverberate through our social networks, affecting entire social groups (Fowler & Christakis, 2008; Rosenquist, Fowler, & Christakis, 2010; Smith, Seger, & Mackie, 2007). Negative emotions that offer advantages for managing threats of the natural world have undeniable survival value, but so do the ones that allow us to effectively conform to group norms, resolve conflict, bond with others, forge cooperation, establish hierarchies and manage threats as groups. Encountering predators is dangerous, but so is encountering an enemy and being unable to count on support and protection from one's tribe due to inability to conform to its social norms.

Although life in social groups has many universal elements, including the centrality of family as a unit of social organization, reliance on kin, reciprocity, and social hierarchy (see Tooby & Cosmides, 1992), there is also considerable cultural variation. Humans are unique among animals in their ability to develop complex cultural systems and contribute to cumulative cultural changes, a process that spans thousands of years. As infants, we arrive into the cultural worlds that are preshaped by previous generations. Due to cultural variation in models of social behavior, the ability

to thrive in one social context does not always translate into thriving in another. Consider recent studies that demonstrate that genetic predispositions linked to emotionality are not functional or dysfunctional in and of themselves. Rather, they are functional in certain social contexts, but not in others (Ellis & Boyce, 2008; Kim et al., 2010).

For instance, the horticulturalist Machiguenga people of the Peruvian Amazon live in a cultural context that values stability and sociability. Anger is discouraged, so much so that Machiguenga prefer social withdrawal to displays of anger. When a Machiguenga feels intense anger, he or she is likely to flee the group (Johnson, 2003; Johnson & Earle, 2000), making it unlikely that one sees displays of anger in this context. In contrast, contexts such as those of the traditional Kaluli of Papua New Guinea, European Americans in the southern regions of the United States, or the Castilian Spanish in Spain encourage and value displays of anger in response to provocations (Cohen, Nisbett, Bowdle, & Schwarz, 1996; Fischer, 1999; Nisbett & Cohen, 1996; Rodriguez-Mosquera, Manstead, & Fischer, 2002). For example, the Kaluli of Papua New Guinea openly express anger, and such displays are generally admired (Schieffelin, 1983). Adaptive emotional functioning in these different cultural contexts is likely to entail different ways of experiencing and expressing anger, with children learning different ways of attending to anger-related cues and of experiencing, expressing, and regulating anger. Indeed, studies suggest that cultural differences in the ways in which young children conceptualize and value emotions emerge relatively early (e.g., Borke & Su, 1972; Tsai, Louie, Chen, & Uchida, 2007). Chinese children between the ages of 3 and 4 recognize sad situations more accurately than American children of the same age (Borke & Su, 1972), a pattern that is thought to be due to greater acceptability of the idea of children feeling sad and ashamed in the Chinese context. This evidence converges to a conception of negative emotions as experience-expectant phenomena (Joseph, 1999) that depend on environmental inputs, including inputs that are culturally shaped.

There is no tension in describing negative emotions as at once biologically driven and cultural. Culture is biologically embedded and human biology is cultural, supporting our ability to function in our sociocultural worlds. Most aspects of physiological functioning, ranging from pubertal timing to susceptibility to disease, depend on contextual factors (Obeidallah, Brennan, Brooks-Gunn, & Earls, 2004; van Vliet, Oates, & Whitelaw, 2007). Cultures and genes can be understood as coevolving (Eisenberg & Hayes, 2011; Laland et al., 2010), with culture shaping environmental threats and rewards as well as modifying the extent to which a given trait conveys adaptive fitness. Recent work in anthropology and population genetics suggests we need to take culture seriously as a factor that can exert selection pressures on physiological and psychological functions,

including negative emotions such as shame (Gintis, 2003; Holden & Mace, 2009; Laland et al., 2010; Richerson & Boyd, 2005). As we have argued elsewhere, culture, mind, and brain can be understood as different and mutually constituted levels of a single system (Ryder et al., 2011). As with psychopathological symptoms, we hold that emotions are best understood as occurring within the system as a whole rather than being reducible to a single level.

Although it is easier to think of cultural shaping manifesting in cultural variation, similarities in cultural worlds can produce similar culturally shaped emotional responses. Negative emotions that engage with universal as well as culturally specific ways of signaling and managing threats allow people to take maximum advantage of the protective function not only of their brains, bodies, and peers but also of their cultural environments. As with human emotions more generally, negative emotions have evolved in large part to allow us to navigate our cultural environments, propagating and transforming meanings and practices (Chentsova-Dutton & Heath, 2009; Nichols, 2002; Bangerter & Heath, 2004; Berger & Milkman, 2012).

Notably, the literature on culture and emotions suggests that cultural variation is more pronounced for positive than negative emotions (e.g., Scollon et al., 2004; Tsai, Chentsova-Dutton, Freire-Bebeau, & Przymus, 2002; Tsai, Levenson & Carstensen, 2000). Although a substantial number of papers do report cultural variations in experiences, models, triggers, and expressions of negative emotions, they may nonetheless provide us with a more conservative domain for examining the extent of cultural shaping (e.g., Eid & Diener, 2001; Matsumoto, 1990; Scherer, Matsumoto, Wallbott, & Kudoh, 1988; Soto, Levenson, & Ebling, 2005; Uchida & Kitayama, 2009; also see Mesquita & Walker, 2003, for a review). One reason for this may be that the North American cultural context, which often serves as cultural reference point, fosters emphasis on positive emotions such as excitement and cheerfulness (Kotchemidova, 2005; Tsai, Knutson, & Fung, 2006).

It is also possible that these results are due to the fact that experimentally elicited negative emotions do not represent the full range of intensity or duration of negative emotions. Clinical studies that report cultural differences in the conception, experience, expression, and consequences of emotional distress may be particularly helpful in uncovering cultural differences in negative emotion (e.g., Dinnel, Kleinknecht, & Tanaka-Matsumi, 2002; Hinton, Um, & Ba, 2001a, 2001b; Lewis-Fernández et al., 2002; Ryder et al., 2008; Zhou et al., 2011). For example, Chentsova-Dutton and colleagues (2007) reported that the association of major depression with experienced and expressed sadness differed for European Americans and Asian Americans. Negative emotions can also have different consequences

in different cultural contexts. Brar and Moneta (2009) found that negative emotions experienced in the context of depression and anxiety predicted levels of alcohol dependence among white British college students, but not among their Indian British counterparts. The authors attributed this finding to the observation that British, but not Indian, cultural contexts tend to emphasize the link between negative emotions and one's overall well-being, thereby promoting efforts to repair negative emotions by drinking. Taken together, the emerging literature in affective and clinical science on culture and negative emotions provides us with a body of evidence focusing on ways in which cultural models constrain and extend meanings of emotions. Let us turn now to the ways in which these processes function.

HOW DOES CULTURE SHAPE NEGATIVE EMOTIONS "IN THE HEAD"?

Cultural models help us make sense of the messy and complex signals that are our negative emotions. Hearts beat, hands tremble, and necks stiffen. Sleep and appetite are lost or, conversely, gained. Past threats come to mind and drive attention to salient cues. Subjective experiences change. Other people notice signs of these feelings and respond to them in real time, requiring behavioral adjustments. Emotion regulation efforts are engaged in order to alter what is felt and what is shown to others. How are we to make sense of these experiences? Cultural contexts foster models of negative emotions that allow people to reduce uncertainty and ambiguity and enable them to respond to emotional cues in culturally adaptive ways. People thereby know what to attend to, what to expect, and how to respond. These models differ from context to context, affecting conceptions of negative emotions, the subjective experience of having them, and their behavioral expression. They are not always accurate (e.g., Philippot & Rimé, 1997). In all cases, though, they help guide attention, organize responses, and ascribe meaning to unpleasant and potentially disturbing experiences.

Over time, these models become culturally reinforced. Negative emotions that are valued are likely to generate interpersonal benefits, such as social approval and ease of communication. For example, expressions of anger are more likely to be accepted in cultural contexts that place a premium on egalitarianism (Matsumoto, Yoo, & Chung, 2010). Studies conducted in these contexts suggest that these expressions garner social approval due to the perceived associations of anger with dominance and credibility (e.g., Hareli et al., 2009; Hess, Blairy, & Kleck, 2000). It is easier to communicate with someone whose emotions, whether positive or negative, match the shared cultural norm. People are more likely to recognize facial expression of emotions from their own cultural context

(Elfenbein, Mandal, Ambady, Harizuka, & Kumar, 2002; Marsh, Elfenbein, & Ambady, 2003). Immigrants arriving in new cultural contexts benefit from adoption of local emotional norms (de Leersnyder, Mesquita, & Kim, 2011), presumably due at least in part to the fact that this adoption of new emotional norms may facilitate communication.

Culturally valued emotions are also likely to garner intrapersonal benefits by virtue of fostering meaning making in the context of stressful events and providing "value from fit" between one's beliefs about how one should ideally feel and one's actual feeling (Higgins, 2005; Park, 2010). For example, Russians who focus on and "suffer through" their negative emotions (Pavlenko, 2002) may have a sense that they are handling stressors in a meaningful way because the very fact that they are suffering fits well with the emphasis in Russian cultural contexts on suffering as a source of meaning. Cultural values regarding emotions are part of the context in which emotions are experienced. An intersubjectively held belief that the experience of negative emotions confers benefits itself becomes part of the experience of having that emotion.

Let us examine cultural differences in the elaboration and extension of meanings of negative emotions, using sadness as an example. Sadness is an unpleasant and deactivating state (Mauro, Sato, & Tucker, 1992; Russell et al., 1989; Tellegen, Watson, & Clark, 1999) that is associated with powerlessness, submission, and withdrawal in the interpersonal sphere (Knutson, 1996; Roseman, Dhawan, Rettek, Naidu, & Thapa, 1995; Wallbott & Scherer, 1986). Evolutionary accounts describe sadness as an evolved and biologically driven response to overwhelming stressors, typically losses, failures, or prolonged inability to escape aversive conditions (Bonanno, Goorin, & Coifman, 2008; Nesse & Ellsworth, 2009).

Sadness is thought to serve a number of intrapersonal and interpersonal functions that can be broadly described as imperatives to *pause* and *engage help* from others (for related research, see Forgas, Chapter 1, this volume). The first imperative (*pause*) signals that one's goals are out of reach, calling for a temporary time-out in order to reassess, process, and accommodate information about oneself in the world that is marked by loss, pain, or failure. This function of sadness is thought to conserve resources and, in humans, foster reflection and careful processing of information about the situation at hand. Sadness can also reduce investment in previously held goals, a functional response in some situations (Wrosch & Miller, 2009). For example, postpartum sadness is thought to reduce maternal investment in a new baby, ensuring continuing engagement with older offspring and recruitment of help and support from others (Hagen & Barrett, 2007). The imperative to pause can affect motivation and behavior, encouraging reconsideration of one's goals and, downstream, bolstering motivation to breach the gap between actual functioning and desired outcomes.

The second imperative (*engage others*) of sadness signals that one is underresourced and needs support. Facial expressions of sadness and sad intonations are recognized across cultures (Elfenbein & Ambady, 2002), although also shaped by the context (Feldman Barrett, Mesquita, & Gendron, 2011). Consistent with the interpersonal meaning, sadness cues are processed as indications of social subordination and lack of agency (Knutson, 1996; Tiedens, 2001). They also signal that the sad person is affiliative and needs care, support, and protection (Hareli & Hess, 2010; Hendriks & Vingerhoets, 2006; Hendriks, Nelson, Cornelius, & Vingerhoets, 2008; Hess et al., 2000). In young children, sadness is thought to serve as a gateway to developing prosocial emotions, such as empathy and sympathy (Hoffman, 1984). The engaging imperative stabilizes social hierarchy and allows people to effectively recruit support and protection in the face of threats. Indeed, some argue that even the prolonged sadness characteristic of minor depression is functional in that it recruits social benefits (e.g., the bargaining model of depression; Hagen, 2003).

These imperatives created by sadness are not entirely unique to humans (Masson & McCarthy, 1996; Seligman, 1975/1992). Sadness also predates enculturation in humans, with infants displaying sad faces that effectively elicit attention and protection from their caregivers (Haviland & Lelwica, 1987; Huebner & Izard, 1988). Yet human sadness is greatly adapted to its sociocultural context, interacting with our higher cognitive capacity and ability to communicate. Taken together, the evolved functions of sadness generate a field of potential interpretations and responses. Sadness can tell many different stories about what happened to the sad person and the effect that this may have on his or her behavior, thoughts, and character.

Sadness can signal to others that the sad person is facing loss or adversity or, put another way, that he or she may be failing to reach desired goals. Sadness can also lead to different behavioral outcomes. On the one hand, slowing down and being more introspective may potentially make sad people less productive and less interpersonally engaged. On the other hand, they may become more careful, thoughtful, and mindful, both in evaluating their attributes and behavior and in interacting with others. In this case, the impact on work and relationships may be beneficial rather than detrimental. We might assume that a sad person needs our support, allowing us to connect with him or her, or we may see an opportunity to influence his or her behavior and, potentially, take charge of the situation. The tendency to use one set of explanations rather than another points to strikingly different models of how sadness informs and colors someone's behavior, personality, and worth as a person. Characteristics associated with sadness can range from laziness, submissiveness, and incompetence to wisdom, perceptiveness, and moral elevation. In a given cultural context, some of these meanings will fit the cultural models of what it means to

be a good person better than others. As these culturally salient meanings are emphasized and elaborated, cultural contexts constrain and extend the potential interpretations of sadness.

Consider the differences between views of sadness in European American and Russian cultural contexts. The European American context fosters the model of a self that is autonomous and independent from others, emphasizing approach motivation or a focus on reaching valued goals and ideal states (Elliot, Chirkov, Kim, & Sheldon, 2001; Higgins, Pierro & Kruglanski, 2008; Lee, Aaker, & Gardner, 2000). Qualities and states that reflect positively on the independent self are also encouraged (Chao, 1995; Haight, 1999; LeVine, Caron, & New, 1980; Wang, 2001). This cultural context places value on the ability to feel high-arousal positive emotions, such as excitement (Tsai et al., 2006). Sadness, in contrast, signals that one is falling short of culturally valued goals. A sad person may feel as though he or she is failing on multiple fronts—not only does he or she feel sad from experiencing loss and/or failing to reach desired goals, but the sadness itself represents a failure in having culturally desirable emotional experiences (D'Andrade, 1984).

Over the course of the last century, sadness has become closely linked with the concept of psychological distress, most notably depression (Horwitz & Wakefield, 2007). It is not surprising that sadness is out of sight in this cultural context, as reflected in the recent finding that European Americans tend to underestimate the extent to which other people feel sad (Jordan et al., 2011). Studies examining mother–infant interactions report that, in contrast to positive facial expressions, European American mothers are unlikely to mirror their babies' sad (or angry) facial expressions (Malatesta et al., 1986). Once triggered, therefore, sadness is a relatively rare signal that is perceived as threatening.

Contrast the European American model of sadness with the one that has been dominant in cultural contexts shaped by Orthodox Christianity, such as Russia (similar models exist in other religious traditions, such as Mediterranean Catholicism, Iranian Shi'ism, and Buddhism; Davies, 2011; Gaines & Farmer, 1986; Good, Good, & Moradi, 1985; Obeyesekere, 1985). This religious tradition places value on physical and emotional suffering generally and on sadness more specifically (Rancour-Laferriere, 1995, 2003; Ries, 1997). How does this cultural model map onto what we know about the evolved functions of sadness? In the domain of pausing, there is emphasis on the ability of sadness to deactivate positive emotions and promote patience, reflection, introspection, humility, and accurate self-knowledge. For example, Ignatius Brianchaninov (1965/2006), a Russian Orthodox bishop and canonized saint, described life's sorrows as one's guide to spiritual wisdom, conferring protection from sinful passions and hubris.

This cultural–religious context also taps into and extends the "engage others" function of sadness to include a widely shared belief that sadness signifies divine attention and represents a test of one's spiritual connection and worth. Certain kinds of sadness can signal spiritual engagement, closeness to God, submission to his will, or even saintliness (Gavrilova, 2009; see also Gaines & Farmer, 1986). Although the influence of the Russian Orthodox church on the larger cultural milieu has fluctuated over the last century, the contemporary Russian cultural context has been historically shaped by this religious tradition. The notion that suffering and sadness have value is widely shared beyond circles of devout believers. Although it is no longer explicitly tied to religion, a Russian model of sadness links this emotion to spirituality, wisdom, sensitivity, responsiveness, moral character, and spiritual growth.

Notably, even within the Russian Orthodox and Catholic religious traditions, the dominant model of sadness has always been contested. An alternative cultural model of excessive sadness taps into perceived costs of pausing. This alternative model conceptualizes sadness as an emotion that impairs function and is accompanied by undesirable levels of self-absorption and disengagement. As such, sadness is viewed as an impediment to a strong relationship with God, problematic at best and sinful at worst. Although both models were historically present in the religious "toolkits," they varied in relative emphasis during different historical periods and in different social contexts. The potential of prolonged sadness, or *unynie*, to encourage idleness was seen as particularly problematic in monastic communities. Gradually, the church promoted this model of sadness to larger circles of believers through its propagation of penitential literature (see a description of the same process in the Catholic church through discussions of *acedia*; Gaines & Farmer, 1986; Jackson, 1985).

Nonetheless, over the course of cultural selection, the model placing value on sadness became relatively more dominant in Russian culture, a salient and readily available "go-to" tool in the cultural toolkit. Although the reasons are unclear, it is possible that this model of sadness gained popularity because of historical events over the last century and a half (i.e., serfdom, revolution, wars, famines, political purges) that shaped the daily lives of Russians to be relatively full of stressful and uncontrollable situations. A model that validated and gave meaning to frequent experiences of powerlessness and loss may have proven particularly useful.

Indeed, although relatively few empirical studies have specifically examined the cultural shaping of sadness, it appears that this emotion is experienced and expressed differently in Russian cultural contexts as compared with the European American contexts in which much emotion research has been conducted. A recurrent puzzle in the well-being literature is that Russian samples consistently report low levels of happiness and high

levels of depressive symptoms relative not only to the U.S. samples but also to their post-Soviet neighbors, such as Hungary (Abbott & Sapsford, 2006; Averina et al., 2005; Balatsky & Diener, 1993; Pikhart et al., 2004; Veenhoven, 2001). Although this pattern is likely due in part to objective life circumstances, it is not fully explained by relevant sociodemographic indicators (see Frijters, Geishecker, Haisken-DeNew, & Shields, 2006). Some of it is in the head and shaped by cultural models of emotions. It appears that the Russian cultural context fosters attention to, experience of, and expression of negative emotions, including sadness and despair.

Indeed, early studies of Soviet expatriates in the United States reported that these migrants judged ambiguous stimuli more negatively and described experiencing more despair than their American counterparts (Inkeles, 1997; Inkeles & Bauer, 1954). Recent studies demonstrate a similar pattern. Students in the United States tend to show a bias in favor of recalling positive life events (Seidlitz & Diener, 1993), whereas Russian students do not show this bias (Balatsky & Diener, 1993). A linguistic study examining descriptions of negative emotions by Russian and English speakers showed evidence of a Russian cultural script emphasizing "giving in" to one's negative emotions and fully "suffering them through" (Pavlenko, 2002). Moreover, dwelling on negative experience has fewer detrimental psychological consequences for Russians than for European Americans (Grossmann & Kross, 2010), suggesting that the positive view of sadness in this cultural context may affect its interpersonal functions.

In a recent study, Russian and American young adults were asked to recall their experiences of sadness and describe the impact of this emotion on their lives (Chentsova-Dutton & Parrott, 2012). Compared with their European American counterparts, Russian participants were more likely to describe sadness as an emotion that is at once pleasant and unpleasant. Moreover, these participants perceived sadness as less dysfunctional and were more likely to express willingness to experience sadness in the future. When asked about these beliefs, they tended to refer to valuable experience gained while feeling sad as a basis for their evaluation of this emotion.

This emergent literature provides an example of the ways in which culture prunes and extends "in-the-head" meanings of negative emotions, thereby adjusting models of these emotions to serve cultural concerns. These findings highlight the ways in which cultural contexts can produce distinct notions of what negative emotions look and feel like, what cues should be attended to or remembered, what one should ideally feel or avoid feeling, and how one should go about doing so (e.g., Eid & Diener, 2001; Matsumoto, 1990; Menon & Shweder, 1994; Soto et al., 2005; Tsai et al., 2006). Although the ability to generate and experience actual emotions is curbed by situational and temperamental factors, cultural models of

negative emotions create widely shared (although not universally endorsed or followed) imperatives to seek or tolerate situations that trigger these emotions, to regulate one's emotional experience in an attempt to feel desired emotions, and to communicate these emotions to others. Culture has less impact on the actual emotional events "in the world." Yes, cultural contexts do differ in terms of the frequency and intensity of emotional responses.

HOW DOES CULTURE SHAPE NEGATIVE EMOTIONS "IN THE WORLD"?

Just as representations of negative emotions in the head differ across cultural contexts, so too does the patterning of negative emotion elicitors in the world. Although people across cultural contexts show substantial agreement in their responses to negative life events (McAndrew, Akande, Turner, & Sharma, 1998), the likelihood of daily hassles and life events that make up typical emotional landscapes differs across cultural contexts. One's chances of encountering an insult or a fight, seeing a reminder of tragedy, injustice, or cruelty, getting stuck in an interminable traffic jam, experiencing poor customer service, or witnessing a traffic accident, illness, and death vary widely. Clearly, occurrence of emotional events depends on many factors, such as random chance, historical context, and differences in health-care and political systems, to name but a few. Yet these differences are also cultural in that cultural norms, values, and practices contribute to them over time (e.g., Cohen & Nisbett, 1994). These patterns of life events become part of culture. It is impossible to cleanly separate, for example, the specific experience of stressful entrance examinations in Japan from the general influence of the Japanese cultural context or the specific experience of serving in the Israeli military from the general influence of the Israeli cultural context.

Indeed, cross-country statistics suggest that the likelihood that a person will experience, witness, or hear about major life events that are stressful, scary, sad, or anger inducing shows striking variability depending on where one lives. Consider exposure to crimes. Statistics such as murder rates and personal experience with crime differ widely across countries (European Institute for Crime Prevention and Control, 2011). For example, people living in Spain have an approximately 10% chance of becoming victims of crime, as compared with approximately 20% for those living in Ireland (Organization for Economic Co-operation and Development, 2009). What about other stressful events? In 2005, death rates ranged from fewer than four deaths per thousand in Middle Eastern countries such as Kuwait to more than twenty in African countries such as Botswana (World Bank,

2012). More than a mere demographic difference, this finding implies that everyday life in these cultural contexts varies substantially in terms of proximity to death. The likelihood of other major life stressors, such as divorces or car accident injuries, also differs (Divorceform, 2012). For example, the number of traffic accident injuries and fatalities is substantially lower in Sweden and Switzerland than in Turkey or Macedonia (United Nations Economic Commission for Europe [UNECE] Transport Division Database, 2012).

Finally, the texture of minor stressors that affect people's daily lives may also depend on locale. For instance, work–life time balance is higher in countries such as Denmark and the Netherlands relative to the United States, presumably contributing to country-level differences in exposure to work-related stressors (Fisher & Layte, 2004). A study comparing Jews and Arabs in Israel revealed that Jewish participants reported greater likelihood of encountering family-related hassles than Arab participants (Ben-Ari & Lavee, 2004). Although the latter findings may be driven by attentional and memory biases, they may also be at least partly grounded in the actual occurrence of the stressors.

In sum, certain cultural contexts are objectively more sad, scary, dangerous, or stressful than others. Cultural models of negative emotions incorporate such realities over time. Although not purely cultural in nature, differences in daily realities contribute to cultural models of negative emotions and are in turn shaped by them. Jointly, cultural models that are in the head and in the world, as well as typical negative events that characterize a particular context, shape cultural environments in which negative emotions vary in terms of how common and visible they are. These variations in turn have important consequences for the functional value of these emotions.

HOW DOES CULTURAL CONTEXT HELP US UNDERSTAND THE SIGNALING VALUE OF NEGATIVE EMOTIONS?

Earlier in this chapter we argued that, at their core, negative emotions are signals that allow us to detect and respond to potentially aversive and dangerous changes in our physical and cultural environments. Over time, as cultural contexts foster the experience and expression of valued emotions and contribute to differences in the likelihood that emotional triggers will occur, these emotions become more common and more normative. Paradoxically, cultural valuation of negative emotions can compromise their ability to serve as clear signals. In order to be effective in shaking us out of our routines and stimulating and coordinating action, negative emotions

need to be triggered and enacted with some degree of discernment. The base rates of events, be they interpersonal losses or cases of flu, affect the likelihood that these events will be accurately detected. Although people are not very skilled at taking base rates into account when making decisions, they are able to do so to some extent, combining this information with factors such as heuristics and source credibility (see Birnbaum, 2001; Birnbaum & Mellers, 1983; Kahneman & Tversky, 1973; Novemsky & Kronzon, 1999; Perham & Oaksford, 2005; Wallsten, 1972). Negative emotions can signal potential threats accurately only if the base rates of real or perceived threats are neither too low nor too high. When cultural models of negative emotions alter these base rates, they shape the information communicated by these emotions.

Take, for example, a recent population survey that asked random samples of people in 28 countries whether they had felt negative emotions the previous day. This survey revealed that in some contexts, such as in Scandinavian countries, very few people admit to feeling negative emotions (Organization for Economic Co-operation and Development, 2009). Less than one-tenth of Finnish respondents reported feeling angry (4.4%) and/ or sad (9.9%) the previous day. Negative emotions are far more common in other cultural contexts. About a third of Turkish respondents reported feeling negatively, with 39.2% experiencing anger and 31.8% experiencing sadness. Consistent with prior anthropological and psychological research, negative emotions were very common (and hence less distinct from normal emotional functioning) in Mediterranean Catholic (e.g., Portugal) and Slavic Eastern European (e.g., Slovakia) countries. What is the likely impact of low or high base rates of negative emotions on their ability to signal threats?

When certain types of threats, whether real or perceived, are very rare in a given context, the ability of negative emotions to communicate accurate information about these threats can be affected. Because of their rarity and memorability, these emotions may successfully propagate through social networks. Yet detection of rare events is difficult, with the inevitable false alarms of emotional responses in the absence of a credible threat. Consider, for example, a story of successful propagation of an urban legend about unknown sadists placing razor blades in apples on Halloween (Best & Horiuchi, 1985). Typical middle-class Americans experience relatively few events that threaten their safety and trigger fear during the course of their typical day. The base rate of sadists harming children in the United States is negligible. There is no reason for people to fear any harm beyond upset stomachs when sending their children out for trick-or-treating. In the handful of known cases in which children did suffer harm on Halloween, the culprits were their own family members, not sadistic neighbors. Yet

fears of razor blades in apples propagated widely and rapidly, affecting shared beliefs about safety. Now, it is a rare American parent who dares to send a young child out alone on Halloween or encourages him or her to accept unwrapped food from strangers.

This is not an isolated example. Other types of unfounded fears and anxieties also propagate in the relatively safe and law-abiding European American cultural context, a phenomenon dubbed the "culture of fear" (Altheide, 2002; Glassner, 2000). One notable characteristic of these fears is that they are experienced vicariously, in response to the media rather than to actual events (Grupp, 2003, as cited in Furedi, 2007). This suggests that when base rates of threats are low, the ties between actual threats and fear are loosened. The United States is not alone in this respect. Chileans also report widespread fears of crime despite the country's relatively efficient police force and low crime rates (Dammert & Malone, 2003, 2006). The authors of these studies argue that these fears have more to tell about the Chileans' political, social, and economic insecurities than about the actual dangers on the streets of Santiago.

Similarly, negative emotions may be more likely to be interpreted as credible and acceptable signals of distress in cultural contexts in which they are generally discouraged. Take the case of working-class women in Northeast Brazil, where expressions of negative emotions (especially by women) are moderated. Within this context, folk ailments such as *nervios* have arisen as socially acceptable avenues for women to express negative emotions. When interpreted as a symptom of these ailments, expression of negative emotions can serve as an effective (and intentional) means of social influence—altering others' behavior and eliciting social support. These studies illustrate that in relatively safe or calm cultural contexts with low base rates of threats and negative outbursts, negative emotions propagate widely but often fail as accurate signals of threats. They may, therefore, be of limited use in accurately signaling uncommon threats.

Conversely, cultural contexts that are oversaturated with negative emotional events or that successfully encourage experience and expression of negative emotions may face the problem of the signal being overwhelmed by noise. If a relatively large number of Turks feel angry on a typical day, and if sad and solemn expressions are normative in a Polish workplace (Bogdanowska-Jakubowska, 2011), what are the chances that these emotions succeed in communicating valuable information about interpersonal relationships? People who are exposed to negative stimuli repeatedly habituate even to the most unpleasant emotions in themselves and others. Thus stressful and objectively dangerous cultural contexts may inhibit the signaling effectiveness of negative emotions. For example, instead of fearful behaviors, dangerous inner-city neighborhoods actually foster risky

behaviors in adolescents (Kruger, Reischl, & Zimmerman, 2008). Although sensitivity to fear cues would appear to be highly functional in these contexts, these cues may be triggered too often to be effective.

Similarly, the clinical literature provides ample evidence of habituation to negative emotions, including severe fear and panic (Foa & Kozak, 1986). The same may happen when we signal negative emotions to others. As we know from the story of the boy who cried wolf, the costs of saturating communication with negative emotions can be grave and counterproductive. Yet, it may not always signal actual losses and threats. For example, when a Brazilian working-class woman's negative expressivity occurs often and to events that others deem trivial, it loses its effective signaling ability to motivate others' behavior (Rebhun, 1993, 1994). Repeated threats of suicide may eventually result in the failure of clinicians to treat these warnings seriously (Gregory, 1998). Frequent national terror level alerts place us at risk of complacency and diminished response to the actual terrorist threats (McDermott & Zimbardo, 2007). Optimal threat warning strategies take into account our prior beliefs and feelings about potential threats (Amegashie & Kutsoati, 2004).

When negative emotions are emphasized in a cultural context, they often take on communicative functions that may have little to do with signaling threats, further decreasing the signal-to-noise ratio. Bogdanowska-Jakubowska (2011) argues that Poles are likely to interpret negative facial expressions as evidence of competence and professionalism or, in some cases, even indirect boasting. These expressions' cultural functions may interfere with the signaling of losses. A similar argument has been made about communication of positive emotions in positively versus negatively oriented cultural contexts. Oettingen and Seligman (1990) observed that nearly 70% of men in West Berlin bars were smiling, whereas only 20% of East Berlin men did the same. The differences between Eastern and Western European contexts have persisted after the fall of communism, as evidenced by rates of smiling in the photographs of Internet users (Szarota, 2010; Wojciszke, 2004). Research in linguistics and communication suggests that smiles may be more effective in signaling good intentions and interpersonal warmth in "nonsmiling" cultural contexts because in such contexts social smiling does not dilute genuine smiling (Bogdanowska-Jakubowska, 2011; Turunen, 2000).

In the clinical domain, the ability of negative emotions to signal severe distress may be compromised in some cultural contexts, replaced by culturally specific meanings. Obeyesekere (1985) observed that in Sri Lanka, a description of clinical depression is very close to the description of a good Buddhist who is aware that losses and sorrows are part of life. Contemplating negative emotions is a necessary part of this spiritual practice; Obeyesekere (1985) argues that expression of severe distress is, "transformed into

publicly accepted sets of meanings and symbols" (pp. 134–152). Similarly, a quantitative study conducted in another Buddhist cultural context, Thailand, found that Thai adults are less concerned about children's emotional problems than American adults are (Weisz et al., 1988), suggesting that the threshold for the ability of negative emotions to signal problems differed in Thailand and the United States.

Further complicating this picture is the fact that the daily landscape of culturally shaped emotional situations does not always match cultural ideas about valued emotions. Because historical events affect daily emotional situations and because cultural values are not always coherent across domains (Chentsova-Dutton & Heath, 2009; Kashima, 2000), culturally shaped environments and culturally shaped values do not always foster the same emotions. For example, the evolving European American cultural environment generates higher and higher levels of stress for a typical American (American Psychological Association, 2010). As this same environment increasingly fosters preference for positive emotions, tension emerges between the actual experiences of daily life—daily commutes, frequent moves, long work hours—and what one is expected to experience.

When scanning a cultural context, therefore, it is necessary to know the ways in which this context shapes models of desirable and undesirable emotions, as well as the ways in which it affects actual and perceived frequency and intensity of experiencing different negative emotions. Furthermore, it is important to track beliefs about emotions and their distribution over time. When cultural preferences for an emotion become widely shared and enacted, they may render this emotion less useful as a signal of threat and require a recalibration of communicating this emotion to issue an alarm. Research in culture and emotions needs to incorporate a historical perspective to fully grasp the dynamic relationship between cultural models of negative emotions and the signaling value of these emotions.

SUMMARY AND CONCLUSION

We have argued that negative emotions have evolved to help us orient to and successfully utilize the protective benefits of our cultural worlds. The key function of negative emotions is to trigger alarms, letting the person experiencing them and people in the immediate vicinity know that their environment is not safe, predictable, or protective. Yet people from different cultural contexts may hear different messages in these alarms. An additional cultural function of these emotions is to help people notice and respond to culturally salient concerns. As such, emotions are experience-expectant and sensitive to cultural inputs.

The full range of possibilities—triggers of emotions and their experience, expression, regulation, and functions—is shaped and constrained by the single integrated system of culture, mind, and brain. We do not fear all of the potentially dangerous situations, feel anger in response to all of the potential interpersonal offenses, or feel disgust in response to a full range of what is potentially unclean and poisonous. Situations that match environments in which humans evolved and that are salient in the current cultural environment are more likely to elicit negative emotions than are other situations that may be equally dangerous or offensive. Cultural models of negative emotions not only constrain but also extend meanings and functions of emotions, shaping the extent to which emotions are valued, how often they are felt, how they are displayed to others and perceived by them, and the functions they take on. These constraints and extensions have consequences for the signaling functions of these emotions. Cultural contexts that deemphasize negative emotions may paradoxically make it more likely that they will propagate across social networks, whereas cultural contexts that foster these emotions may make it harder for these emotions to do so, as the signal becomes overwhelmed by noise.

We opened with a specific illustration of a particular cultural model promoting the acceptance of negative emotions, infusing them with significance. The character of "Stalker's wife" continues in this soliloquy, revealing that the practice of acceptance is itself a reflection of an even more deeply held belief. Negative emotions are not merely to be accepted when they occur. They must be understood as an integral part of life—upon which the positive crucially depends:

> If there were no sorrow in our lives, it wouldn't be better. It would be worse. Because then there'd be no happiness, either. And there'd be no hope.

REFERENCES

Abbott, P., & Sapsford, R. (2006). Life satisfaction in post-Soviet Russia and Ukraine. *Journal of Happiness Studies, 7*(2), 251–287.

Altheide, D. L. (2002). *Creating fear: News and the construction of crisis.* Hawthorne, NY: Aldine.

Amegashie, A. J., & Kutsoati, E. (2004). *Terror alerts and beliefs about terrorism.* Retrieved from *www.uoguelph.ca/~jamegash/terrorism_beliefs.pdf.*

American Psychological Association. (2010). *Stress in America 2009.* Retrieved from *www.apa.org/news/press/releases/stress/national-report.pdf.*

Averina, M., Nilssen, O., Brenn, T., Brox, J., Arkhipovsky, V. L., & Kalinin, A. G. (2005). Social and lifestyle determinants of depression, anxiety, sleeping

disorders and self-evaluated quality of life in Russia. *Social Psychiatry and Psychiatric Epidemiology, 40*(7), 511–518.

Balatsky, G., & Diener, E. (1993). Subjective well-being among Russian students. *Social Indicators Research, 28*(3), 225–243.

Bangerter, A., & Heath, C. (2004). The Mozart effect: Tracking the evolution of a scientific legend. *British Journal of Social Psychology, 43*(4), 605–623.

Ben-Ari, A., & Lavee, Y. (2004). Cultural orientation, ethnic affiliation, and negative daily occurrences: A multidimensional cross-cultural analysis. *American Journal of Orthopsychiatry, 74*(2), 102–111.

Berger, J. (2011). Arousal increases social transmission of information. *Psychological Science, 22*(7), 891–893.

Berger, J., & Milkman, K. L. (2012). What makes online content viral? *Journal of Marketing Research, 49*(2), 192–205.

Best, J., & Horiuchi, G. T. (1985). The razor blade in the apple: The social construction of urban legends. *Social Problems, 32*(5), 488–499.

Birnbaum, M. H. (2001). *Introduction to behavioral research on the Internet.* Upper Saddle River, NJ: Prentice Hall.

Birnbaum, M. H., & Mellers, B. A. (1983). Bayesian inference: Combining base rates with opinions of sources who vary in credibility. *Journal of Personality and Social Psychology, 45*(4), 792–804.

Bogdanowska-Jakubowska, E. (2011). Getting rid of the modesty stigma. In J. Arabski & A. Wojtaszek (Eds.), *Aspects of culture in second-language acquisition and foreign-language learning* (pp. 167–181). Berlin and Heidelberg: Springer.

Bonanno, G. A., Goorin, L., & Coifman, K. G. (2008). Sadness and grief. In M. Lewis, J. M. Haviland-Jones, & L. F. Barrett (Eds.), *Handbook of emotions* (3rd ed., pp. 797–810). New York: Guilford Press.

Borke, H., & Su, S. (1972). Perception of emotional responses to social interactions by Chinese and American children. *Journal of Cross-Cultural Psychology, 3*(3), 309–314.

Boyd, R., & Richerson, P. J. (1992). Punishment allows the evolution of cooperation (or anything else) in sizable groups. *Ethology and Sociobiology, 13*(3), 171–195.

Brar, A., & Moneta, G. B. (2009). Negative emotions and alcohol dependence symptoms in British Indian and White college students. *Addictive Behaviors, 34*(3), 292–296.

Brianchaninov, I. (2006). *On the prayer of Jesus* (Fr. Lazarus, Trans.). Boston: New Seed Books. (Original work published 1965)

Chang, E. C. (1996). Cultural differences in optimism, pessimism, and coping: Predictors of subsequent adjustment in Asian American and Caucasian American college students. *Journal of Counseling Psychology, 43*(1), 113–123.

Chansky, T. (2004). *Freeing your child from anxiety: Powerful, practical solutions to overcome your child's fears, worries, and phobias.* New York: Random House Digital.

Chao, R. K. (1995). Chinese and European American cultural models of the self reflected in mothers' childrearing beliefs. *Ethos, 23*(3), 328–354.

Chentsova-Dutton, Y. E., Chu, J. P., Tsai, J. L., Rottenberg, J., Gross, J. J., & Gotlib, I. H. (2007). Depression and emotional reactivity: Variation among Asian Americans of East Asian descent and European Americans. *Journal of Abnormal Psychology, 116*(4), 776–785.

Chentsova-Dutton, Y. E., & Heath, C. (2009). Cultural evolution: Why are some cultural variants more successful than others? In M. Schaller, S. J. Heine, T. Yamagishi, & T. Kameda (Eds.), *Evolution, culture, and the human mind* (pp. 49–70). Mahwah, NJ: Erlbaum.

Chentsova-Dutton, Y. E., & Parrott, G. (2012, January). *Culture and perceived functions of sadness.* Poster presented at the annual cultural psychology pre-conference meeting of the Society for Personality and Social Psychology, San Diego, CA.

Childre, D. L., Rozman, D., & McKay, M. (2003). *Transforming anger: The Heart-Math solution for letting go of rage, frustration, and irritation.* Oakland, CA: New Harbinger.

Church, A. T., Katigbak, M. S., Reyes, J. A. S., & Jensen, S. M. (1999). The structure of affect in a non-Western culture: Evidence for cross-cultural comparability. *Journal of Personality, 67*(3), 505–534.

Cohen, D., & Nisbett, R. E. (1994). Self-protection and the culture of honor: Explaining Southern violence. *Personality and Social Psychology Bulletin, 20*(5), 551–567.

Cohen, D., Nisbett, R. E., Bowdle, B. F., & Schwarz, N. (1996). Insult, aggression, and the Southern culture of honor: An "experimental ethnography." *Journal of Personality and Social Psychology, 70*(5), 945–960.

Cole, P. M., Bruschi, C. J., & Tamang, B. L. (2002). Cultural differences in children's emotional reactions to difficult situations. *Child Development, 73*(3), 983–996.

Cosmides, L., & Tooby, J. (2000). Evolutionary psychology and the emotions. In M. Lewis & J. M. Haviland-Jones (Eds.), *Handbook of emotions* (2nd ed., pp. 91–115). New York: Guilford Press.

Dammert, L., & Malone, M. F. T. (2003). Fear of crime or fear of life?: Public insecurities in Chile. *Bulletin of Latin American Research, 22*(1), 79–101.

Dammert, L., & Malone, M. F. T. (2006). Does it take a village?: Policing strategies and fear of crime in Latin America. *Latin American Politics and Society, 48*(4), 27–51.

D'Andrade, R. G. (1984). Cultural meaning systems. In R. A. Shweder & R. A. LeVine (Eds.), *Culture theory: Essays on mind, self, and emotion* (pp. 88–119). New York: Cambridge University Press.

Davies, J. (2011). Positive and negative models of suffering: An anthropology of our shifting cultural consciousness of emotional discontent. *Anthropology of Consciousness, 22*(2), 188–208.

de Leersnyder, J., Mesquita, B., & Kim, H. S. (2011). Where do my emotions belong?: A study of immigrants' emotional acculturation. *Personality and Social Psychology Bulletin, 37*(4), 451–463.

Demidova, A. (Producer), & Tarkovsky, A. A. (Director). (1979). *Stalker* [Motion picture]. USSR: Mosfilm.

Dickerson, S. S., Gruenewald, T. L., & Kemeny, M. E. (2004). When the social self

is threatened: Shame, physiology, and health. *Journal of Personality, 72*(6), 1191–1216.

Dinnel, D. L., Kleinknecht, R. A., & Tanaka-Matsumi, J. (2002). A cross-cultural comparison of social phobia symptoms. *Journal of Psychopathology and Behavioral Assessment, 24*(2), 75–84.

Divorceform. (2012). *Divorce rate by country.* Retrieved from *www.nationmaster. com/graph/peo_div_rat-people-divorce-rate.*

Eid, M., & Diener, E. (2001). Norms for experiencing emotions in different cultures: Inter- and intranational differences. *Journal of Personality and Social Psychology, 81*(5), 869–885.

Eisenberg, D. T. A., & Hayes, M. G. (2011). Testing the null hypothesis: Comments on "Culture-gene coevolution of individualism-collectivism and the serotonin transporter gene." *Proceedings of the Royal Society B: Biological Sciences, 278*(1704), 329–332.

Ekman, P., Friesen, W. V., & Ellsworth, P. (1972). *Emotion in the human face: Guidelines for research and an integration of findings* (Vol. 12). Oxford, UK: Pergamon Press.

Elfenbein, H. A., & Ambady, N. (2002). On the universality and cultural specificity of emotion recognition: A meta-analysis. *Psychological Bulletin, 128*(2), 203–235.

Elfenbein, H. A., Mandal, M. K., Ambady, N., Harizuka, S., & Kumar, S. (2002). Cross-cultural patterns in emotion recognition: Highlighting design and analytical techniques. *Emotion, 2*(1), 75–84.

Elliot, A. J., Chirkov, V. I., Kim, Y., & Sheldon, K. M. (2001). A cross-cultural analysis of avoidance (relative to approach) personal goals. *Psychological Science, 12*(6), 505–510.

Ellis, B. J., & Boyce, W. T. (2008). Biological sensitivity to context. *Current Directions in Psychological Science, 17*(3), 183–187.

European Institute for Crime Prevention and Control. (2011). *Murders (per capita) by country.* Retrieved from *www.nationmaster.com/graph/cri_mur_percap-crime-murders-per-capita.*

Feldman Barrett, L. (2006). Are emotions natural kinds? *Perspectives on Psychological Science, 1*(1), 28–58.

Feldman Barrett, L., Mesquita, B., & Gendron, M. (2011). Context in emotion perception. *Current Directions in Psychological Science, 20*(5), 286–290.

Fessler, D. M. T. (2007). From appeasement to conformity: Evolutionary and cultural perspectives on shame, competition, and cooperation. In J. L. Tracy, R. W. Robins, & J. P. Tangney (Eds.), *The self-conscious emotions: Theory and research* (pp. 174–193). New York: Guilford Press.

Fischer, A. H. (1999). The role of honour-related vs. individualistic values in conceptualizing pride, shame, and anger: Spanish and Dutch cultural prototypes. *Cognition and Emotion, 13*(2), 149–179.

Fisher, K., & Layte, R. (2004). Measuring work–life balance using time diary data. *Electronic International Journal of Time Use Research, 1*(1), 1–13.

Foa, E. B., & Kozak, M. J. (1986). Emotional processing of fear: Exposure to corrective information. *Psychological Bulletin, 99*(1), 20–35.

Folkman, S., & Moskowitz, J. T. (2000). Positive affect and the other side of coping. *American Psychologist, 55*(6), 647–654.

Fowler, J. H., & Christakis, N. A. (2008). Dynamic spread of happiness in a large social network: Longitudinal analysis over 20 years in the Framingham Heart Study. *British Medical Journal, 337.*

Fredrickson, B. L. (1998). What good are positive emotions? *Review of General Psychology, 2*(3), 300–319.

Fredrickson, B. L. (2000). Cultivating positive emotions to optimize health and well-being. *Prevention and Treatment, 3.*

Fredrickson, B. L., & Levenson, R. W. (1998). Positive emotions speed recovery from the cardiovascular sequelae of negative emotions. *Cognition and Emotion, 12*(2), 191–220.

Frijda, N. H. (1989). The function of emotional expression. In J. P. Forgas & J. M. Innes (Eds.), *Recent advances in social psychology: An international perspective* (pp. 205–217). Amsterdam: North-Holland. Retrieved from *http://dare. uva.nl/record/117994.*

Frijters, P., Geishecker, I., Haisken-DeNew, J. P., & Shields, M. A. (2006). Can the large swings in Russian life satisfaction be explained by ups and downs in real incomes? *Scandinavian Journal of Economics, 108*(3), 433–458.

Fung, H. (1999). Becoming a moral child: The socialization of shame among young Chinese children. *Ethos, 27*(2), 180–209.

Furedi, F. (2007, April). The only thing we have to fear is the "culture of fear" itself. *Spiked Online, 4.* Retrieved from *www.spiked-online.com/index.php?/ site/article/3053.*

Gaines, A. D., & Farmer, P. E. (1986). Visible saints: Social cynosures and dysphoria in the Mediterranean tradition. *Culture, Medicine and Psychiatry, 10*(4), 295–330.

Gavrilova, T.P. (2009). Popytka sopostavleniya bogoslovkih i nauchno-psihologicheskih ponyatij [An attempt to relate concepts from theology and psychological science]. *Trudy po psihologicheskomy konsultirovaniyu and psihoterapii, 2,* 195–213.

Gintis, H. (2003). The hitchhiker's guide to altruism: Gene–culture coevolution, and the internalization of norms. *Journal of Theoretical Biology, 220*(4), 407–418.

Glassner, B. (2000). *The culture of fear: Why Americans are afraid of the wrong things.* New York: Basic Books.

Good, B. J., Good, M. D., & Moradi, R. (1985). The interpretation of Iranian depressive illness and dysphoric affect. In A. Kleinman & B. Good (Eds.), *Culture and depression: Studies in the anthropology and cross-cultural psychiatry of affect and disorder* (pp. 134–152). Berkeley: University of California Press.

Gottman, J. M., & Levenson, R. W. (1992). Marital processes predictive of later dissolution: Behavior, physiology, and health. *Journal of Personality and Social Psychology, 63*(2), 221–233.

Graham, S. M., Huang, J. Y., Clark, M. S., & Helgeson, V. S. (2008). The positives of negative emotions: Willingness to express negative emotions promotes relationships. *Personality and Social Psychology Bulletin, 34*(3), 394–406.

Gregory, R. J. (1998). Managing suicide risk in borderline personality disorder: Distinguishing real risk from attention seeking. *Psychiatric Times, 29*(5).

Grossmann, I., & Kross, E. (2010). The impact of culture on adaptive versus maladaptive self-reflection. *Psychological Science, 21*(8), 1150–1157.

Gruber, J., Mauss, I. B., & Tamir, M. (2011). A dark side of happiness?: How, when, and why happiness is not always good. *Perspectives on Psychological Science, 6*(3), 222–233.

Hagen, E. H. (2003). The bargaining model of depression. In P. Hammerstein (Ed.), *The genetic and cultural evolution of cooperation*. Retrieved from *http://cogprints.org/4135/1/hagen_2003.pdf*.

Hagen, E. H., & Barrett, H. C. (2007). Perinatal sadness among Shuar women: Support for an evolutionary theory of psychic pain. *Medical Anthropology Quarterly, 21*(1), 22–40.

Haight, W. L. (1999). The pragmatics of caregiver–child pretending at home: Understanding culturally specific socialization practices. *Children's engagement in the world: Sociocultural perspectives* (pp. 128–147). Cambridge, UK: Cambridge University Press.

Hanh, T. N. (2002). *Anger: Wisdom for cooling the flames*. New York: Riverhead Books.

Hareli, S., Harush, R., Suleiman, R., Cossette, M., Bergeron, S., Lavoie, V., et al. (2009). When scowling may be a good thing: The influence of anger expressions on credibility. *European Journal of Social Psychology, 39*(4), 631–638.

Hareli, S., & Hess, U. (2010). What emotional reactions can tell us about the nature of others: An appraisal perspective on person perception. *Cognition and Emotion, 24*(1), 128–140.

Haviland, J. M., & Lelwica, M. (1987). The induced affect response: 10-week-old infants' responses to three emotion expressions. *Developmental Psychology, 23*(1), 97–104.

Hayashi, A., Karasawa, M., & Tobin, J. (2009). The Japanese preschool's pedagogy of feeling: Cultural strategies for supporting young children's emotional development. *Ethos, 37*(1), 32–49.

Hendriks, M. C. P., Nelson, J. K., Cornelius, R. R., & Vingerhoets, A. J. J. M. (2008). Why crying improves our well-being: An attachment-theory perspective on the functions of adult crying. In A. J. J. M. Vingerhoets, I. Nyklíček, & J. Denollet (Eds.), *Emotion regulation* (pp. 87–96). New York: Springer. Retrieved from *www.springerlink.com/content/wn5p75g442620594/abstract*.

Hendriks, M. C. P., & Vingerhoets, A. J. J. M. (2006). Social messages of crying faces: Their influence on anticipated person perception, emotions and behavioural responses. *Cognition and Emotion, 20*(6), 878–886.

Hershfield, H. E., Scheibe, S., Sims, T. L., & Carstensen, L. L. (2012). When feeling bad can be good: Mixed emotions benefit physical health across adulthood. *Social Psychological and Personality Science, 4*(1), 54–61.

Hess, U., Blairy, S., & Kleck, R. E. (2000). The influence of facial emotion displays, gender, and ethnicity on judgments of dominance and affiliation. *Journal of Nonverbal Behavior, 24*(4), 265–283.

Higgins, E. T. (2005). Value from regulatory fit. *Current Directions in Psychological Science, 14*(4), 209–213.

Higgins, E. T., Pierro, A., & Kruglanski, A. W. (2008). Re-thinking culture and personality: How self-regulatory universals create cross-cultural differences. In R. M. Sorrentino & E. T. Higgins (Eds.), *Handbook of motivation and cognition* (pp. 161–190). New York: Guilford Press.

Hinton, D., Um, K., & Ba, P. (2001a). KyolGoeu ("Wind Overload"): Part I. A cultural syndrome of orthostatic panic among Khmer refugees. *Transcultural Psychiatry, 38*(4), 403–432.

Hinton, D., Um, K., & Ba, P. (2001b). KyolGoeu ("Wind Overload"): Part II. Prevalence, characteristics, and mechanisms of KyolGoeu and near-KyolGoeu episodes of Khmer patients attending a psychiatric clinic. *Transcultural Psychiatry, 38*(4), 433–460.

Hoffman, M. L. (1984). Interaction of affect and cognition in empathy. In C. E. Izard, J. Kagan, & R. B. Zajonc (Eds.), *Emotion, cognition, and behavior* (pp. 103–131). Cambridge, UK: Cambridge University Press.

Holden, C., & Mace, R. (2009). Phylogenetic analysis of the evolution of lactose digestion in adults. *Human Biology, 81*(5–6), 597–619.

Horwitz, A. V., & Wakefield, J. C. (2007). *The loss of sadness: How psychiatry transformed normal sorrow into depressive disorder.* New York: Oxford University Press.

Huebner, R. R., & Izard, C. E. (1988). Mothers' responses to infants' facial expressions of sadness, anger, and physical distress. *Motivation and Emotion, 12*(2), 185–196.

Inkeles, A. (1997). *National character: A psycho-social perspective.* New Brunswick, NJ: Transaction.

Inkeles, A., & Bauer, R. (1954). *Patterns of life experiences and attitudes under the Soviet system.* Cambridge, MA: Russian Research Center.

Izard, C. E. (1992). Basic emotions, relations among emotions, and emotion–cognition relations. *Psychological Review, 99*(3), 561–565.

Jackson, S. W. (1985). Acedia the sin and its relationship to sorrow and melancholia. In A. Kleinman & B. Good (Eds.), *Culture and depression: Studies in the anthropology and cross-cultural psychiatry of affect and disorder* (pp. 43–62). Berkeley: University of California Press.

James, W. (2007). *The principles of psychology.* New York: Cosimo. (Original work published 1890)

Johnson, A. (2003). *Families of the forest: The Matsigenka Indians of the Peruvian Amazon.* Berkeley and Los Angeles: University of California Press.

Johnson, A., & Earle, T. (2000). *The evolution of human societies: From foraging group to agrarian state* (2nd ed.). Stanford, CA: Stanford University Press.

Jordan, A. H., Monin, B., Dweck, C. S., Lovett, B. J., John, O. P., & Gross, J. J. (2011). Misery has more company than people think: Underestimating the prevalence of others' negative emotions. *Personality and Social Psychology Bulletin, 37*(1), 120–135.

Joseph, R. (1999). Environmental influences on neural plasticity, the limbic system, emotional development and attachment: A review. *Child Psychiatry and Human Development, 29*(3), 189–208.

Kahneman, D., & Tversky, A. (1973). On the psychology of prediction. *Psychological Review, 80*(4), 237–251.

Kashima, Y. (2000). Conceptions of culture and person for psychology. *Journal of Cross-Cultural Psychology, 31,* 14–32.

Keltner, D., & Haidt, J. (2001). Social functions of emotions. In T. J. Mayne & G. A. Bonanno (Eds.), *Emotions: Current issues and future directions* (pp. 192–213). New York: Guilford Press.

Keltner, D., Haidt, J., & Shiota, M. N. (2006). Social functionalism and the evolution of emotions. In M. Schaller, J. A. Simpson, & D. T. Kenrick (Eds.), *Evolution and social psychology* (pp. 115–142). Madison, CT: Psychosocial Press.

Kim, H. S., Sherman, D. K., Sasaki, J. Y., Xu, J., Chu, T. Q., Ryu, C., et al. (2010). Culture, distress, and oxytocin receptor polymorphism (OXTR) interact to influence emotional support seeking. *Proceedings of the National Academy of Sciences, 107*(36), 15717–15721.

Kitayama, S., Markus, H. R., & Kurokawa, M. (2000). Culture, emotion, and well-being: Good feelings in Japan and the United States. *Cognition and Emotion, 14*(1), 93–124.

Knutson, B. (1996). Facial expressions of emotion influence interpersonal trait inferences. *Journal of Nonverbal Behavior, 20*(3), 165–182.

Kotchemidova, C. (2005). From good cheer to "drive-by smiling": A social history of cheerfulness. *Journal of Social History, 39*(1), 5–37.

Kruger, D. J., Reischl, T., & Zimmerman, M. A. (2008). Time perspective as a mechanism for functional developmental adaptation. *Journal of Social, Evolutionary, and Cultural Psychology, 2*(1), 1–22.

Kubzansky, L. D., & Kawachi, I. (2000). Going to the heart of the matter: Do negative emotions cause coronary heart disease? *Journal of Psychosomatic Research, 48*(4), 323–337.

Laland, K. N., Odling-Smee, J., & Myles, S. (2010). How culture shaped the human genome: Bringing genetics and the human sciences together. *Nature Reviews Genetics, 11*(2), 137–148.

LeDoux, J. E. (2000). Emotion circuits in the brain. *Annual Review of Neuroscience, 23*(1), 155–184.

Lee, A. Y., Aaker, J. L., & Gardner, W. L. (2000). The pleasures and pains of distinct self-construals: The role of interdependence in regulatory focus. *Journal of Personality and Social Psychology, 78*(6), 1122–1134.

Levenson, R. W. (2003). Blood, sweat, and fears. *Annals of the New York Academy of Sciences, 1000*(1), 348–366.

LeVine, R. A., Caron, J., & New, R. (1980). Anthropology and child development. *New Directions for Child and Adolescent Development, 1980*(8), 71–86.

Lewis-Fernández, R., Guarnaccia, P. J., Martínez, I. E., Salmán, E., Schmidt, A., & Liebowitz, M. (2002). Comparative phenomenology of *ataques de nervios,* panic attacks, and panic disorder. *Culture, Medicine and Psychiatry, 26*(2), 199–223.

Lock, M. (1995). Contesting the natural in Japan: Moral dilemmas and technologies of dying. *Culture, Medicine and Psychiatry, 19*(1), 1–38.

Lucado, M. (2009). *Fearless: Imagine your life without fear.* Nashville, TN: Nelson.

Lutz, C. A. (1988). *Unnatural emotions: Everyday sentiments on a Micronesian atoll and their challenge to Western theory.* Chicago: University of Chicago Press.

Malatesta, C. Z., Grigoryev, P., Lamb, C., Albin, M., & Culver, C. (1986). Emotion socialization and expressive development in preterm and full-term infants. *Child Development*, *57*(2), 316–330.

Marsh, A. A., Elfenbein, H. A., & Ambady, N. (2003). Nonverbal "accents": Cultural differences in facial expressions of emotion. *Psychological Science*, *14*(4), 373–376.

Masson, J. M., & McCarthy, S. (1996). *When elephants weep: The emotional lives of animals*. New York: Random House Digital.

Masuda, T., Ellsworth, P. C., Mesquita, B., Leu, J., Tanida, S., & Van de Veerdonk, E. (2008). Placing the face in context: Cultural differences in the perception of facial emotion. *Journal of Personality and Social Psychology*, *94*(3), 365–381.

Matsumoto, D. (1990). Cultural similarities and differences in display rules. *Motivation and Emotion*, *14*(3), 195–214.

Matsumoto, D., Yoo, S. H., & Chung, J. (2010). The expression of anger across cultures. In M. Potegal, G. Stemmler, & C. Spielberger (Eds.), *International handbook of anger* (pp. 125–137). New York: Springer. Retrieved from *www.springerlink.com/content/m223375631618762/abstract*.

Mauro, R., Sato, K., & Tucker, J. (1992). The role of appraisal in human emotions: A cross-cultural study. *Journal of Personality and Social Psychology*, *62*(2), 301–317.

McAndrew, F. T., Akande, A., Turner, S., & Sharma, Y. (1998). A cross-cultural ranking of stressful life events in Germany, India, South Africa, and the United States. *Journal of Cross-Cultural Psychology*, *29*(6), 717–727.

McDermott, R., & Zimbardo, P.G. (2007). The psychological consequences of terrorist alerts. In B. Bongar, L. M. Brown, L. E. Beutler, J. N. Breckenridge, & P. G. Zimbardo (Eds.), *Psychology of terrorism* (pp. 357–370). New York: Oxford University Press.

Menon, U., & Shweder, R. A. (1994). Kali's tongue: Cultural psychology and the power of shame in Orissa, India. In S. Kitayama & H. R. Markus (Eds.), *Emotion and culture: Empirical studies of mutual influence* (pp. 241–282). Washington, DC: American Psychological Association.

Mesquita, B., & Karasawa, M. (2002). Different emotional lives. *Cognition and Emotion*, *16*(1), 127–141.

Mesquita, B, & Walker, R. (2003). Cultural differences in emotions: A context for interpreting emotional experiences. *Behaviour Research and Therapy*, *41*(7), 777–793.

Miller, P., & Sperry, L. L. (1987). The socialization of anger and aggression. *Merrill–Palmer Quarterly*, *33*(1), 1–31.

Miyamoto, Y., Uchida, Y., & Ellsworth, P. C. (2010). Culture and mixed emotions: Co-occurrence of positive and negative emotions in Japan and the U.S. *Emotion*, *10*(3), 404–415.

Moskowitz, J. T., & Epel, E. S. (2006). Benefit finding and diurnal cortisol slope in maternal caregivers: A moderating role for positive emotion. *Journal of Positive Psychology*, *1*(2), 83–91.

Nesse, R. M., & Ellsworth, P. C. (2009). Evolution, emotions, and emotional disorders. *American Psychologist*, *64*(2), 129–139.

Nichols, S. (2002). On the genealogy of norms: A case for the role of emotion in cultural evolution. *Philosophy of Science, 69*(2), 234–255.

Nisbett, R. E., & Cohen, D. (1996). *Culture of honor: The psychology of violence in the South.* Boulder, CO: Westview Press.

Novemsky, N., & Kronzon, S. (1999). How are base-rates used, when they are used: A comparison of additive and Bayesian models of base-rate use. *Journal of Behavioral Decision Making, 12*(1), 55–67.

Obeidallah, D., Brennan, R.T., Brooks-Gunn, J., & Earls, F. (2004). Links between pubertal timing and neighborhood contexts: Implications for girls' violent behavior. *Journal of the American Academy of Child and Adolescent Psychiatry, 43*(12), 1460–1468.

Obeyesekere, G. (1985). Depression, Buddhism, and the work of culture in Sri Lanka. In A. Kleinman & B. Good (Eds.), *Culture and depression* (pp. 134–152). Berkeley & Los Angeles: University of California Press.

Oettingen, G., & Seligman, M. E. P. (1990). Pessimism and behavioural signs of depression in East versus West Berlin. *European Journal of Social Psychology, 20*(3), 207–220.

Organization for Economic Co-operation and Development. (2009). *Negative experience index by country.* Retrieved from *www.nationmaster.com/graph/lif_soc_sub_wel_neg_exp_ind-well-being-negative-experience-index.*

Panksepp, J. (2004). Emerging neuroscience of fear and anxiety: Therapeutic practice and clinical implications. In J. Panksepp (Ed.), *Textbook of biological psychiatry* (pp. 489–519). Hoboken, NJ: Wiley.

Park, C. L. (2010). Making sense of the meaning literature: An integrative review of meaning making and its effects on adjustment to stressful life events. *Psychological Bulletin, 136*(2), 257–301.

Pavlenko, A. (2002). Emotions and the body in Russian and English. *Pragmatics and Cognition, 10*(1), 207–241.

Perham, N., & Oaksford, M. (2005). Deontic reasoning with emotional content: Evolutionary psychology or decision theory? *Cognitive Science, 29*(5), 681–718.

Philippot, P., & Rimé, B. (1997). The perception of bodily sensations during emotion: A cross-cultural perspective. *Polish Psychological Bulletin, 28*(2), 175–188.

Pikhart, H., Bobak, M., Pajak, A., Malyutina, S., Kubinova, R., Topor, R., et al. (2004). Psychosocial factors at work and depression in three countries of Central and Eastern Europe. *Social Science and Medicine, 58*(8), 1475–1482.

Rancour-Laferriere, D. (1995). *The slave soul of Russia: Moral masochism and the cult of suffering.* New York: New York University Press.

Rancour-Laferriere, D. (2003). The moral masochism at the heart of Christianity: Evidence from Russian Orthodox iconography and icon veneration. *Journal for the Psychoanalysis of Culture and Society, 8*(1), 12–22.

Rebhun, L. A. (1993). Nerves and emotional play in Northeast Brazil. *Medical Anthropology Quarterly, 7*(2), 131–151.

Rebhun, L. A. (1994). Swallowing frogs: Anger and illness in northeast Brazil. *Medical Anthropology Quarterly, 8*(4), 360–382.

Richerson, P. J., & Boyd, R. (2005). *Not by genes alone: How culture transformed human biology.* Chicago: University of Chicago Press.

Ries, N. (1997). *Russian talk: Culture and conversation during perestroika.* Cornell, NY: Cornell University Press.

Rimé, B., Mesquita, B., Boca, S., & Philippot, P. (1991). Beyond the emotional event: Six studies on the social sharing of emotion. *Cognition and Emotion, 5*(5–6), 435–465.

Rodriguez-Mosquera, P. M., Manstead, A. S. R., & Fischer, A. H. (2002). Honor in the Mediterranean and northern Europe. *Journal of Cross-Cultural Psychology, 33*(1), 16–36.

Roseman, I. J., Dhawan, N., Rettek, S. I., Naidu, R. K., & Thapa, K. (1995). Cultural differences and cross-cultural similarities in appraisals and emotional responses. *Journal of Cross-Cultural Psychology, 26*(1), 23–48.

Rosenquist, J. N., Fowler, J. H., & Christakis, N. A. (2010). Social network determinants of depression. *Molecular Psychiatry, 16*(3), 273–281.

Russell, J. A., Lewicka, M., & Niit, T. (1989). A cross-cultural study of a circumplex model of affect. *Journal of Personality and Social Psychology, 57*(5), 848–856.

Ryder, A. G., Ban, L. M., & Chentsova-Dutton, Y. E. (2011). Towards a cultural-clinical psychology. *Social and Personality Psychology Compass, 5*(12), 960–975.

Ryder, A. G., Yang, J., Zhu, X., Yao, S., Yi, J., Heine, S. J., et al. (2008). The cultural shaping of depression: Somatic symptoms in China, psychological symptoms in North America? *Journal of Abnormal Psychology, 117*(2), 300–313.

Scherer, K. R., Matsumoto, D., Wallbott, H. G., & Kudoh, T. (1988). Emotional experience in cultural context: A comparison between Europe, Japan, and the United States. In K. R. Scherer (Ed.), *Facets of emotion: Recent research* (pp. 5–30). Hillsdale, NJ: Erlbaum.

Schieffelin, E. (1983). Anger and shame in the tropical forest: On affect as a cultural system in Papua New Guinea. *Ethos, 11*(3), 181–191.

Schimmack, U., Oishi, S., & Diener, E. (2002). Cultural influences on the relation between pleasant emotions and unpleasant emotions: Asian dialectic philosophies or individualism–collectivism? *Cognition and Emotion, 16*(6), 705–719.

Scollon, C. N., Diener, E., Oishi, S., & Biswas-Diener, R. (2004). Emotions across cultures and methods. *Journal of Cross-Cultural Psychology, 35*(3), 304–326.

Seidlitz, L., & Diener, E. (1993). Memory for positive versus negative life events: Theories for the differences between happy and unhappy persons. *Journal of Personality and Social Psychology, 64*(4), 654–663.

Seligman, M. E. P. (1992). *Helplessness: On depression, development, and death.* San Francisco: Freeman. (Original work published 1975)

Simon, H. A. (1990). A mechanism for social selection and successful altruism. *Science, 250*(4988), 1665–1668.

Smith, E. R., Seger, C. R., & Mackie, D. M. (2007). Can emotions be truly group level?: Evidence regarding four conceptual criteria. *Journal of Personality and Social Psychology, 93*(3), 431–446.

Soto, J. A., Levenson, R. W., & Ebling, R. (2005). Cultures of moderation and expression: Emotional experience, behavior, and physiology in Chinese Americans and Mexican Americans. *Emotion, 5*(2), 154–165.

Stearns, C. Z., & Stearns, P. N. (1989). *Anger: The struggle for emotional control in America's history.* Chicago: University of Chicago Press.

Szarota, P. (2010). The mystery of the European smile: A comparison based on individual photographs provided by Internet users. *Journal of Nonverbal Behavior, 34*(4), 249–256.

Tellegen, A., Watson, D., & Clark, L. A. (1999). On the dimensional and hierarchical structure of affect. *Psychological Science, 10*(4), 297–303.

Thompson, E. R. (2007). Development and validation of an internationally reliable short-form of the Positive and Negative Affect Schedule (PANAS). *Journal of Cross-Cultural Psychology, 38*(2), 227–242.

Tiedens, L. Z. (2001). Anger and advancement versus sadness and subjugation: The effect of negative emotion expressions on social status conferral. *Journal of Personality and Social Psychology, 80*(1), 86–94.

Tooby, J., & Cosmides, L. (1990). The past explains the present: Emotional adaptations and the structure of ancestral environments. *Ethology and Sociobiology, 11*(4–5), 375–424.

Tooby, J., & Cosmides, L. (1992). The psychological foundations of culture. In J. H. Barkow, L. Cosmides, & J. Tooby (Eds.), *The adapted mind: Evolutionary psychology and the generation of culture* (pp. 19–136). New York: Oxford University Press.

Tsai, J. L., Chentsova-Dutton, Y., Freire-Bebeau, L., & Przymus, D. E. (2002). Emotional expression and physiology in European Americans and Hmong Americans. *Emotion, 2*(4), 380–397.

Tsai, J. L., Knutson, B., & Fung, H. H. (2006). Cultural variation in affect valuation. *Journal of Personality and Social Psychology, 90*(2), 288–307.

Tsai, J. L., Levenson, R. W., & Carstensen, L. L. (2000). Autonomic, subjective, and expressive responses to emotional films in older and younger Chinese Americans and European Americans. *Psychology and Aging, 15*(4), 684–693.

Tsai, J. L., Louie, J. Y., Chen, E. E., & Uchida, Y. (2007). Learning what feelings to desire: Socialization of ideal affect through children's storybooks. *Personality and Social Psychology Bulletin, 33*(1), 17–30.

Turner, J. (2000). *On the origins of human emotions: A sociological inquiry into the evolution of human affect.* Stanford, CA: Stanford University Press.

Turunen, N. (2000). *Russkoe i finskoe kommunikativnoe povedenie* [Russian and Finnish communicative behavior]. Voronezh, Russia: Voronezh State University.

Uchida, Y., & Kitayama, S. (2009). Happiness and unhappiness in east and west: Themes and variations. *Emotion, 9*(4), 441–456.

United Nations Economic Commission for Europe Transport Division Database. (2012). *Statistics of road traffic accidents in Europe and North America.* Retrieved from *www.unece.org/trans/main/wp6/wp6.html.*

vanVliet, J., Oates, N., & Whitelaw, E. (2007). Epigenetic mechanisms in the context of complex diseases. *Cellular and Molecular Life Sciences, 64*(12), 1531–1538.

Veenhoven, R. (2001). Are the Russians as unhappy as they say they are? *Journal of Happiness Studies, 2*(2), 111–136.

Verdick, E., & Lisovskis, M. (2002). *How to take the grrrr out of anger.* Minneapolis, MN: Free Spirit.

Wallbott, H. G., & Scherer, K. R. (1986). Cues and channels in emotion recognition. *Journal of Personality and Social Psychology, 51*(4), 690–699.

Wallsten, T. S. (1972). Conjoint-measurement framework for the study of probabilistic information processing. *Psychological Review, 79*(3), 245–260.

Wang, Q. (2001). "Did you have fun?": American and Chinese mother–child conversations about shared emotional experiences. *Cognitive Development, 16*(2), 693–715.

Weisz, J. R., Suwanlert, S., Chaiyasit, W., Weiss, B., Walter, B. R., & Anderson, W. W. (1988). Thai and American perspectives on over- and undercontrolled child behavior problems: Exploring the threshold model among parents, teachers, and psychologists. *Journal of Consulting and Clinical Psychology, 56*(4), 601–609.

Wierzbicka, A. (1998). Russian emotional expression. *Ethos, 26*(4), 456–483.

Wierzbicka, A. (1999). *Emotions across languages and cultures: Diversity and universals.* Cambridge, UK: Cambridge University Press.

Wojciszke, B. (2004). The negative social world: The Polish culture of complaining. *International Journal of Sociology, 34*(4), 38–59.

World Bank. (2012). *Death rate, crude (per 1,000 people by country).* Retrieved from *http://data.worldbank.org/indicator/sp.dyn.cdrt.in.*

Wrosch, C., & Miller, G. E. (2009). Depressive symptoms can be useful: Self-regulatory and emotional benefits of dysphoric mood in adolescence. *Journal of Personality and Social Psychology, 96*(6), 1181–1190.

Xu, J., & Roberts, R. E. (2010). The power of positive emotions: It's a matter of life or death: Subjective well-being and longevity over 28 years in a general population. *Health Psychology, 29*(1), 9–19.

Yuki, M., Maddux, W. W., & Masuda, T. (2007). Are the windows to the soul the same in the East and West? Cultural differences in using the eyes and mouth as cues to recognize emotions in Japan and the United States. *Journal of Experimental Social Psychology, 43*(2), 303–311.

Zhou, X., Dere, J., Zhu, X., Yao, S., Chentsova-Dutton, Y. E., & Ryder, A. G. (2011). Anxiety symptom presentations in Han Chinese and Euro-Canadian outpatients: Is distress always somatized in China? *Journal of Affective Disorders, 135*(1–3), 111–114.

8

The Function of Negative Emotions in the Confucian Tradition

LOUISE SUNDARARAJAN

The sixth-century literary critic Chung Hung recommended the following scenarios for the poet's contemplation:

At festive gatherings he turns to poetry to express his feelings of intimacy; at separations he expresses his grief in verse. The exiling of the minister of Ch'u [who drowned himself to express his loyalty for the king who misunderstood him], the Han concubine taking leave of the palace [as she was to live the rest of her life with the barbarian ruler, far away from the civilized world], or skeletons spread out over the northern wilderness, or the soul flown away among the tangled grasses, or spears carried to the far-flung regions, the spirit of combat flooding the borderlands [where soldiers were dispatched far away from home to which they might never return], the traveler on the frontier with clothes too thin, the lady in her chamber with tears run dry, or the scholar-official who gives up his office and takes leave of the court with no thought of ever returning, or the woman who wins favor by the raising of a brow, and topples a kingdom with a mere second glance [the famed beauty ordered to kill herself by the reluctant emperor, who was forced to do so by the rioting

troops]—all these things touch the heart and stir the soul. How else can one give vent to these feelings than by expressing them in poetry? How else can one give free reign to his emotions than through the Long Song? (in Yeh & Walls, 1978, pp. 51–52)

With the exception of festive gatherings, all the social scenarios suggested by Chung Hung are episodes of negative emotions.

The negative focus of East Asians (Chinese and Japanese people) is well documented in cross-cultural psychology. Explanations for this phenomenon have been offered along the lines of the match hypothesis (Higgins, 2005), which claims that the fit between behavior and cultural context is the reason that potentially harmful effects of the negative focus are neutralized in collectivistic cultures. One variant of this theme is that collectivists are interested in self-improvement, which can benefit from a negative focus, such as is the case with self-criticism (Heine, Lehman, Markus, & Kitayama, 1999). Another variant of the theme is that collectivism privileges the pursuit of avoidance personal goals, which revolve around the hub of the negative as an attempt to eliminate deviance in order to fit in and maintain group harmony (Elliot, Chirkov, Kim, & Sheldon, 2001).

These cross-cultural data are intrinsically constrained by a research bias toward comparison for contrast, such as the self-improvement focus of collectivists versus self-promotion focus of individualists (Heine et al., 1999), or avoidance personal goals of the former versus approach personal goals of the latter (Elliot et al., 2001). This chapter follows the advice of Fiske (2002) that "we [Western psychology] must transcend our ethnocentric framework and not just study how other cultures differ from the United States but explore what they are intrinsically" (p. 87). The intention of this indigenous turn to the study of a culture on its own terms is to spell out the reasons that the negative focus in Chinese emotions contributes to thriving, not just for collectivists but potentially for all human beings.

My investigation of the negative focus in Chinese emotions proceeds in two steps: First, I adumbrate the epistemological universe behind the Chinese compound *qing gan*, which is usually translated as "emotion." Next, I explore the language game (Wittgenstein, 1953) of a key negative emotion, *chi*, which is usually translated as "shame." By *language game* Wittgenstein (1953) refers to the fact that the meaning of a term typically is not to be found in its referent but in its use and that its use is part of a game-like activity. Thus the meaning of legal terms must be sought in the games lawyers play; that of culinary terms, in games cooks play; and so on. Exploring the language game of *chi* (shame), I examine its usage in both classical and contemporary texts.

QING GAN: THE CHINESE
CONCEPTION OF EMOTION

A Definition of Terms

The modern Chinese term that comes closest to *emotion* is the compound *qing gan* or *gan qing*, with *qing* often serving as a shorthand for it. Although *qing* by itself is often taken as the Chinese term for *emotion* (Hansen, 1995), it is well to remember that the Chinese notion of emotion has two tributaries, *qing* and *gan*, which warrant separate treatment.

The term *qing*, as documented in preHan texts (500–200 B.C.E.), means primarily "genuine," "the facts," or "what essentially is" (Graham, 1986, p. 63). The truth connotation of *qing* has two registers—world and mind. Pertaining to the world, *qing* means the true condition of a situation; pertaining to the mind, the term, according to Harbsmeier (2004), means "essential sensibilities and sentiments" (p. 94) or "individual deep convictions, responses, feelings" (p. 101).

Emotion Is for Truth

There is a long tradition in the West, from Plato to Sartre (with the exception of Heidegger), that considers emotions to be somehow distorting of reality. The Chinese believe, on the contrary, that emotion (*qing*) discloses something that is true about the person and the world. Feng Meng-leng (1574–1645), the eminent compiler and writer of folktales, claimed that *qing*, rendered *ch'ing* in the translation of Mowry (Feng, 1983), "never misleads man; but man sometimes causes *ch'ing* to mislead him" (p. 109); and again, "*ch'ing* never fails man, although man at times obscures his *ch'ing*" (p. 147). On this view, it is *qing* that grounds us in reality; it is humans who distort reality when they fail to be true to their *qing*.

The idea that humans distort reality when they fail to be true to their *qing* finds an eloquent expression in the following statements of Mencius (371–289 B.C.E.), one of the major philosophers in Confucianism:

> Now, when men suddenly see a child about to fall into a well, they all have a feeling of alarm and distress, not to gain friendship with the child's parents, nor to seek the praise of their neighbors and friends, nor because they dislike the reputation [of lack of humanity if they did not rescue the child]. From such a case, we see that a man without the feeling of commiseration is not a man. . . . The feeling of commiseration is the beginning of humanity. (Chan, 1963, p. 65)

Drawing a distinction between empathy (commiseration) and the appraisals of personal loss and gain ("not to gain . . . nor to seek . . . nor

because . . . "), Mencius suggested the possibility that self-related appraisals can interfere with our being true to our emotions, which in turn prevents us from being truly human.

Concern with the "true" condition of things (which pertains to both the self and the world) is sustained in the tradition of mindfulness awareness. One of the earliest references to mindful self-reflection is the following passage from *The Doctrine of the Mean* (1971):

> There is nothing more visible than what is secret, and nothing more manifest than what is minute. Therefore the superior man is watchful over himself, when he is alone. (p. 384)

Because, to the Chinese, the self and the world are inextricably connected in a way best described by Heidegger (1962) as "being in the world" (p. 107), the self-examination showcased here does not share with Western introspection the liability of being preoccupied with the intrapsychic to the extent of compromising an outward responsiveness. Tu's (1989) exegesis says it all:

> "Self-watchfulness" . . . is . . . personal but not subjectivistic. The assumption is that when a person is perceptive of the subtle manifestations of his inner feelings, he is, at the same time, particularly sensitive to the world out there. Indeed, "self-watchfulness," according to this view, opens one's mind and heart to the outside. (p. 26)

It is in the same vein that Brown and Cordon (2009) claim that mindful awareness shares with phenomenology an outward intentional orientation: "For Husserl, our most fundamental intentional activity is to be actively receptive to reality, to take notice by giving attention to that which affects us" (p. 63). This outward orientation contrasts sharply with cognitive appraisal theories that privilege appraisals of self-related loss and gain based on subjective, intrapsychic experiences. For instance, according to Lazarus and Folkman (1984), emotions revolve around the "main evaluative issues" of personal stake, such as "Am I in trouble or being benefited, now or in the future, and in what way?" (p. 31). Mindfulness researchers, by contrast, tend to emphasize receptivity and openness to the world: Williams (2010) claims that "emotions evolved as signaling systems that need to be sensitive to environmental contingencies" (p. 1). Similarly, Siegel (2007) avers that "the aim of our attention is primarily on the outer world—but the self is a full participant" (p. 255).

So far as negative focus is concerned, the most relevant form of mindful awareness is the Buddhist practice known as self-compassion (Barnard

& Curry, 2011). Two out of three of the essential ingredients of self-compassion, as outlined by Barnard and Curry (2011), concern negative emotions: "(b) perceiving one's own suffering as part of a larger human experience, and (c) holding painful feelings and thoughts in mindful awareness" (p. 289, abstract). Consistent with the concern with the true condition of things in the mindfulness tradition, research found that individuals rated high in self-compassion tend to be relatively more accurate in self-assessment (Barnard & Curry, 2011). In addition to accuracy in perception, holding painful feelings and thoughts in mindful awareness serves another function, namely, the development of empathy. To understand the centrality of empathy in Chinese conceptualizations of emotion, we turn to the second term of the emotion (*qing gan*) compound—*gan*, which refers to the capacity to be moved.

Gan and Other-Centeredness

Gan refers to affectivity in both of its tenses—stirring or being stirred. One of the earliest treatises in Chinese poetics, the Great Preface (date uncertain, but no later than the first century C.E.) to the *Odes*, stated that: "to move Heaven and Earth, to stir [*gan*] the gods and spirits, there is nothing more apposite than poetry" (Owen, 1992, p. 45). Reiterating the Confucian emphasis, Owen (1992) claims that "stirring in itself is less significant than developing the capacity to be stirred" (p. 89).

For illustration, consider the following lines by the Tang poet Zhang Ji (768–830):

> My husband died in the battlefield, and my child
> Still in my womb,
> Surviving, I burn like a candle in the daylight. (Yan, 2000, p. 148)

This poem is not an autobiographical narrative. Exegesis by the Chinese commentator (Yan, 2000) suggests that the poet, perturbed by the cruelty of wars, used the young widow's plight as a means to protest against war. This drives home an important point about Chinese poetics, namely, that the feelings poets write about usually refer not to a subjective so much as an intersubjective event—feeling *for* the other. Consistent with the subjective and intersubjective divide is the distinction between two factors of embarrassability, found by Singelis, Bond, Sharkey, and Lai (1999): Self-embarrassability versus empathetic embarrassability. The former refers to the individual as the center of attention in an embarrassing situation (e.g., you fall getting on a bus); the latter on a second person as the center of attention (e.g., an actor forgets his lines; see also Miller, 1987). Note that

all the negative scenarios recommended by Chung Hung for the poet's contemplation, cited in the beginning of this chapter, were emotions in the empathetic, not self-, register.

Thus consistent with the outward orientedness of mindful awareness, the Chinese notion of affectivity (*gan*) is other-centered (Bråten, 2007). This other-centeredness presupposes an intersubjective openness, which is a "pre-reflective couplings of self and other" that Thompson (2001, p. 12) claims to be borne out by the mirror-neuron findings (Gallese, 2001). With *gan*, this intersubjective openness gains a negative focus on suffering *for* the other.

Heart-Aching Love

When one of his favorite disciples, Yen Hui, died, Confucius mourned for him: The disciples noticed that the wailing of Confucius went beyond the limits of ritual decorum (just as the recluse noticed that his chime beating was improperly impetuous). "Master," they said, "You are afflicted," to which Confucius replied, "Am I afflicted? If I am not to be afflicted *for* this man, *for* whom am I to be afflicted?" (*Confucian Analects*, 11/9, cited in Henry, 1987, p. 23; emphasis added). In the preceding scenario, the subjectivity of Confucius was shot through and through by an Other: The crucial question for him was not whether he was having positive or negative emotions so much as *"for* whom" he was having his passions/afflictions.

Shaver and colleagues made the astute observation that "sad aspects of love and attachment are hypercognized in China (i.e., are frequently noticed, emphasized, thought about, and articulated)" (Shaver, Wu, & Schwartz, 1992, p. 196). A case in point is the "heart aching love" (*xin teng*) rendered "sorrow/love" by Shaver et al. (1992), who found that 70% of the Chinese mothers of 30- to 35-month-olds claimed that their children could understand this term (p. 199). This is not surprising, because Chinese children are often teased with the question, "does your mother's heart ache (*xin teng*) for you?" It is also common for mothers to say "my heart aches" (*xin teng*) in reference to the afflictions that befall their children. Unmistakable in this common household expression of love is the ethos of intersubjective openness with its characteristic other-centeredness, an ethos that measures love and attachment primarily in terms of the extent to which one is willing to be afflicted *by* the Other and *for* the Other.

Sensitivity to the plight of the Other constitutes the foundation of Confucian ethics. According to Mencius, the roots of our humane treatment of others lies in an innate inability to screen out the painful experience of others, which he refers to as the unbearing mind. In his own words: "all men have the mind which cannot bear to see the suffering of others"

(Chan,1963, p. 65). The Confucian emphasis on the unbearing mind finds support in contemporary psychology, in which there is growing evidence of the connection between a lack of empathy and psychopathy (Blair, Mitchell, & Blair, 2005).

Stephan, Stephan, and De Vargas (1996, p. 151) created four subscales of emotions, out of which three are relevant to empathy-related emotions:

- Positive-interdependent: sympathetic, considerate, and so forth;
- Negative-independent: ashamed and so forth;
- Negative-interdependent: remorseful and so forth.

This neat partition of the affective space does not hold in the Chinese language game of empathy-related emotions. Contrary to the assumption, prevalent in the field, that positive emotions are to be promoted and negative ones down-regulated, the Chinese approach to empathy seems to play up the negative, as evidenced by the predominance of the negative sign in the Confucian formulations of empathy, such as "the *inability* to bear" other's *suffering*. Furthermore, positive and negative emotions seem to be intertwined in the Chinese mind. For instance, closely related to empathy or commiseration is a cluster of emotions associated with *chi*, usually translated as shame, as Mencius put it: "One is not a human without the feeling of sympathy; one is not a human without the feeling of shame [*chi*]" (Liu, 2002, p. 101).

CHI: CASE STUDY OF A CHINESE NEGATIVE EMOTION

"Unlike American children, Chinese children use the term *shame* as one of their first emotion words early in development" (Mascolo, Fischer, & Li, 2003, p. 38; emphasis in the original). Shame is a negative emotion, of which the Chinese seem to have an especially large repertoire, which serves to capitalize on conformity and adherence to group norms as characteristic of a collectivistic culture—so we are told in numerous cross-cultural studies. A close examination of the language game based on *chi* and related terms suggests a more nuanced story.

Chi: Shame, Guilt, and Much More

In mainstream psychology, shame and guilt are differentiated along the distinction between external and internal norms (Fontaine, 2009). According to conventional wisdom in the field, individualistic cultures, being

intrapersonally oriented, privilege guilt, which signifies a breach of personal norms, whereas collectivistic cultures, being externally governed by social norms, privilege shame. Implicit in this partitioning of guilt and shame along the individualism and collectivism divide is the individual-versus-group dichotomy, a dichotomy that no longer holds in the other-centered register. A case in point is the Chinese notion of *chi*, which can be examined at both the individual and the group levels.

At the individual level of self-evaluation, the Confucian tradition differentiates between two types of *chi* along the distinction between internal versus external norms—intrinsic and circumstantial shame—with an unmistakable bias in favor of the former. Intrinsic shame concerns one's moral character; circumstantial shame concerns social norms such as position, appearance, wealth, and so on. Confucius said, "When internal examination discovers nothing wrong, what is there to be anxious about, what is there to fear?" (*Confucian Analects*, 1971, p. 252). A Confucian gentleman is not supposed to let circumstantial shame bother him—only intrinsic shame counts (Cua, 1996, p. 183). In the Chinese tradition, the ability to withstand extrinsic shame is the hallmark of a crowd-defying, creative individual, such as Mao Zedong (Fang & Faure, 2011) and countless poets and statesmen before him.

That the function of *chi* serves the purpose of moral autonomy, rather than conformity to group norms, is consistent with the Confucian pedagogy in which it is benevolent guidance, not fear of punishment, that motivates one's self-correction. Confucius said:

> If the people be led by laws, and uniformity sought to be given them by punishments, they will try to avoid *the punishment*, but have no sense of shame. If they be led by virtue, and uniformity sought to be given them by the rules of propriety, they will have the sense of shame, and moreover will become good. (*Confucian Analects*, 1971, p. 146; emphasis in the original)

Although *chi* has significant overlap and affinity with guilt at the level of self-evaluation, it encompasses more fully the notion of shame at the group level of other-evaluation. Here *chi* could be either embarrassment (*xiu*) or humiliation (*ru*), depending on the ingroup or outgroup context. For illustration, consider the following scenario (Mascolo et al., 2003): A young child refuses to comply with mother's request to share candy with grandma. Mother says with a sad voice and expression, "Aiya [my goodness], Lin won't share her candy," or "I have a child who won't share with Grandma" (p. 395).

Why is food sharing so important in educating the young? One study

(Aknin, Hamlin, & Dunn, 2012) found that young Canadian children under the age of 2 exhibited greater happiness when giving treats to others than when receiving treats and that they were happier after engaging in costly giving, forfeiting their own resources, than when giving treats at no cost. In a blog from Taiwan, Zhu Taixiang's (2011) mother-in-law (see later in the chapter) seemed to be capitalizing on this insight into child psychology when she stated that children have a natural tendency to share food with those close to them, but if you keep refusing their offers, they will not think of you next time they enjoy something delicious. Missing is this potentially nurturing intent behind the Confucian pedagogy in Mascolo and colleagues' (2003) observation of the candy-sharing episode:

> To encourage respect to elders, caregiver tries to coax unwilling infant to share her candy with her grandma. Caregiver's coaxing directs child's attention to her failure to give up candy. Caregiver's words, emotion, and vocal tone convey disapproval; child looks away. (p. 396)

One important factor was missing from the preceding report: the grandmother's reaction. This is an important omission. As the authors pointed out, the Chinese family interactions are not dyadic (mother and child) so much as triadic—interactions that include the ingroup of friends and relatives. Thus it is the response of the third party—the grandmother—that will determine the nature of *chi* for the child: If the grandmother is nurturing enough, she might plead in attenuation for the child, saying something like "That's OK, I don't need any candy," or even offer to give the child some candy so as to model the act of sharing. If the grandmother shows no response or even joins the mother to scold the child—both scenarios deviate from the normal expectations of the ingroup, to be elaborated later—then and only then would the child experience shaming (*ru*).

The Chinese parent's tendency to comment on the child's failure in front of others has been interpreted by Mascolo et al. (2003) as shaming, which is interpreted as public exposure of failure in order to motivate self-improvement. Usually, the other-evaluation in shaming and humiliation pertains to the outgroup of strangers. An important detail that was overlooked by Mascolo et al. (2003) is the fact that the "others" in the Chinese scenarios under discussion are usually not strangers, but members of the ingroup—relatives and friends. What the child learns in this situation is not necessarily the discrepancy between mother and others (Mascolo et al., 2003) so much as the dynamic exchange in social transactions, in which mother and others balance each other out with their opposite behavioral appraisals of the child. The key to this intricate exchange lies in the art of modesty or embarrassment (*xiu*) that the mother is modeling for the child.

"Embarrassment results from a concern that people have about their observable behavior and a desire to conform and please others" (Singelis et al., 1999, p. 320). Although this mild form of social sanction used to regulate public behavior (Miller, 1996) seems to be a good candidate for the cultural-match hypothesis of collectivistic cultures, there is growing evidence that embarrassment is effective in garnering affection from others even in Western cultures. In one study by Feinberg, Willer, and Keltner (2012), the researchers found that observers recognized the expression of embarrassment as a signal of prosociality and commitment to social relationships. In turn, observers responded with affiliative behaviors toward the signaler, including greater trust and desire to share resources and to affiliate with the embarrassed individual. In the context of the Chinese ingroup interactions, the mother's self-induced embarrassment may be understood as such a strategy to garner social affection. And her strategy worked very well to the advantage of the child: Mascolo et al. (2003) reported effusive praises of the child by others, as if to counteract the mother's disparaging statements. This scenario is a far cry from the notion of shaming (*ru*) as public exposure of failure used to create a heightened consciousness of the self as being intrinsically flawed (Tangney & Dearing, 2002).

The differences between the ingroup and outgroup accounts of embarrassment seem to fall along the divide between two types of attachment, secure and insecure (Rothbaum, Morelli, & Rusk, 2011). The cross-cultural narrative about collectivistic cultures tends to cast *chi* and related terms in the framework of insecure attachment, characterized by the defensive coping of loss of face and its restoration. By contrast, the traditional Confucian account capitalizes on secure attachment, with an emphasis on the constructive coping of compassion, perspective taking, and self-correction. This secure-attachment version of *chi* warrants further exploration.

A Secure Attachment Version of *Chi*

Another account of food sharing is found in a talk by Zhu Taixiang (Zhu, 2011), the principal of an elementary school in Taiwan, retrieved from a blog titled "Teach children to love us" (*http://blog.udn.com/juie3087/5845122*). Zhu's ideas revolve around two anecdotes. The first anecdote concerns a friend undergoing cancer treatment in a hospital who told her family not to wait on her, saying that she would call if she needed them. To this independent-minded woman, Zhu recommended letting herself be cared for by her son. We should teach our children how to love us, lest they be plagued by remorse in the future and lest they be rendered unrighteous (*bu-yi*, to be elaborated later) by us, said Zhu. Furthermore, she added, learning to care for us will enhance their capacity to love their wives and children in a "heart-aching" way.

Zhu went on to illustrate her point with an anecdote of her own son. She has been following the advice of her mother-in-law to always accept the offer from a child—be it a piece of candy, a cookie, or a sip of juice—with a sincere "thank you, it's delicious," regardless of whether she really enjoyed it or not. One day when she picked up her 3-year-old son, the kindergarten teacher reminded the little boy that he had something for his mother. The boy took out of his pocket a bundle of napkins, wrapped under which was one shrimp-flavored chip, which he had saved from his snack. The chip was soggy and tasted awful, but under the teacher's gaze, she felt the need to honor her son ("give him face"). She quickly gobbled up the chip and thanked her son: "It is delicious!" The important point is not food, said Zhu, so much as "being responsive to the heart/mind that is being mindful of you." The main themes of this scenario can be traced back to Confucian classics.

Chi as the Epicenter of Empathy-Related Emotions

Chi is integral to a cluster of empathy-related sensibilities that revolve around two cardinal virtues of Confucianism—ren (love/benevolence) and yi (righteousness). These two terms are defined by Mencius as follows: "The feeling of commiseration is the principle of benevolence [ren]. The feeling of shame and dislike is the principle of righteousness [yi]" (1971, pp. 202–203). Liu (2002) explains:

> ren is from the feeling of empathy and love, and yi from the feeling of shame and dislike. The feeling of sympathy and love underlies the feeling of shame and dislike: The latter does not occur until one sees the neglecting or trampling of the former. To be accurate, we can say that the feeling of shame and dislike is a particular modification or configuration of the feeling of sympathy and love. (p. 107)

The principles of benevolence (ren) and righteousness (yi) are intimately related through a negative sign—violation of the former results in unrighteousness (bu-yi), with associated feelings of remorse, shame, and dislike (repulsion). This exegesis brings to light the proactive nature of chi. The food-sharing practices have a prevention focus—namely, to prevent the violation of reciprocity in the child–parent relationship, a violation that renders the child unrighteousness (bu-yi). Thus Zhu summed up the take-home lesson of her talk as follows: Teach our children how to love us, lest they be rendered unrighteous; lest they lament forever the lost opportunity of repaying us our love when we are no more. In this regard, chi is more akin to guilt than shame for the following reasons: (1) it entails a violation of personal and moral standard; (2) it entails agency in the sense

of taking responsibility for a blameworthy action, associated with a sense of remorse that motivates repair of damage caused by one's violation of the principle of reciprocity. In the case of adult children, the remorse is the more poignantly felt when the opportunity for repair is denied by the parent's death.

This Confucian pedagogy may be formulated as follows:

(Anticipated) negation of *ren* (love) → negation of *yi* (righteousness) → negative emotions associated with *chi* (guilt/shame) → pursuit of virtue (*ren* and *yi*).

Note that in this scheme, the pursuit of virtue is propelled through a negative focus, as evidenced by the extensive use of negative signs such as negation and negative valence.

Prevention Focus Revisited

Higgins, Grant, and Shah (1999) postulate two different self-regulation systems—one with a promotion focus, the other a prevention focus. The neuropsychological underpinnings of the promotion-focus regulation correspond to, in very general terms, the reward system, which manages incentive motivation and approach; those of the prevention-focus system correspond to the fear system, which manages aversive motivation and avoidance (Gray, 1990). Personal goals, approach, and avoidance are not created equal, according to Elliot and colleagues (2012). Creating an absence of undesirable outcome by moving away from it (avoidance) is not as effective in guiding behavior and informing goal progress as moving toward an incentive (approach). Negative consequences of avoidance of personal goals for subjective well-being have been found in a U.S. sample (Elliot, Sheldon, & Church, 1997), but not for collectivistic countries such as South Korea and Russia (Elliot et al., 2001). In explanation, Elliot et al. (2001) invoked the match hypothesis, which states that motivation goals that serve cultural emphasis are adaptive, such that avoidance goals are adaptive in collectivistic cultures because they "seem more concordant with the collectivistic emphasis on fitting in, which fosters a bias toward negative information and a desire to avoid negative outcomes" (p. 506). But a second study by Elliot et al. (2012) did find some negative consequences of avoidance goals in both the U.S. and the Japanese samples. The authors managed to save the match hypothesis to some extent by showing that the negative consequences of avoidance goals were culture-specific for individualistic and collectivistic samples, respectively. Saving one's pet theory is one thing; shedding light on culture and emotion is another. To sort out the tangled relationship between negative focus in

Chinese emotions and approach–avoidance theories, we do well to go back to the drawing board and start over with the other-centeredness of Chinese emotions.

In mainstream psychology, avoidance goals are cast in the individualistic framework of concern with the security and safety of oneself (Higgins et al.,1999). Shifting to the other-centered framework of *gan*, the avoidance goals entail a very different language game, in which the prototype of the prevention-focus regulation is the securely attached infant's being cared for by caretakers who show good qualities of *gan*, such as sensitivity and responsivity, qualities consistent with Bowlby's (1988) classic definition of the attachment figure.

The commitment to protection and the vigilance that goes along with it help to explain why worry tends to loom large in the attachment narratives of the Chinese. Meng Wubo asked about filial piety. Confucius said, "Parents are anxious lest their children should be sick" (*Confucian Analects*, 1971, p. 148). According to another rendition of the text, Confucius replied, "Give your mother and father nothing to worry about beyond your physical well-being" (Ames & Rosemont, 1998, p. 77). Either version speaks of the anxiety-prone caretaker. Consistent with the notion of *gan* as the capacity to be stirred, the good caretaker is one who has the sympathetic sensitivity or intersubjective vulnerability to detect stress in others and thereby provide timely relief. Consistent with this observation is the finding of Rothbaum, Weisz, Pott, Miyake, and Morelli (2000) that Japanese parents prefer to anticipate their infants' needs and take anticipatory measures to minimize the stress.

Cast into the other-centered context of Chinese emotions, the avoidance motivation has two versions, consistent with the two harmony motives identified by Leung (1997)—harmony enhancement and disintegration avoidance. Disintegration avoidance is motivated by a prevention focus that puts a premium on keeping the status quo and fitting in. By contrast, harmony in the classical Chinese texts (Sundararajan, 2013) is conceptualized along the lines of promotion focus, in which interpersonal harmony is pursued as an end in and of itself (Leung, 1997). The need to fit in was found to be a contributing factor to the Asian preference for usefulness and conformity over novelty (Leung & Morris, 2011). The classical view of harmony, on the contrary, was found to be beneficial in creative conflict management (Leung, Koch & Lu, 2002).

The major difference between these two versions of harmony lies in the promotion or avoidance of the negative focus. Disintegration avoidance—defined by items such as "avoid relational discord"—is geared toward avoidance of the negative stimuli (such as conflict). The harmony enhancement goal, by contrast, promotes the negative focus by anticipating the negative outcome as a prevention strategy, very much in line with the ideal caretaker

in China and Japan. This difference in anticipation or avoidance of the negative outcome can be traced back to the definition of harmony according to Confucius. In the context of relational harmony, difference may be considered the root cause of all conflicts. But elimination of difference, according to Confucius, is the way of the petty person. The superior person, by contrast, would anticipate difference and conflict so as to build a harmony that has the capacity for creative conflict management. Thus said Confucius: "Exemplary persons seek harmony not sameness; petty persons, then, are the opposite" (*Confucian Analects*, quoted in Ames & Rosemont, 1998, p. 169).

SUMMARY AND CONCLUSION

Qing is a language game that plays out in the other-centered register, which is an intersubjective space opened up by *gan*, the capacity to be moved. Consequences of this particular orientation for the language game of emotions have been identified by the foregoing analysis, as follows:

1. Negative emotions are not avoided in the affective landscape of a decentered self. This observation is consistent with the nonavoidant attitude toward negative emotions in the discourses on *rasa* (Indian theory of aesthetic tasting; Sundararajan, 2010) and self-compassion (Barnard & Curry, 2011)—in both traditions emotion is a language game that plays out in the empathetic, or other-centered, register. Further investigations of this uniquely Asian approach to emotions can make a significant contribution to research in self-distancing, a processing strategy that has been found to be associated with effective emotion regulation (Kross & Ayduk, 2008; Kross, Duckworth, Ayduk, Tsukayama, & Mischel, 2011).

2. Contrary to the widespread assumption of the suppression of negative emotions in collectivistic cultures (for a more nuanced account, see Sundararajan, 2002), the foregoing analysis brings to light a nonsuppressive and nonavoidant approach to negative emotions, an approach that does not capitalize on the mechanisms of self-control (Sundararajan, 2013). Given the ego depletion and other costs of self-control (Muraven & Baumeister, 2000) that loom large in Western notions of emotion regulation, it is worthwhile to investigate further the alternative emotion regulation strategies broached here and explained elsewhere in more detail under the rubric of emotion refinement (Frijda & Sundararajan, 2007).

3. Combined with a proactive imagination, negative emotions can even be promoted as a motivating factor toward the pursuit of virtue. The

use of negative focus for positive results needs not be the monopoly of collectivistic cultures. The legendary basketball coach Bob Knight (Knight & Hammel, 2013) claims that his coaching philosophy is to focus on preventing the things that could go wrong and that this negative focus produces positive results in sports, daily life, and business.

4. Who is the Other? The degree of aversiveness of *chi* (shame) depends on whether the shame-related scenario takes place in front of the ingroup or the outgroup. Why is it that the robust correlation between negative health outcome and shaming (Randles & Tracy, 2013) is not found in China (Mascolo et al., 2003)? Might it not be that the researchers neglected to distinguish between ingroup and outgroup contexts, thereby mixing different subtypes of *chi* (shame) in their analysis?

In conclusion, with a nondefensive openness to negative emotions, one can be expected to take full advantage of the function of emotion as information (Clore & Storbeck, 2006), thereby increasing the accuracy of one's assessment of self and the world. This point is summed up succinctly by the Chinese term *qing*, which refers to both emotion and the true condition of a situation.

REFERENCES

Aknin, L. B., Hamlin, J. K., & Dunn, E. W. (2012). Giving leads to happiness in young children. *PLoS One, 7*(6), e39211.

Ames, R. T., & Rosemont, H., Jr. (1998). *The analects of Confucius: A philosophical translation*. New York: Ballantine.

Barnard, L. K., & Curry, J. F. (2011). Self-compassion: Conceptualizations, correlates, and interventions. *Review of General Psychology, 15*, 289–303.

Blair, J., Mitchell, D., & Blair, K. (2005). *The psychopath*. Malden, MA: Blackwell.

Bowlby, J. (1988). *A secure base: Parent–child attachment and healthy human development*. New York: Basic Books.

Bråten, S. (Ed.). (2007). *On being moved: From mirror neurons to empathy*. Amsterdam: Benjamins.

Brown, K. W., & Cordon, S. (2009). Toward a phenomenology of mindfulness: Subjective experience and emotional correlates. In F. Didonna (Ed.), *Clinical handbook of mindfulness* (pp. 59–81). New York: Springer.

Chan, W.-T. (1963). *A source book in Chinese philosophy*. Princeton, NJ: Princeton University Press.

Clore, G. L., & Storbeck, J. (2006). Affect as information about liking, efficacy, and importance. In J. Forgas (Ed.), *Affect in social thinking and behavior* (pp. 123–142). New York: Psychology Press.

Confucian analects. (1971). In J. Legge (Trans.), *The Chinese classics* (Vol. I, pp. 1–354). Taipei: Wen Shih Chi. (Translation first published 1893)

Cua, A. S. (1996). A Confucian perspective on self-deception. In R. T. Ames & W. Dissanayake (Eds.), *Self and deception: A cross-cultural philosophical enquiry* (pp. 177–199). Albany: State University of New York.

The doctrine of the mean. (1971). In J. Legge (Trans.), *The Chinese classics* (Vol. I, pp. 382–434). Taipei, Republic of China: Wen Shih Chi. (Translation first published 1893)

Elliot, A. J., Chirkov, V. I., Kim, Y., & Sheldon, K. M. (2001). A cross-cultural analysis of avoidance (relative to approach) personal goals. *Psychological Science, 12,* 505–510.

Elliot, A. J., Sedikides, C., Murayama, K., Tanaka, A., Thrash, T. M., & Mapes, R. R. (2012). Cross-cultural generality and specificity in self-regulation: Avoidance personal goals and multiple aspects of well-being in the United States and Japan. *Emotion, 12,* 1031–1040.

Elliot, A. J., Sheldon, K. M., & Church, M. A. (1997). Avoidance personal goals and subjective well-being. *Personality and Social Psychology Bulletin, 23,* 915–927.

Fang, T., & Faure, G. L. (2011). Chinese communication characteristics: A yin–yang perspective. *International Journal of Intercultural Relations, 35,* 320–333.

Feinberg, M., Willer, R., & Keltner, D. (2012). Flustered and faithful: Embarrassment as a signal of prosociality. *Journal of Personality and Social Psychology, 102,* 81–97.

Feng, M. (1983). *Chinese love stories from "Ch'ing-shih"* (H. L. Mowry, Trans.). Hamden, CT: Archon Books.

Fiske, A. P. (2002). Using individualism and collectivism to compare cultures: A critique of the validity and measurement of the constructs: Comment on Oyserman et al. (2002). *Psychological Bulletin, 128,* 78–88.

Fontaine, J. R. J. (2009). Shame. In D. Sander & K. Scherer (Eds.), *Oxford companion to the affective sciences* (pp. 367–368). Oxford, UK: Oxford University Press.

Frijda, N. H., & Sundararajan, L. (2007). Emotion refinement: A theory inspired by Chinese poetics. *Perspectives on Psychological Science, 2,* 227–241.

Gallese, V. (2001). The "shared manifold" hypothesis: From mirror neurons to empathy. In E. Thompson, *Between ourselves: Second-person issues in the study of consciousness* (pp. 33–50). New York: Imprint Academic.

Graham, A. C. (1986). *Studies in Chinese philosophy and philosophical literature.* Albany: State University of New York Press.

Gray, J. A. (1990). Brain systems that mediate both emotion and cognition. *Cognition and Emotion, 4,* 269–288.

Hansen, C. (1995). *Qing* (emotions) in pre-Buddhist Chinese thought. In J. Marks & R. T. Ames (Eds.), *Emotions in Asian thought* (pp. 181–209). Albany: State University of New York Press.

Harbsmeier, C. (2004). The semantics of *qing* in pre-Buddhist Chinese. In H.

Eifring (Ed.), *Love and emotions in traditional Chinese literature* (pp. 69–148). Leiden, The Netherlands: Brill.

Heidegger, M. (1962). *Being and time* (J. Macquarrie & E. Robinson, Trans.). New York: Harper & Row.

Heine, S. J., Lehman, D., Markus, H., & Kitayama, S. (1999). Is there a universal need for positive regard? *Psychological Review, 106*, 766–794.

Henry, E. (1987). The motif of recognition in early China. *Harvard Journal of Asiatic Studies, 47*, 5–30.

Higgins, E. T. (2005). Value from regulatory fit. *Current Directions in Psychological Science, 14*, 209–213.

Higgins, E. T., Grant, H., & Shah, J. (1999). Self-regulation and the quality of life: Emotional and non-emotional life experiences. In D. Kahneman, E. Diener, & N. Schwarz (Eds.), *Well-being: The foundations of hedonic psychology* (pp. 244–266). New York: Russell Sage Foundation.

Knight, B., & Hammel, B. (2013). *The power of negative thinking.* New York: New Harvest.

Kross, E., & Ayduk, O. (2008). Facilitating adaptive emotional analysis: Distinguishing distanced analysis of depressive experiences from immersed analysis and distraction. *Personality and Social Psychology Bulletin, 34*, 924–938.

Kross, E., Duckworth, A., Ayduk, O., Tsukayama, E., & Mischel, W. (2011). The effect of self-distancing on adaptive versus maladaptive self reflection in children. *Emotion, 11*, 1032–1039.

Lazarus, R. S., & Folkman, S. (1984). *Stress, appraisal, and coping.* New York: Springer.

Leung, K. (1997). Negotiation and reward allocations across cultures. In P. C. Early & M. Erez (Eds.), *New perspectives on international industrial and organizational psychology* (pp. 640–675). San Francisco: New Lexington.

Leung, K., Koch, P. T., & Lu, L. (2002). A dualistic model of harmony and its implications for conflict management in Asia. *Asia Pacific Journal of Management, 19*, 201–220.

Leung, K., & Morris, M. W. (2011). Culture and creativity: A social psychological analysis. In D. D. Cremer, R. V. Dick, & I. K. Murnighan (Eds.), *Social psychology and organizations* (pp. 371–395). New York: Routledge.

Liu, X. S. (2002). Mengzian internalism. In X. S. Liu & P. J. Ivanhoe (Eds.), *Essays on the moral philosophy of Mengzi* (pp. 101–131). Cambridge, MA: Hackett.

Mascolo, M. F., Fischer, K. W., & Li, J. (2003). Dynamic development of component systems of emotions: Pride, shame, and guilt in China and the United States. In R. J. Davidson (Ed.), *Handbook of affective sciences* (pp. 375–408). Oxford, UK: Oxford University Press.

Miller, R. S. (1987). Empathic embarrassment: Situational and personal determinants of reactions to the embarrassment of another. *Journal of Personality and Social Psychology, 53*, 1061–1069.

Miller, R. S. (1996). *Embarrassment: Poise and peril in everyday life.* New York: Guilford Press.

Muraven, M., & Baumeister, R. F. (2000). Self-regulation and depletion of limited

resources: Does self-control resemble a muscle? *Psychological Bulletin, 126,* 247–259.

Owen, S. (1992). *Readings in Chinese literary thought.* Cambridge, MA: Harvard University, Council of East Asian Studies.

Randles, D., & Tracy, J. L. (2013). Nonverbal displays of shame predict relapse and declining health in recovering alcoholics. *Clinical Psychological Science, 1*(2), 149–155.

Rothbaum, F., Morelli, G., & Rusk, N. (2011). Attachment, learning, and coping. In M. J. Gelfand, C.-Y. Chiu, & Y.-Y. Hong (Eds.), *Advances in culture and psychology* (pp. 153–215). Oxford, UK: Oxford University Press.

Rothbaum, F., Weisz, J., Pott, M., Miyake, K., & Morelli, G. (2000). Attachment and culture: Security in the United States and Japan. *American Psychologist, 55,* 1093–1104.

Shaver, P. R., Wu, S., & Schwartz, J. C. (1992). Cross-cultural similarities and differences in emotion and its representation: A prototype approach. In M. S. Clark (Ed.), *Review of personality and social psychology: Vol. 13. Emotion* (pp. 175–212). Beverly Hills, CA: Sage.

Siegel, D. J. (2007). *The mindful brain.* New York: Norton.

Singelis, T. M., Bond, M. H., Sharkey, W. F., & Lai, C. S. Y. (1999). Unpacking culture's influence on self-esteem and embarrassability. *Journal of Cross-Cultural Psychology, 30,* 315–341.

Stephan, W. G., Stephan, C. W., & De Vargas, M. C. (1996). Emotional expression in Costa Rica and the United States. *Journal of Cross-Cultural Psychology, 27,* 147–160.

Sundararajan, L. (2002). The veil and veracity of passion in Chinese poetics. *Consciousness and Emotion, 3*(2), 197–228.

Sundararajan, L. (2010). Two flavors of aesthetic tasting: *Rasa* and savoring: A cross-cultural study with implications for psychology of emotion. *Review of General Psychology, 14,* 22–30.

Sundararajan, L. (2013). The Chinese notions of harmony, with special focus on implications for cross-cultural and global psychology. *Humanistic Psychologist, 41,* 1–10.

Tangney, J. P., & Dearing, R. L. (2002). *Shame and guilt.* New York: Guilford Press.

Thompson, E. (2001). Empathy and consciousness. In E. Thompson, *Between ourselves: Second-person issues in the study of consciousness* (pp. 1–32). New York: Imprint Academic.

Tu, W. M. (1989). *Centrality and commonality.* Albany: State University of New York Press.

Williams, J. M. G. (2010). Commentary: Mindfulness and psychological process. *Emotion, 10,* 1–7.

Wittgenstein, L. (1953). *Philosophical investigations* (G. E. M. Anscombe, Trans.). New York: Macmillan.

The works of Mencius. (1971). In J. Legge (Trans.), *The Chinese classics* (Vol. II, pp. 125–502). Taipei, Republic of China: Wen Shih Chi. (Translation first published 1894)

Yan, K. Y. (2000). *Joy, anger, sadness, and happiness* (in Chinese). Taipei, Republic of China: Xin Zi Ran Zu Yi.

Yeh, C.-Y., & Walls, J. W. (1978). Theory, standards, and practice of criticizing poetry in Chung Hung's Shih-P'in. In R. C. Miao (Ed.), *Chinese poetry and poetics* (Vol. 1, pp. 43–80). San Francisco: Chinese Materials Center.

Zhu, T. (2011, November 16). *Teach children to love us* (in Chinese) [Talk downloaded from blog]. Retrieved from *http://blog.udn.com/juie3087/5845122*.

PART III

THE DESIRABILITY OF NEGATIVE EMOTIONS

9

Why Might People Want to Feel Bad?

Motives in Contrahedonic
Emotion Regulation

MAYA TAMIR
YOCHANAN BIGMAN

Unlike thoughts, motives, and other mental states, emotions feel good or bad. Indeed, the phenomenology of emotions is one of their identifying features. The powerful hedonic implications of emotions make them a common target of self-regulation. People often engage in hedonic emotion regulation. That is, they often want to rid themselves of unpleasant emotions and amplify pleasant ones. Often, but not always. There are times when people want to maintain or even increase unpleasant emotions and decrease pleasant ones. In such cases, people engage in contrahedonic emotion regulation. Although such cases are less frequent, they are important because they expose a latent range of motives in emotion regulation that is otherwise difficult to detect. Identifying the range of motives that underlie emotion regulation is critical because such motives determine the direction and the course of emotion regulation.

This chapter, therefore, focuses on cases of contrahedonic emotion regulation. Integrating existing theoretical and empirical advances, we try to offer a taxonomy of motives for experiencing unpleasant emotions and

decreasing pleasant ones. In what follows, we first examine what people want in general, and then discuss whether people ever want to feel unpleasant. We then present a taxonomy of motives in contrahedonic emotion regulation. We provide examples for each proposed motive and review related empirical evidence. We conclude by highlighting some theoretical implications and remaining challenges.

WHAT DO PEOPLE WANT?

Human beings have evolved a unique capacity for self-regulation. Rather than merely responding to the environment, we can anticipate possible futures and exert control in an attempt to shape our own. These efforts are directed toward the achievement of desired end states, which are hierarchically organized, from the specific to the more abstract. As discussed by Thrash and Elliot (2001), goals reflect specific desired end states and refer to *what* people want to achieve as they engage in self-regulation (e.g., losing weight). Motives, on the other hand, reflect an orientation toward a type of desired outcome and refer to *why* people engage in self-regulation (e.g., gaining social acceptance or being healthy). Because a particular goal can serve more than one motive, goals point to the specific direction of regulation but do not necessarily explain why it is pursued. Because a particular motive can be served by multiple goals, motives point to a general rather than a specific direction of regulation but identify the reason for pursuing it (McClelland, 1987).

At any given moment, people are driven by multiple motives. Motives can complement each other (e.g., as when a person wants to do well at work and get along with work colleagues) or conflict with each other (e.g., as when a person wants to work harder and spend more time with her romantic partner). The relative importance of specific motives depends on the superordinate motives that they serve.

Perhaps the strongest superordinate motive that shapes animal behavior is the desire to experience pleasure and avoid pain. According to Epicurus, people naturally strive to optimize hedonic experience, especially by reducing pain (Rist, 1972). According to this approach, self-regulation is geared toward maximizing pleasure and minimizing pain. According to Aristotle, on the other hand, people strive to maximize moral and intellectual excellence, which are not always commensurate with pleasure (Ross, 1995). According to this approach, self-regulation is geared toward maximizing excellence. These approaches differ in the importance they attribute to pleasure, but they converge in highlighting the desirability of virtue. For Epicurus virtue leads to pleasure, but pleasure is the desired end state. For Plato and Aristotle, virtue may or may not lead to pleasure, but virtue is the desired end state.

There seems to be an agreement, therefore, that humans want more than to maximize immediate hedonic pleasure. Instead, they are motivated to optimize future benefits (hedonic or otherwise) as well. Indeed, the desire to attain future benefits is what triggers the process of self-regulation—a process designed to modify current experiences in order to alter the likelihood of future events (see Barkley, 2004). In an attempt to maximize future benefits, self-regulation can even lead people to forego immediate pleasure (Mischel, Shoda, & Rodriguez, 1989).

DO PEOPLE EVER WANT TO FEEL BAD?

All forms of self-regulation involve moving from a current state to a desired end state. Whereas the regulation of behavior is directed toward desired behaviors (i.e., behavioral goals), the regulation of emotion is directed toward desired emotions (i.e., emotional goals). Behavioral and emotional goals are incorporated in a larger goal hierarchy, in which they operate together to serve various motives.

Unlike behaviors, emotions are inherently hedonic states (i.e., they are either pleasant or unpleasant to experience). Given their hedonic nature, emotional goals contribute to pleasure or pain (e.g., Spinoza, 1677/1982). Increasing pleasant emotions promotes greater pleasure, and decreasing unpleasant emotions promotes less pain. Understandably, therefore, research on emotion regulation was initially guided by the assumption that emotional goals operate exclusively in the service of the hedonic motive (e.g., Larsen, 2000). It quickly became clear, however, that seeking pleasure and avoiding pain cannot account for all instances of emotion regulation.

Building on functional approaches to emotion, researchers highlighted the fact that emotions are not just hedonic states. Because they can influence behavior in a desirable or undesirable manner, emotions can be pursued not only for how they feel but for what they do (e.g., Bonanno, 2001; Fischer, Rodriguez Mosquera, van Vianen, & Manstead, 2004). Within this theoretical approach, it seems likely that pleasant emotions serve the hedonic motive, yet they may serve other motives as well. In contrast, it seems unlikely that unpleasant emotions serve the hedonic motive, yet they may serve other motives instead. To support this idea, researchers have suggested possible motives other than the hedonic one in emotion regulation (e.g., Augustine, Hemenover, Larsen, & Shulman, 2010; Parrott, 1993; Vastfjall & Garling, 2006). To empirically test whether emotion regulation can indeed be driven by motives other than the hedonic one, it was essential to demonstrate that people do sometimes want to feel bad (or avoid feeling good).

Gradually, evidence for cases of emotion regulation that do not adhere

to a simple hedonic motive began to accumulate. Riediger, Schmiedek, Wagner, and Lindenberger (2009) demonstrated that in daily life people can regulate their emotions in ways that impair rather than promote hedonic benefits. In a week-long experience sampling study, participants reported on their emotional goals six times a day. On 15% of the measurements, participants reported contrahedonic emotional goals (i.e., trying to maintain or increase unpleasant emotions and decrease pleasant emotions). Other studies provided evidence for cases that reflect contrahedonic emotion regulation, showing that people did not want to increase happiness (Wood, Heimpel, Manwell, & Whitting, 2009) and that people wanted to increase anger (Tamir, Mitchell, & Gross, 2008), fear (Tamir & Ford, 2009), or sadness (Hackenbracht & Tamir, 2010).

Such research demonstrated that there are motives other than increasing pleasure that drive emotion regulation. But what might they be? People can be motivated to experience unpleasant emotions or to avoid pleasant ones for various reasons. In the next section, we describe what we see as the main categories of motives that underlie such cases of emotion regulation. The categories are organized in a taxonomy that is depicted in Figure 9.1. Although they differ from each other, these categories are not mutually exclusive. Also, our proposed taxonomy refers to motives that underlie the regulation of emotion experience rather than expression. The reason is that the regulation of emotion expression targets behavior, whereas the regulation of emotion experience targets subjective experiences, which is the focus of our chapter.

A TAXONOMY OF MOTIVES

Epicurus distinguished between two types of value (Rist, 1972). Activities that have *intrinsic value* are those that are inherently pleasant (e.g., a person may order a salad because he or she enjoys the taste of fresh salad greens). Activities that have *instrumental value* are those that serve as means to attain future intrinsic value (e.g., a person may order a salad not because it is inherently pleasant to eat but because it is healthy and feeling healthy is pleasant). An experience or an activity, therefore, can be pursued either for its intrinsic or for its instrumental value. Building on this distinction, we propose that, similarly, emotions can be pursued for their intrinsic or for their instrumental value. When emotions are pursued for their intrinsic value, people are motivated to experience an emotion for its immediate hedonic implications, whereas its nonhedonic implications (e.g., cognitive or behavioral) are something they either benefit or suffer from in the process. In contrast, when emotions are pursued for their instrumental value, people are motivated to experience them to attain some future

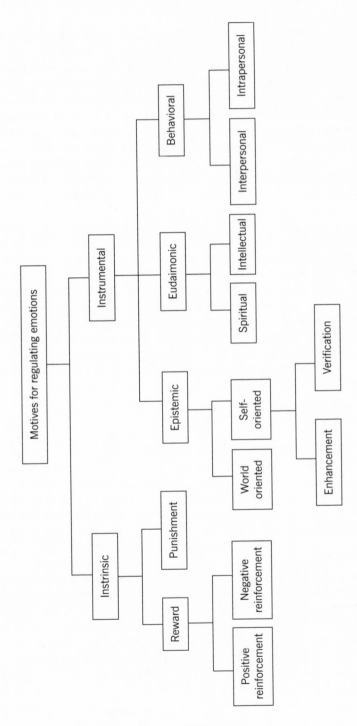

FIGURE 9.1. A taxonomy of motives for increasing unpleasant emotions or decreasing pleasant emotions.

benefit, whereas their immediate hedonic implications are something that they either benefit or suffer from in the process.

Our first distinction, therefore, is between intrinsic and instrumental motives in contrahedonic emotion regulation. Because people are generally guided by the hedonic principle (Freud, 1920/1952), it seems less likely that people can be motivated to increase unpleasant emotions for their immediate hedonic implications. Because people are sometimes willing to forego immediate pleasure to maximize future benefits, it seems more likely that people can be motivated to increase unpleasant emotions for their subsequent instrumental benefits. We begin, therefore, by discussing instrumental motives and follow with a discussion of intrinsic motives.

Instrumental Motives

People may choose to engage in an activity that carries an immediate hedonic cost if it is expected to yield future benefits (Mischel et al., 1989). To the extent that unpleasant emotional states can yield future benefits, people may be motivated to experience them for instrumental reasons. Emotion regulation is driven by *instrumental motives* when people are motivated to experience an emotion in order to maximize future benefits. Different motives can target different types of benefits. We distinguish between three types of instrumental motives: behavioral, epistemic, and eudaimonic. We describe each of these next.

Behavioral Motives

According to functional approaches to emotion, emotions shape behavior in a goal-consistent manner (e.g., Frijda, 1986). That is, emotions can lead people to behave in desirable ways (e.g., as when worrying about lung cancer leads a person to stop smoking; McCaul, Mullens, Romanek, Erickson, & Gatheridge, 2007). Therefore, emotions can be recruited to promote the successful pursuit of behavioral goals. Fear, for example, bolsters avoidance, whereas anger bolsters confrontation. Therefore, fear can be recruited to promote successful avoidance, and anger can be recruited to promote successful confrontation. Emotion regulation is driven by *instrumental behavioral goals* when people are motivated to experience an emotion to increase the likelihood of desirable behaviors.

There is considerable evidence in support of instrumental behavioral motives in emotion regulation. Our own work demonstrates that emotional goals (i.e., what people want to feel) can be shaped by higher order behavioral goals (e.g., Tamir et al., 2008; Tamir & Ford, 2009; Tamir & Ford, 2012). People actively tried to increase fear when they needed to avoid threats (Tamir & Ford, 2009), anger when they needed to confront others

(e.g., Tamir et al., 2008; Tamir & Ford, 2012), and sadness when they wanted to elicit help from others (Hackenbracht & Tamir, 2010). Importantly, such motives appear to influence behavior only when people expect the immediate hedonic cost to lead to future benefits (Tamir, Ford, & Gilliam, 2013).

Behavioral motives can be further divided into *intrapersonal* and *interpersonal* motives, depending on the source of the behavior the emotions are intended to modulate. Emotions can modulate the behavior of the person experiencing them by shaping the person's cognition, motivation, physiology, or behavior. Therefore, people may be motivated to experience emotions to change the likelihood of their own states. In such cases, emotion regulation is motivated by *intrapersonal behavioral motives*. For instance, if sadness promotes analytical thinking (see Martin & Clore, 2001), people may try to increase sadness when facing an important analytical task. In support of this hypothesis, participants were more motivated to feel sad when instructed to perform an analytical (vs. a creative) task (Cohen & Andrade, 2004). Similarly, if empathy and compassion motivate people to help others (e.g., Batson, 1991), people may try to decrease empathy or compassion when helping others necessitates personal sacrifice. In support of this hypothesis, when helping others was costly to the self, participants were motivated to decrease their empathy or compassion to avoid their motivational implications (Cameron & Payne, 2011; Shaw, Batson, & Todd, 1994). These examples demonstrate that people want to increase emotional experiences that are likely to lead to desirable behaviors and decrease emotional experiences that are likely to lead to undesirable ones.

In addition to influencing the self, emotions influence others. Emotions influence others by influencing their feelings, thoughts, and behaviors. Because one's social environment is a prominent contributor to one's well-being, a person may be motivated to experience emotions that are likely to lead others to behave in a way that benefits him or her. In such cases, emotion regulation is motivated by *interpersonal behavioral motives*. For example, happiness can make others more likely to collaborate, whereas anger can make others more likely to concede (Van Kleef, Van Dijk, Steinel, Harinck, & Van Beest, 2008; see Van Kleef & Côté, Chapter 6, this volume). We found that participants were motivated to increase happiness when their goal was to collaborate with others but increase anger when their goal was to confront others (Tamir & Ford, 2012). Similarly, Tsai, Miao, Seppala, Fung, and Yeung (2007) found that when people wanted others to follow their lead, they were more motivated to experience high- (vs. low-) arousal pleasant emotions but that these preferences reversed when people wanted others to lead them.

Interpersonal behavioral motives can also lead people to increase an emotional state that is likely to promote affiliation or other social functions.

For instance, if emotional congruence promotes affiliation, people who want to affiliate with their partners may be motivated to assimilate their emotional states into their partners'. In support of this hypothesis, participants who expected to interact with a stranger whose emotional state was unknown tended to neutralize their emotional experiences before the interaction (Erber, Wegner, & Therriault, 1996). Participants who expected to interact with strangers whose emotional states were known tended to match their emotional states to those of their partners (Huntsinger, Lun, Sinclair, & Clore, 2009). Participants who expected to interact with less happy partners reported less positive emotional experiences than those who expected to interact with happier partners. In the latter case, these patterns of regulation were evident only among participants who wanted to affiliate with their partners (i.e., those for whom emotional matching was instrumental).

Interpersonal motives in emotion regulation can also operate at the group level. According to intergroup emotion theory (Mackie, Devos, & Smith, 2000; Smith, 1993), group-level emotions play an important role in group cohesion and collective action. Just as congruent emotions among two partners can promote successful dyadic interaction, there is evidence that congruent emotions among group members (i.e., emotion convergence; Smith, Seger, & Mackie, 2007) promote group cohesion and facilitate political action. Therefore, people may be motivated to experience normative group emotions, pleasant or unpleasant, to signal group membership and promote successful interactions at the group level (Thomas, McGarty & Mavor, 2009).

Regulating group-based emotions can serve both interpersonal and intrapersonal instrumental motives. With respect to intrapersonal benefits, increasing group-based emotions can increase the likelihood of the person experiencing those emotions behaving in accordance with his or her values by taking collective action. For instance, anger about unfair treatment of women was associated with female participants' willingness to take action to promote women's rights (Leonard, Moons, Mackie, & Smith, 2011). With respect to interpersonal benefits, to the extent to which they promote collective action, group-based emotions can promote the achievement of group goals. Increasing group-based emotions can also promote group cohesion by influencing other members of the group. This occurs because group-based emotions highlight group concerns and signal the individuals' commitment to those concerns.

In summary, behavioral motives in emotion regulation involve attempts to modify one's emotions in ways that promote desired behaviors in oneself, in others, or in both. Because instrumental motives depend on the anticipated behavioral implications of emotions, they are shaped by people's expectations regarding such effects. People want to feel sadder when performing analytical tasks, but that is likely because they expect

sadness to lead to more analytical thinking (Cohen & Andrade, 2004). People are motivated to increase their anger before a confrontation, but only to the extent to which they expect anger to promote successful confrontation (Tamir & Ford, 2012). Similarly, runners who expect to run faster when angry or anxious try to amplify these emotions before a run, whereas runners who expect to run faster when they don't feel angry or anxious try to decrease these emotions before a run (Lane, Beedie, Devonport, & Stanley, 2011). Such findings show that people are motivated to experience unpleasant emotions that they expect to promote desirable behaviors (in themselves or in others).

Epistemic Motives

Emotions can influence behavior, but they have other implications, as well. One important function of emotion is to provide information (Schwarz & Clore, 1983). Such information is valuable, in part, because it can affect subsequent behavior. Such information, however, is also valuable in its own right. Emotion regulation is driven by *epistemic motives* when people are motivated to experience emotions to attain certain information. Emotions provide information about oneself and about the world. Therefore, people may be motivated to regulate their emotions to attain certain information about themselves or about the world around them, as detailed in this section.

To function adaptively in the world, individuals need a coherent sense of self (Festinger, 1957). Because individuals constantly construct, monitor, and evaluate their sense of self, information about the self is valuable. Emotion regulation is driven by *self-epistemic motives* when people are motivated to experience emotions to attain certain information about themselves. In particular, people are motivated to attain two different types of information about themselves (for a recent review, see Alicke & Sedikides, 2011). First, given the need for positive self-regard, people seek out information that enhances their self-images (Rogers, 1951). Second, given the need for consistency and predictability, people seek out information that verifies their self-images (Swann, 1987). As we discuss, emotions can provide information that can enhance as well as verify self-perceptions.

When emotional experiences reflect negatively on themselves, people may be motivated to avoid these experiences, and when emotional experiences reflect positively on themselves, people may be motivated to approach these experiences to enhance their sense of self. The implications of our emotional experiences for our self-images are the focus of research on meta-emotion and emotional acceptance. Because emotions reflect aspects of the self, people can react emotionally to their emotions (Gottman, Katz, & Hooven, 1997). For instance, people can feel ashamed for having certain

emotional experiences (Mayer & Stevens, 1994). Negative self-evaluations on account of emotional experiences are common among individuals who suffer from depression or anxiety and may contribute to maintaining the disorder (Hayes, Luoma, Bond, Masuda, & Lillis, 2006).

More generally, people judge themselves for experiencing any emotion that is deemed inappropriate or undesirable in a particular context. Unpleasant emotions can be inappropriate in some contexts, but appropriate in others. Therefore, people may be motivated to experience unpleasant emotions when they reflect positively on themselves. For example, feeling angry in the face of moral injustice reflects a moral self. To the extent that morality is a desirable attribute of themselves, people may be motivated to feel angry in the face of injustice (see Hess, Chapter 3, this volume). In support of this hypothesis, Greene, Sedikides, Barbera, and Van Tongerena (2013) found that participants were motivated to maintain anger in the face of moral injustice and that such feelings directly contributed to the perception of the self as moral. Similarly, Stearns and Parrott (2012) found that people were evaluated more positively if they expressed guilt and shame following their misconduct. Such favorable evaluations can arise from external or internal sources and may motivate people to experience shame and guilt in some contexts.

Of course, what is desirable is determined by one's cultural context (see Chentsova-Dutton, Senft, & Ryder, Chapter 7, this volume). People are motivated to experience those emotions that are deemed appropriate by their culture (e.g., Tsai, Knutson, & Fung, 2006). Although pleasant emotions are universally more desirable than unpleasant emotions, the desirability of specific pleasant and unpleasant emotions differs dramatically across cultures (e.g., Eid & Diener, 2001). Seeking to experience emotions that are normative in one's culture could be driven by behavioral motives when doing so is designed to achieve specific goals (e.g., promoting the pursuit of culturally meaningful goals or gaining social approval), but it can be motivated by epistemic motives when doing so is designed to enhance one's evaluation of the self in accordance with cultural standards. Doing so, in turn, is likely to enhance one's evaluation of oneself.

Self-enhancement is a powerful motive but not the only motive for seeking information regarding the self. People can also be motivated to self-verify (e.g., Swann, 1987). That is, people seek information that confirms their existing self-perceptions. This applies to both positive and negative aspects of the self. For instance, people with low self-esteem preferred to receive more negative feedback about themselves from others (Swann, Stein-Seroussi, & Giesler, 1992). Similarly, people may be motivated to experience emotions that provide information that is consistent with their sense of self.

Emotional experiences inform people about their emotional selves (see

Robinson & Clore, 2002). Indeed, emotional experiences lie at the core of nearly all theories of personality. People rely, in part, on their emotional experiences to construct their self-images (e.g., "I often feel anxious, therefore I am an anxious person"). If emotional experiences inform people about their emotional selves, it may be that people are motivated, at least to some extent, to experience those emotions that they view as most typical of them, whether they are pleasant or unpleasant to experience. There are now several sources of evidence that support this hypothesis. People are inclined to maintain emotional experiences that they view as typical for them or more familiar (e.g., Mayer & Stevens, 1994; Wood et al., 2009). Individuals higher in extraversion report stronger preferences for pleasant emotions (e.g., Augustine et al., 2010; Rusting & Larsen, 1995), whereas individuals higher in neuroticism tend to report stronger preferences for unpleasant emotions (Kampfe & Mitte, 2009). We recently found that people who reported more (vs. less) frequent experiences of happiness were more motivated to experience happiness, that people who reported more (vs. less) frequent experiences of anger were more motivated to experience anger, and that people who reported more (vs. less) frequent experiences of fear were more motivated to experience fear (Ford & Tamir, 2012). These patterns are consistent with self-verifying motives in emotion regulation.

Emotional experiences can also inform people about nonemotional aspects of their personalities. For instance, experiencing anger or compassion in the face of injustice informs people about their moral nature. People who view themselves as moral may be motivated to experience anger or compassion in the face of injustice because it confirms their moral sense of self (Cameron & Payne, 2011; Greene et al., 2012). However, this may not be true for people who do not view themselves as moral. Similar patterns with regard to other emotions remain to be tested. For instance, people who view themselves as intellectual may be motivated to experience interest and excitement rather than boredom in certain contexts, people who see themselves as low in agreeableness may be motivated to feel less empathy for others, and so forth.

One type of epistemic motive in emotion regulation, therefore, concerns knowledge about the self. Another type of epistemic motive concerns knowledge about the social world. People tend to seek out information that supports their goals, values, and beliefs (Kruglanski, 1996). Given that emotions provide information, it is possible that people seek emotional experiences that support their views of the social world. Emotion regulation is driven by *world epistemic motives* when people are motivated to experience emotions to attain certain information about the social world or things external to themselves.

If people are motivated to see the world in particular ways, they may be motivated to experience emotions that are consistent with these views.

For instance, some people distrust close relationships. The experience of love and attachment may be inconsistent with this basic view. It is possible that to maintain their basic assumptions about close relationships, such people may be motivated to decrease feelings of trust and love, particularly when relationships go awry. Similar ideas have been proposed within the framework of attachment theory. For example, people who are avoidantly attached believe that significant others are unreliable and cannot be trusted. Suppressing feelings of love and attachment confirms the belief that others have relatively low value and should be kept at a distance (Shaver & Mikulincer, 2007).

The motivation to experience emotions that help maintain particular worldviews may also contribute to the experience of group emotions. We recently examined whether people are motivated to experience emotions that reflect appraisals consistent with their political ideology (Halperin, Wayne, Porat, & Tamir, 2012). We found that ideology was significantly linked to the motivation to experience anger in political contexts and that such motives mediated emotional experiences and behavior in response to a politically relevant event. Such findings demonstrate that people are motivated to experience emotions that reinforce a particular interpretation of the world that is consistent with their goals and values.

In summary, emotions can be pursued to attain desirable information about the self or the social world. Obviously, epistemic and behavioral motives are not independent of each other. It is likely that access to particular information about the self or the world propels certain behaviors that help people attain their goals. For instance, decreasing feelings of love and attachment confirms the view of avoidantly attached individuals that others are untrustworthy, and this, in turn, can lead them to maintain their distance and protect themselves from possible pain (Shaver & Mikulincer, 2007). Similarly, decreasing the experience of anger toward outgroup members can help confirm the political worldviews of doves, and this, in turn, can increase support for humanitarian action (e.g., Halperin, Porat, Tamir, & Gross, 2013). As these examples demonstrate, epistemic motives for contrahedonic emotion regulation can (but do not necessarily) subserve behavioral motives.

Eudaimonic Motives

According to Aristotle, people strive to actualize their *daimon*, or "true self," through moral, spiritual, and intellectual excellence (Ackrill, 1973). Such motives are referred to as *eudaimonic* (e.g., Waterman, 1993). Eudaimonic approaches to happiness have broadened the definition of eudaimonic motives to include various forms of self-actualization, including successful goal pursuit and authenticity (see Ryan & Deci, 2001). In the

present context, however, we use the term in its narrower original meaning, as reflecting the motivation to excel spiritually or intellectually. Within this narrower conceptualization, eudaimonic motives are distinct from behavioral motives because they do not target desirable behaviors, and they are distinct from epistemic motives because they do not target desirable information. Instead, eudaimonic motives target spiritual and intellectual improvement. Emotion regulation is driven by *eudaimonic motives* when people are motivated to experience emotions to attain spiritual or intellectual growth.

Emotions can have spiritual value. Indeed, religious traditions prescribe specific pleasant as well as unpleasant, emotional experiences (Davies, 2011). Empirical support for this claim was recently provided by Kim-Prieto and Diener (2009), who asked members of different religions from around the world to rate the desirability of different emotional states. They found that the desirability of various emotions differed substantially as a function of religious affiliation. For instance, pride was very desirable to Jews (M = 7.44 on a scale ranging from 1–9) but somewhat undesirable to Christians (M = 4.26); shame was desirable to Muslims (M = 6.50) but undesirable to Hindus (M = 3.77); sadness was desirable to Muslims (M = 6.60) but undesirable to Buddhists (M = 4.09). It is possible that religions cultivate emotional experiences that reinforce religious values (Vishkin, Bigman, & Tamir, in press). Thus emotions carry spiritual value to the extent that certain emotional experiences can bring people closer to their faith.

Emotions can also have intellectual value. Outside the domain of emotion, people are motivated to do things out of interest or curiosity. There is an intellectual benefit in exposure to the novel or the unknown. Just as curiosity leads people to seek out certain behaviors, perhaps it could also lead people to seek out certain emotions. Curiosity or interest might explain why people are often drawn to works of art or entertainment that elicit unpleasant emotions (e.g., Oliver & Raney, 2011; Eskine, Kacinik, & Prinz, 2012). These ideas are theoretically compelling, and there is some evidence consistent with them. However, to date there is no direct evidence confirming that people are motivated to experience unpleasant emotions for purely intellectual reasons.

Intrinsic Motives

Emotions can be pursued as means of attaining a higher order goal (behavioral, epistemic, or eudaimonic), in which case emotion regulation is motivated by instrumental motives. However, emotions are often sought as an end in themselves. We refer to emotion regulation as driven by *intrinsic motives* when people are motivated to experience an emotion for its

immediate subjective hedonic consequences. Hedonic motives typically refer to the motivation to feel pleasure and avoid pain and, by inference, the motivation to increase pleasant and decrease unpleasant emotions. The focus on preferences for pleasure is based on the assumption that people always want to feel pleasure and avoid pain. The focus on the desire to minimize unpleasant emotions to attain pleasure is based on the assumption that unpleasant emotions are inherently unpleasant. In the discussion that follows, we probe both of these assumptions.

Punishment Motives

People reward themselves when they wish to increase the likelihood of things they attribute to themselves. For instance, to reward themselves people buy themselves gifts or treat themselves to pampering massages. However, people are also willing to punish themselves when they wish to decrease the likelihood of things they attribute to themselves. In a decision-making task, for instance, participants who felt guilty for past behavior chose to punish themselves financially (Nelissen & Zeelenberg, 2009). There are even extreme cases in which, to punish themselves, people go so far as to inflict physical harm on themselves. At least one motivation for causing physical self-injury is the desire to punish oneself (for a review, see Klonsky, 2007). Such evidence suggests that people do not always seek to increase pleasure and minimize pain. There are times when people are, in fact, motivated to experience pain as such.

Unpleasant emotions are painful, and so, at least theoretically, people may be motivated to experience unpleasant emotions as a form of self-punishment. In these cases, emotion regulation is driven by *hedonic punishment motives*. Preliminary support for this hypothesis comes from research by Joanne Wood and her colleagues. They found that individuals low in self-esteem failed to repair their unpleasant emotional experiences specifically because they believed they deserved to suffer (Wood et al., 2009). Although more empirical research is needed, such evidence suggests that at least some people may be motivated to experience unpleasant emotions as a form of self-punishment. In these cases, people use unpleasant emotions to decrease their overall hedonic balance.

Reward Motives

Because unpleasant emotions are painful and pain is a form of punishment, it seems plausible that people can be motivated to experience unpleasant emotions as a form of punishment. It seems less plausible, however, that people can be motivated to experience unpleasant emotions as a form of reward. Nonetheless, we argue that there might be cases in which, perhaps

ironically, unpleasant emotions may increase overall hedonic balance. We offer two possible cases in which people may be motivated to increase unpleasant emotions as a form of reward, either as negative reinforcers or as positive reinforcers, as detailed next.

Pleasure and pain are relative. They are always experienced in reference to another state. This is reflected in the process of habituation, in which experiences of pleasure or pain lose their hedonic impact as their frequency increases (Groves & Thompson, 1970). Because pleasure and pain are relative, less intense pain can be considered pleasant in comparison with more intense pain. This has been shown empirically in research on the temporal dynamics of pleasure. Kahneman, Fredrickson, Schreiber, and Redelmeier (1993), for example, have shown that people prefer to endure longer periods of pain when the intensity of pain at the end of the period was low than to endure a shorter period of pain when the pain at the end of the period was high, even though the total amount of pain was lower. Therefore, it appears that people seek relatively less intense pain when it eliminates worse pain (see also Fredrickson, 2000). Indeed, this idea originated with Epicurus himself, who argued that people may choose to avoid pleasure when, by doing so, they avoid greater pain and to accept pain when, by doing so, they attain greater pleasure (Rist, 1972).

People prefer less intense to more intense pain of the same quality. However, different types of pain may be painful to a different degree. In such cases, people may prefer one type of pain when it diminishes the likelihood of another, more subjectively intense type of pain. For instance, some have argued that individuals engage in physical self-harm partly because this allows them to escape from even less desirable emotional experiences (Chapman, Gratz, & Brown, 2006; Franklin et al., 2010; Klonsky, 2007). For example, Pip, the main character in Dickens's *Great Expectations* (1969/1861), is described hitting the wall and pulling his hair after realizing that Estella saw him cry. He says: "I got rid of my injured feelings for a time by kicking them into the brewery wall, and twisting them out of my hair" (p. 70).

If people are sometimes motivated to endure physical pain to avoid worse emotional pain, perhaps there are times when people are motivated to endure one type of emotional pain to avoid worse emotional pain. In this case, unpleasant emotions may serve as *negative reinforcement*, because the experience of the unpleasant emotion diminishes a relatively more aversive emotional experience. These ideas are incorporated in the avoidance theory of worry and generalized anxiety disorder (Borkovec, Alcaine, & Behar, 2004). According to this theory, individuals who suffer from generalized anxiety disorder are often motivated to experience worry because it helps them avoid the far worse experience of fear.

Although there is little empirical research that directly tests this idea, it

could potentially be extended to other emotional contexts. For instance, to the extent that jealousy is less painful for a person than rejection, a person who believes that the likelihood of rejection is high may be motivated to experience jealousy. Similarly, to the extent that fear is less painful than despair, a person who believes that the likelihood of despair is high may be motivated to experience fear.

These ideas have struck a chord with clinicians and some researchers of emotion regulation (Campos, Frankel, & Camras, 2004). Although they are certainly plausible, we suggest that without further empirical support they should be considered cautiously. The reason is that when applied broadly, this account of contrahedonic emotion regulation may be in danger of becoming tautological. One could argue, for instance, that any time a person seeks to increase an unpleasant emotional state the goal is ultimately to prevent worse hedonic states. For instance, perhaps when soldiers amplify their anger as they prepare to go to battle, they do so because they expect the fear of death or the sadness of defeat to be more painful. Such explanations may not always be the most parsimonious or useful. To promote the understanding of emotion regulation, we encourage researchers to consider proximal goals in emotion regulation and the direct superordinate motives that they serve.

Unpleasant emotions may be pursued as negative reinforcement. However, if people can derive pleasure from unpleasant emotions, they may be motivated to experience unpleasant emotions as a form of *positive reinforcement*. At this point, this possibility is highly speculative and, if supported, could lead one to question basic assumptions in emotion research. Nonetheless, we believe it is worth exploring at least tentatively. Could pain ever be pleasant?

Masochism is generally viewed as the tendency to derive pleasure from one's own pain (e.g., Glick & Meyers, 1988). If some people derive pleasure from physical pain, might it be that some people can also derive pleasure from emotional pain? To the extent that some people find fear, sadness, or anger pleasant to some extent, they may be motivated to experience such emotions as a form of reward. Some support for these ideas comes from research on emotions derived from art and entertainment. For instance, Andrade and Cohen (2007) found that the more intense the fear participants experienced when watching horror films, the more pleasure they reported deriving from it. Similar propositions have been made in the context of preferences for sad music (e.g., Huron, 2011; Schubert, 1996). These findings suggest that fear and sadness may be pleasant in certain contexts. Therefore, at least in these contexts they may be rewarding. It remains to be tested whether, when, and for whom personally relevant, naturally occurring unpleasant emotions elicit pleasure, and, if they do, whether they are pursued for that reason.

SHOULD PEOPLE PURSUE UNPLEASANT EMOTIONS?

Our understanding of emotion regulation has advanced dramatically in the last few decades, and this has been particularly pronounced in the study of motives in emotion regulation. Whereas research initially focused only on cases in which people want to increase pleasant emotions and decrease unpleasant ones, it is now evident that there is a broad range of motives in emotion regulation that can lead people to increase unpleasant emotions or decrease pleasant ones. In this chapter, we highlighted the main categories of motives for doing so. We also reviewed the empirical literature, which is relatively extant with respect to some motives (e.g., instrumental) but scarce with respect to others (e.g., hedonic). Although there is a growing number of studies that examine contrahedonic emotion regulation, such studies are still few and far between. There are many motives that are yet to be empirically tested, and there are many questions that await empirical examination.

Perhaps the most important question that remains is whether contrahedonic emotion regulation is harmful or perhaps useful. Ultimately, the answer depends on how these motives are pursued and on the consequences of the experiences and behaviors they give rise to. From a psychological standpoint, the question can be answered by setting clear empirical standards for psychological health. On the one hand, following the principles set forth in DSM-5 (American Psychiatric Association, 2013), pursuing unpleasant emotions should be considered harmful when doing so leads to "significant distress or impairment in social, occupational, or other important areas of functioning." Certainly, there are cases in which the motivation to maintain or increase unpleasant emotions can lead to such impairments. For instance, if maintaining worry prevents people with generalized anxiety disorder from exposing themselves to the stimuli they fear, extinction would not be possible, and the disorder would be maintained (Borkovec et al., 2004).

On the other hand, following the principles set forth by certain theories of well-being (e.g., Seligman, 2011), pursuing unpleasant emotions should be considered useful when it leads to "engagement, positive relationships, meaning and purpose, and a sense of accomplishment." Certainly, there are cases in which the motivation to maintain unpleasant emotion can lead to such benefits. Maintaining some level of worry, for instance, can propel hard work and contribute to professional success and a sense of accomplishment (Perkins & Corr, 2005; see Perkins & Corr, Chapter 2, this volume). Therefore, we believe that contrahedonic emotion regulation can be either harmful or useful, depending on the specific case in question and on the context in which it occurs (for related arguments, see Coifman & Bonanno, 2010; Kashdan & Rottenberg, 2010).

From a philosophical standpoint, however, the question is more difficult to address. It brings us back to the debate between Aristotle and Epicurus, a debate that reverberates throughout the philosophical and scientific study of well-being. From an Aristotelian perspective, the pursuit of unpleasant emotions is desirable to the extent that it leads to excellence. From this perspective, pursuing unpleasant emotions can be right or wrong depending on its objective consequences. For instance, maintaining fear to avoid making mistakes at work may be good if it results in professional excellence. On the other hand, from an Epicurean perspective, the pursuit of unpleasant emotions is desirable to the extent that it leads to future pleasure. From this perspective, pursuing unpleasant emotions can be right or wrong depending on its subjective hedonic consequences. For instance, maintaining fear to avoid making mistakes at work is good if professional excellence leads to a sense of pride and accomplishment, but it may not be good to the extent that professional excellence comes at the cost of constant stress and worry. We leave the resolution of these issues in the trusted hands of philosophers.

ACKNOWLEDGMENTS

This work was supported by a National Science Foundation grant (No. SES 0920918) to Maya Tamir.

REFERENCES

Ackrill, J. L. (1973). *Aristotle's ethics*. London: Faber & Faber.
Alicke, M. D., & Sedikides, C. (Eds.). (2011). *Handbook of self-enhancement and self-protection*. New York: Guilford Press.
Andrade, E. B., & Cohen, J. D. (2007). On the consumption of negative feelings. *Journal of Consumer Research, 34*, 283–300.
American Psychiatric Association. (2013). *Diagnostic and statistical manual of mental disorders* (5th ed.). Arlington, VA: Author.
Augustine, A. A., Hemenover, S. H., Larsen, R. J., & Shulman, T. E. (2010). Composition and consistency of the desired affective state: The role of personality and motivation. *Motivation and Emotion, 34*, 133–143.
Barkley, R. A. (2004). Attention-deficit/hyperactivity disorder and self-regulation: Taking an evolutionary perspective on executive functioning. In R. F. Baumeister & K. D. Vohs (Eds.), *Handbook of self-regulation: Research, theory, and applications* (pp. 301–323). New York: Guilford Press
Batson, C. D. (1991). *The altruism question: Toward a social-psychological answer*. Hillsdale, NJ: Erlbaum.
Bonanno, G. A. (2001). Emotion self-regulation. In T. J. Mayne & G. A. Bonanno

(Eds.), *Emotions: Current issues and future directions* (pp. 251–285). New York: Guilford Press.

Borkovec, T. D., Alcaine, O., & Behar, E. (2004). Avoidance theory of worry and generalized anxiety disorder. In R. G. Heimberg, C. L. Turk, & D. S. Mennin (Eds.), *Generalized anxiety disorder: Advances in research and practice* (pp. 77–108). New York: Guilford Press.

Cameron, C. D., & Payne, B. K. (2011). Escaping affect: How motivated emotion regulation creates insensitivity to mass suffering. *Journal of Personality and Social Psychology, 100,* 1–15.

Campos, J. J., Frankel, C. B., & Camras, L. (2004). On the nature of emotion regulation. *Child Development, 75,* 377–394.

Chapman, A. L., Gratz, K. L., & Brown, M. Z. (2006). Solving the puzzle of deliberate self-harm: The experiential avoidance model. *Behaviour Research and Therapy, 44,* 371–394.

Cohen, J. B., & Andrade, E. B. (2004). Affective intuition and task-contingent affect regulation. *Journal of Consumer Research, 31,* 358–367.

Coifman, K. G., & Bonanno, G. A. (2010).When distress does not become depression: Emotion context sensitivity and adjustment to bereavement. *Journal of Abnormal Psychology, 119,* 479–490.

Davies, D. J. (2011). *Emotion, identity and religion: Hope, reciprocity, and otherness.* Oxford, UK: Oxford University Press.

Dickens, C. (1969). *Great expectations.* London: Heron Books. (Original work published 1861)

Eid, D., & Diener, E. (2001). Norms for experiencing emotions in different cultures: Inter- and intranational differences. *Journal of Personality and Social Psychology, 81,* 869–885.

Erber, R., Wegner, D. M., & Therriault, N. (1996). On being cool and collected: Mood regulation in anticipation of social interaction. *Journal of Personality and Social Psychology, 70,* 757–766.

Eskine, K. J., Kacinik, N. A., & Prinz, J. J. (2012). Stirring images: Fear, not happiness or arousal, makes art more sublime. *Emotion, 12,* 1071–1074.

Festinger, L. (1957). *A theory of cognitive dissonance.* Stanford, CA: Stanford University Press.

Fischer, A. H., Rodriguez Mosquera, P. M., van Vianen, A. E. M., & Manstead, A. S. R. (2004). Gender and culture differences in emotion. *Emotion, 4,* 87–94.

Ford, B. Q., & Tamir, M. (2012). When getting angry is smart: Emotional preferences and emotional intelligence. *Emotion, 12,* 685–689.

Franklin, J. C., Hessel, E. T., Aaron, R. V., Arthur, M. S., Heilbron, N., & Prinstein, M. J. (2010). The functions of nonsuicidal self-injury: Support for cognitive–affective regulation and opponent processes from a novel psychophysiological paradigm. *Journal of Abnormal Psychology, 119,* 850–862.

Fredrickson, B. L. (2000). Extracting meaning from past affective experiences: The importance of peaks, ends, and specific emotions. *Cognition and Emotion, 14,* 577–606.

Freud, S. (1952). *A general introduction to psychoanalysis.* New York: Washington Square Press. (Original work published 1920)

Frijda, N. (1986). *The emotions.* New York: Cambridge University Press.

Glick, R. A., & Meyers, D. I. (Eds.). (1988). *Masochism: Current psychoanalytic perspectives.* Hillsdale, NJ: Analytic Press.

Gottman, J. M., Katz, L. F., & Hooven, C. (1997). *Meta-emotion: How families communicate emotionally.* Mahwah, NJ: Erlbaum.

Greene, J. D., Sedikides, C., Barbera, J. M., & Van Tongerena, D. R. (2012). *Righteous anger and moral grandiosity.* Manuscript submitted for publication.

Groves, P. M., & Thompson, R. F. (1970). Habituation: A dual-process theory. *Psychological Review, 77,* 419–450.

Hackenbracht, J., & Tamir, M. (2010). Preferences for sadness when eliciting help: Instrumental motives in sadness regulation. *Motivation and Emotion, 34,* 306–315.

Halperin, E., Porat, R., Tamir, M., & Gross, J. J. (2013). Can emotion regulation change political attitudes in intractable conflict?: From the laboratory to the field. *Psychological Science, 24,* 106–111.

Halperin, E., Wayne, C., Porat, R., & Tamir, M. (2012, July). *Motivation to regulate emotion in political-conflict decision making: The role of accountability and beliefs about emotions.* Paper presented at the International Society of Political Psychology meeting, Chicago.

Hayes, S. C., Luoma, J. B., Bond, F. W., Masuda, A., & Lillis, J. (2006). Acceptance and commitment therapy: Model, processes and outcomes. *Behaviour Research and Therapy, 44,* 1–25.

Huntsinger, J. R., Lun, J., Sinclair, S., & Clore, G. L. (2009). Contagion without contact: Anticipatory mood matching in response to affiliative motivation. *Personality and Social Psychology Bulletin, 35,* 909–922.

Huron, D. (2011). Why is sad music pleasurable?: A possible role for prolactin. *Musicae Scientiae, 15,* 146–158.

Kahneman, D., Fredrickson, B. L., Schreiber, C. A., & Redelmeier, D. A. (1993). When more pain is preferred to less: Adding a better end. *Psychological Science, 4,* 401–405.

Kampfe, N., & Mitte, K. (2009). What you wish is what you get?: The meaning of individual variability in desired affect and affective discrepancy. *Journal of Research in Personality, 43,* 409–418.

Kashdan, T. B., & Rottenberg, J. (2010). Psychological flexibility as a fundamental aspect of health. *Clinical Psychology Review, 30,* 865–878.

Kim-Prieto, C., & Diener, E. (2009). Religion as a source of variation in the experience of positive and negative emotions. *Journal of Positive Psychology, 4,* 447–460.

Klonsky, E. D. (2007). The functions of deliberate self-injury: A review of the evidence. *Clinical Psychology Review, 27,* 226–239.

Kruglanski, A. W. (1996). Motivated social cognition: Principles of the interface. In E. T. Higgins & A. W. Kruglanski (Eds.), *Social psychology: Handbook of basic principles* (pp. 493–520). New York: Guilford Press.

Lane, A. M., Beedie, C. J., Devonport, T. J., & Stanley, D. M. (2011). Instrumental emotion regulation in sport: Relationships between beliefs about emotion

and emotion regulation strategies used by athletes. *Scandinavian Journal of Medicine and Science in Sports, 21,* 445–451.

Larsen, R. J. (2000). Toward a science of mood regulation. *Psychological Inquiry, 11,* 129–141.

Leonard, D. J., Moons, W. G., Mackie, D. M., & Smith E. R. (2011). We're mad as hell and we're not going to take it anymore: Anger, self-stereotyping and collective action. *Group Processes and Intergroup Relations, 14,* 99–111.

Mackie, D. M., Devos, T., & Smith, E. R. (2000). Intergroup emotions: Explaining offensive action tendencies in an intergroup context. *Journal of Personality and Social Psychology, 79,* 602–616.

Martin, L. L., & Clore, G. L. (Eds.). (2001). *Theories of mood and cognition: A user's guidebook.* Mahwah, NJ: Erlbaum.

Mayer, J. D., & Stevens, A. A. (1994). An emerging understanding of the reflective (meta) experience of mood. *Journal of Research in Personality, 28,* 351–373.

McCaul, K. D., Mullens, A. B., Romanek, K. M., Erickson, S. C., & Gatheridge, B. J. (2007). The motivational effects of thinking and worrying about the effects of smoking cigarettes. *Cognition and Emotion, 21,* 1780–1798.

McClelland, D. C. (1987). *Human motivation.* New York: Cambridge University Press.

Mischel, W., Shoda, Y., & Rodriguez, M. L. (1989). Delay of gratification in children. *Science, 244*(4907), 933–938.

Nelissen, R. M., & Zeelenberg, M. (2009). When guilt evokes self-punishment: Evidence for the existence of a Dobby effect. *Emotion, 9,* 118–122.

Oliver, M. B., & Raney, A. A. (2011). Entertainment as pleasurable and meaningful: Identifying hedonic and eudaimonic motivations for entertainment consumption. *Journal of Communication, 61,* 984–1004.

Parrott, W. G. (1993). Beyond hedonism: Motives for inhibiting good moods and for maintaining bad moods. In D. M. Wegner & J. W. Pennebaker (Eds.), *Handbook of mental control* (pp. 278–305). Englewood Cliffs, NJ: Prentice-Hall.

Perkins, A. M., & Corr, P. J. (2005). Can worriers be winners?: The association between worrying and job performance. *Personality and Individual Differences, 38,* 25–31.

Riediger, M., Schmiedek, F., Wagner, G. G., & Lindenberger, U. (2009). Seeking pleasure and seeking pain: Differences in prohedonic and contra-hedonic motivation from adolescence to old age. *Psychological Science, 20,* 1529–1535.

Rist, J. M. (1972). *Epicurus: An introduction.* Cambridge, UK: Cambridge University Press.

Robinson, M. D., & Clore, G. L. (2002). Belief and feeling: Evidence for an accessibility model of emotional self-report. *Psychological Bulletin, 128,* 934–960.

Rogers, C. R. (1951). *Client-centered therapy: Its current practice, implications, and theory.* Boston: Houghton Mifflin.

Ross, D. (1995). *Aristotle* (6th ed.). London: Routledge.

Rusting, C. L., & Larsen, R. J. (1995). Moods as sources of stimulation: Relationships between personality and desired mood states. *Personality and Individual Differences, 18,* 321–329.

Ryan, R. M., & Deci, E. L. (2001). On happiness and human potentials: A review of research on hedonic and eudaimonic well-being. *Annual Review of Psychology, 52,* 141–166.

Schubert, E. (1996). Enjoyment of negative emotions in music: An associative network explanation. *Psychology of Music, 24,* 18–28.

Schwarz, N., & Clore, G. L. (1983). Mood, misattribution, and judgments of well-being: Informative and directive functions of affective states. *Journal of Personality and Social Psychology, 45,* 513–523.

Seligman, M. E. P. (2011). *Flourish: A visionary new understanding of happiness and well-being.* New York: Free Press.

Shaver, P. R., & Mikulincer, M. (2007). Adult attachment strategies and the regulation of emotion. In J. J. Gross (Ed.), *Handbook of emotion regulation* (pp. 446–465). New York: Guilford Press.

Shaw, L. L., Batson, C. D., & Todd, R. M. (1994). Empathy avoidance: Forestalling feeling for another in order to escape the motivational consequences. *Journal of Personality and Social Psychology, 67,* 879–887.

Smith, E. R. (1993). Social identity and social emotions: Toward new conceptualizations of prejudice. In D. M. Mackie & D. L. Hamilton (Eds.), *Affect, cognition, and stereotyping: Interactive processes in group perception* (pp. 297–315). San Diego, CA: Academic Press.

Smith, E. R., Seger, C. R., & Mackie, D. M. (2007). Can emotions be truly group level?: Evidence regarding four conceptual criteria. *Journal of Personality and Social Psychology, 93,* 431–446.

Spinoza, B. (1982). *Ethics* (S. Shirley, Trans.). Indianapolis, IN: Hackett. (Original work published 1677)

Stearns, D. C., & Parrott, W. G. (2012). When feeling bad makes you look good: Guilt, shame, and person perception. *Cognition and Emotion, 26,* 407–430.

Swann, W. B. (1987). Identity negotiation: Where two roads meet. *Journal of Personality and Social Psychology, 53,* 1038–1051.

Swann, W. B., Stein-Seroussi, A., & Giesler, B. R. (1992). Why people self-verify. *Journal of Personality and Social Psychology, 62,* 392–401.

Tamir, M., & Ford, B. Q. (2009). Choosing to be afraid: Preferences for fear as a function of goal pursuit. *Emotion, 9,* 488–497.

Tamir, M., & Ford, B. Q. (2012). When feeling bad is expected to be good: Emotion regulation and outcome expectancies in social conflicts. *Emotion, 12,* 807–816.

Tamir, M., Ford, B. Q., & Gilliam, M. (2013). Evidence for utilitarian emotion regulation. *Cognition and Emotion, 27,* 483–491.

Tamir, M., Mitchell, C., & Gross, J. J. (2008). Hedonic and instrumental motives in anger regulation. *Psychological Science, 19,* 324–328.

Thomas, E. F., McGarty, C., & Mavor, I. (2009). Aligning identities, emotions, and beliefs to create commitment to sustainable social and political action. *Personality and Social Psychology Review, 13,* 194–217.

Thrash, T. M., & Elliot, A. J. (2001). Delimiting and integrating the goal and motive constructs in achievement motivation. In A. Efklides, J. Kuhl, & R. M. Sorrentino (Eds.), *Trends and prospects in motivation research* (pp. 3–21). Amsterdam: Kluwer Academic.

Tsai, J. L., Knutson, B., & Fung, H. H. (2006). Cultural variation in affect valuation. *Journal of Personality and Social Psychology, 90*, 288–307.

Tsai, J. L., Miao, F. F., Seppala, E., Fung, H. H., & Yeung, D. Y. (2007). Influence and adjustment goals: Sources of cultural differences in ideal affect. *Journal of Personality and Social Psychology, 92*, 1102–1117.

Van Kleef, G. A., Van Dijk, E., Steinel, W., Harinck, F., & Van Beest, I. (2008). Anger in social conflict: Cross-situational comparisons and suggestions for the future. *Group Decision and Negotiation, 17*, 13–30.

Vastfjall, D., & Garling, T. (2006). Preference for negative emotions. *Emotion, 6*, 326–329.

Vishkin, A., Bigman, Y., & Tamir, M. (in press). Emotion regulation and religion. In C. Kim-Prieto (Ed.), *Positive psychology of religion and spirituality across cultures*. New York: Springer.

Waterman, A. S. (1993). Two conceptions of happiness: Contrasts of personal expressiveness (eudaimonia) and hedonic enjoyment. *Journal of Personality and Social Psychology, 64*, 678–691.

Wood, J. V., Heimpel, S. A., Manwell, L. A., & Whitting, E. J. (2009). This mood is familiar and I don't deserve to feel better anyway: Mechanisms underlying self-esteem differences in motivation to repair sad moods. *Journal of Personality and Social Psychology, 96*, 363–380.

10

Negative Emotions and the Meaningful Sides of Media Entertainment

MARY BETH OLIVER
ANNE BARTSCH
TILO HARTMANN

The landscape of media entertainment is obviously broad and diverse, with variations in topics and themes wide enough to appeal to almost any person, regardless of disposition or personal experience. With this diversity in mind, though, the most typical characterization of media entertainment is arguably one that focuses on the trivial and superficial. That is, media entertainment is frequently understood in terms of providing viewers with silly slapstick comedies, banal melodramas, or, in more recent times, "reality" programs that depict human beings in what might be their lowest moments of greed, shamelessness, or vulgarity. In short, entertainment is often perceived to be a prime example of what might be called a "guilty pleasure."

To identify an activity as a "guilty pleasure" makes two assumptions, both of which seem apt in most discussions of media entertainment. First, the word *pleasure* seems to assume that the activity is associated with positive valence. Second, the word *guilty* implies that the activity has little or no value or that any value that may be present is short-lived, shallow, or

inconsequential. Together, then, the consumption of media entertainment as a guilty pleasure fits with popular (and many scholarly) views that characterize this activity as, though perhaps pleasurable, one with little intrinsic value or benefit (Postman, 1986).

In this chapter we do not want to argue against the general view of entertainment as a guilty pleasure. Rather, we do want to suggest that with this conceptualization in mind, there are many notable counterexamples. Specifically, it may seem odd to characterize many examples of valued films, epic poetry, plays, or even some television programs as "pleasures," as many of the most notable and prized forms of entertainment provoke feelings that are far from positively valanced. Likewise, these types of entertainment offerings likely elicit little to no "guilt," as they are perceived by individuals to be particularly intrinsically valuable or meaningful.

In short, although much entertainment undoubtedly consists of diversions that are pleasant but arguably shallow, there are numerous examples of entertainment that are notable and highly valued. Interestingly, these examples are ones that appear to give rise to more negative affective experiences—a phenomenon that has attracted considerable theorizing and speculation regarding the seemingly paradoxical nature of the "enjoyment" of "sad" entertainment (see, e.g., Zillmann, 1998). In this chapter, we provide an overview of such research, noting some of the primary means by which extant scholarship has tried to address this paradox. We then turn to our more recent work that shifts the focus to provide a greater emphasis on additional gratifications associated with meaningfulness, as well as the unique cognitive and affective components that appear to accompany this experience. We end our chapter by outlining potential directions for future research, including the need for greater attention to individual differences and state-like variations, the potential outcomes associated with the consumption of meaningful entertainment, and finally, the possible implications that newer media technologies may have for entertainment experiences.

THE PARADOX OF THE ENJOYMENT
OF TRAGIC ENTERTAINMENT

Although the subject of tragedy has a long and distinguished history of philosophical discussion (e.g., Aristotle, 1961), social science has only recently begun to explore this particular type of entertainment. Perhaps the lack of attention given to tragic entertainment is a reflection of the paradox that it presents. Namely, why do people enjoy entertainment that is designed to evoke negative emotions? Why do we spend money and leisure time on heart-wrenching stories when instead we could simply have a good

time using the abundant choice of fun and cheerful content that modern entertainment media make available to us at all times?

Mood Management

From a social science perspective, the paradox of tragedy is perhaps best illustrated in Zillmann and his colleagues' work on mood-management theory (Zillmann, 1988; Zillmann, 2000; Zillmann, Hezel, & Medoff, 1980). Briefly, this theory of selective exposure to media content is based on the assumption that hedonistic motivations govern much of human behavior. Acting in accord with hedonistic goals, people will choose entertainment that serves to enhance or prolong positive moods or that helps to terminate or diminish negative moods. More precisely, mood management-theory assumes that individuals prefer an intermediate level of arousal that is experienced as pleasant, compared with suboptimal levels of arousal such as boredom or stress. In addition to balanced arousal, mood-management theory highlights the appeal of positive valence and the absorption potential of strong emotions that can help distract individuals from ruminating on distressing thoughts. Empirical research has revealed abundant and robust support for the general propositions of this theory. For example, studies support the idea that individuals use media content to regulate suboptimal levels of arousal and that they show a preference for comedy when in negative mood states (for reviews, see Knobloch-Westerwick, 2006; Oliver, 2003).

Affective Disposition Theory

The hedonistic conceptualization of entertainment as pleasure is also echoed in affective disposition theory (Bryant & Miron, 2002; Raney, 2003; Zillmann & Bryant, 1986), another prominent model in entertainment research that focuses on viewers' *responses* to media content rather than on their *selection* of such content. This model argues that while viewing entertainment, individuals make moral judgments concerning the "goodness" or "badness" of the characters depicted. With these judgments in mind, viewers tend to experience the greatest level of positive affect when good outcomes occur for liked characters and when bad outcomes befall disliked characters. Research on disposition theory supports these assumptions across a variety of genres, suggesting that viewers experience the greatest level of enjoyment when the portrayed outcomes in media entertainment are perceived as "just" or "correct" (Raney & Bryant, 2002; Weber, Tamborini, Lee, & Stipp, 2008; Zillmann & Cantor, 1977).

Although the majority of media entertainment appears to conform to the good-person-wins–bad-person-loses formula, there are several genres

that deviate from this standard. Suspenseful entertainment is one such example, as these types of films typically feature portrayals of supposedly liked characters in distressing, if not horrifying, situations. In the case of the drama genre, the paradox is even more striking, given the numerous examples of popular movies that end on decidedly tragic notes (e.g., *Titanic, Gone with the Wind, Dancer in the Dark*). Not all sad films intend to leave viewers feeling melancholy or depressed. However, the substantial number of examples of films that conspicuously lack optimistic or cheerful conclusions suggest that many sad films or tearjerkers never intend to create positive affect but, instead, attempt to arouse feelings of sorrow or grief. Given the assumptions of mood-management theory, one would expect that negative affective reactions induced by viewing these types of tearjerkers would be inversely related to enjoyment, and therefore to exposure. However, this is clearly not the case. Further, and perhaps more seemingly at odds with mood-management predictions, some research suggests that attraction to sad or tragic entertainment is most pronounced when individuals are experiencing negative affect themselves—sad people preferring sad entertainment. For example, Mares and Cantor (1992) reported that among the lonely participants in their study, the greatest reported interest was in viewing negatively valenced entertainment, and particularly when the entertainment featured similar (i.e., older) characters. Likewise, Gibson, Aust, and Zillmann (2000) found that lovesick individuals showed a preference for love-lamenting pop songs.

Sad Films as Ultimately Positively Valenced

Perhaps one of the most common and straightforward approaches to address the paradox of individuals' attraction to sad entertainment is the concept of delayed gratification. In some cases, individuals may forgo hedonic gratifications in the present in the interest of future goals that promise even higher levels of positive mood or that serve to avoid or alleviate negative experiences. Thus the paradox may boil down to individuals' willingness to endure negative affect in the present as a necessary evil to gain future hedonistic rewards.

Excitation Transfer

Research on excitation transfer (Zillmann, 1980) provides an interesting example of how entertainment that is seemingly negative may ultimately be experienced in positive terms. Excitation transfer explains how negative affect experienced during suspenseful episodes when audiences are made to fear bad outcomes for liked characters can contribute to entertainment gratification, nevertheless. Based on Schachter and Singer's (1962)

two-factor theory of emotions, the concept of excitation transfer assumes that residual arousal that stems from the experience of empathic distress can spill over and can be reframed with positive thoughts and feelings when the suspenseful episode comes to a happy end. Thus excitation transfer can give rise to euphoric feelings that are characterized by high levels of both arousal and positive valence (for an overview, see Bryant & Miron, 2003). Given that such experiences of euphoric relief are relatively rare in everyday life, it seems plausible that individuals are willing to endure some level of empathic distress during exposure to sad or suspenseful entertainment in order to be rewarded with the experience of excitation transfer at the happy end. Some sad movies have a narrative structure that seems to promote excitation transfer, such as *The Piano*, for example, in which the heroine nearly drowns attached to her sinking piano but narrowly manages to escape harm. However, as noted before, a number of sad films end on more tragic or even depressing notes.

Downward Social Comparison

Another example of how "sad" entertainment may elicit positive valance is via downward social comparison. Based on Festinger's (1954) theory of social comparison, Mares and Cantor (1992) hypothesized that, rather than avoiding negatively valenced portrayals that remind them of their own problems (as suggested by mood-management theory), individuals may find comfort and gratification in such content because it shows that others are worse off than themselves. In line with this reasoning, Mares and Cantor (1992) predicted and found that among older viewers, lonely individuals preferred a film about a lonely old man, whereas their counterparts who were not lonely preferred a film about a happy and well-integrated old man. Of particular note, the mood states of lonely individuals was improved after exposure to the film about the lonely old man, whereas the opposite was true for nonlonely participants (Knobloch, Weisbach, & Zillmann, 2004; Nabi, Finnerty, Domschke, & Hull, 2006).

In sum, excitation transfer and social comparison suggests that individuals' exposure to negatively valenced media content may, under some circumstances, result in positive affect. Against the background of these findings, it seems plausible that viewers take the experience of negative affect into account as a necessary evil to obtain a desired outcome, such as excitation transfer at the happy end, or the opportunity to engage in downward comparison with the deplorable fate of a character who is worse off than themselves. It is important to note in this context that individuals need not be consciously aware that they expect a specific, hedonically pleasant outcome resulting from their media-selection behavior. As Zillmann and Bryant (1986) have argued, selective exposure to media content

can be driven by implicit learning processes such as operant conditioning or reinforcement learning. If a certain behavior, such as watching sad or suspenseful films, has been repeatedly rewarded with hedonically positive outcomes in the past, then this behavior will be reinforced and will serve as an implicit motivation for future entertainment choices.

Meta-Emotions

A related concept that deals with the conditions under which the experience of sad films can be ultimately positively valenced is the notion of meta-emotions, or the meta-experience of mood (cf., Bartsch, Vorderer, Mangold, & Reinhold, 2008; Oliver, 1993; Schramm & Wirth, 2010). Mayer and Gaschke (1988) define meta-mood as "the possible outcome of a regulatory process that monitors, evaluates, and changes mood" (p. 109). This concept has attracted particular interest in sad-film research because it provides a theoretical description of individual differences in the experience of sad films (Bartsch, Appel, & Storch, 2010; Oliver, 1993). For some viewers, the monitoring and evaluation of their own sadness may be associated with positive thoughts and feelings, leading them to embrace and sustain the sad experience, whereas other viewers might be uncomfortable with the experience of sadness, leading them to avoid or suppress such feelings. Consistent with this line of reasoning, Oliver (1993) found that among individuals who scored high on a measure of preference for sad films, sadness and enjoyment of a sad movie were positively related; in contrast, sadness and enjoyment were inversely related for individuals scoring low on the measure of sad-film preference (see also Mills, 1993).

Bartsch et al. (2008; cf., Schramm & Wirth, 2010) have recently argued that meta-emotions can be explained within the general framework of appraisal theories of emotion (Lazarus, 1991; Scherer, 2001). Through the lens of appraisal theories, it seems that emotions can be appraised using the same set of appraisal criteria that are usually applied to environmental situations: Is the emotion novel? Is it pleasant? Is it goal conducive? Is it controllable? Is it normatively adequate? Is it in accord with the person's self-ideal? Based on these appraisals, meta-emotions can be understood as affective reactions about the primary emotion. For example, some viewers may enjoy a "good cry" because they appraise the emotion as pleasant and normatively adequate, whereas others embarrassedly wipe off a tear because they appraise their sadness as a loss of control that is incompatible with their self-ideal. Again, viewers need not be consciously aware that they are making these kinds of judgments about their own feelings. In line with general appraisal theories of emotion (Lazarus, 1991; Scherer, 2001), emotion-eliciting appraisals can also be based on implicit schemata and reinforcement learning.

Such a broader conceptualization of meta-emotions in terms of appraisal theories does not contribute to solving the sad-film paradox in a direct manner, because this framework leaves open the question of why and under what conditions feelings of sadness can be associated with positive appraisals. To provide more detailed explanations of the appeal of tragic entertainment, meta-emotions need to be broken down to domain-specific appraisal processes. For example, models that employ concepts associated with delayed gratification (such as excitation transfer) might help explain appraisals via goal conduciveness, whereas gender stereotypes concerning the appropriateness of displays of sadness in response to sad entertainment (cf., Oliver, 1993; Mills, 1993) might explain appraisals via normative adequacy. What is most helpful about the theoretical framework of meta-emotions, perhaps, is that it draws attention to the diversity of appraisal processes that can transform the predominantly negative valence of sadness into something more positive, or even desirable. Thus the concept of meta-emotions has contributed to a theoretical integration of earlier work on the sad-film paradox, and it has paved the way for more recent approaches that focus on nonhedonistic gratifications, such as individuals' sense of meaning and purpose in life.

RECONCEPTUALIZING THE ENJOYMENT OF SAD ENTERTAINMENT

Past approaches trying to solve the paradox of sad emotions in entertainment deserve merit, because they have illuminated how sadness experienced during film exposure may be turned into enjoyment. However, enjoyment—or hedonistic pleasure—may neither be the sole nor the primary reason that viewers find sad movies gratifying. Similarly, sadness experienced during entertainment exposure may not be gratifying only if it is turned into enjoyment but may be gratifying for other reasons. Obviously, some films provide nonhedonistic entertainment experiences that users still perceive as gratifying. It may be odd to say, for example, that viewers typically enjoy tragic or disturbing movies such as The Piano or Schindler's List. Obviously, many people endorse these and similar movies for reasons that are not sufficiently captured by the concept of enjoyment.

Accordingly, scholars have started to broaden the notion of the entertainment experience by moving beyond hedonistic pleasure and exploring emotionally ambivalent, meaningful, and thought-provoking experiences that are typically triggered by film genres such as drama, tragedies, war movies, or documentaries (Oliver, 2003, 2008; Oliver, Ash, & Woolley, 2012; Oliver & Bartsch, 2010, 2011; Oliver & Hartmann, 2010; Oliver, Hartmann, & Woolley, 2012; Oliver & Raney, 2011; Schramm &

Wirth, 2010; Wirth, Hofer, & Schramm, 2012). Specifically, much of the recent theorizing in entertainment psychology draws a distinction between hedonic motivations and gratifications that tend to be associated with positive affect and *eudaimonic* motivations that tend to be associated with greater insight and psychological well-being (Ryan & Deci, 2001; Ryff, 1989; Waterman, 1993). Oliver and Bartsch (2010, 2011) summarized viewer responses that are akin to eudaimonic considerations as gratifying experiences that entail painful sensations or inconvenient insights and that users, therefore, eventually *appreciate* rather than simply enjoy. Appreciation can be understood as a positive appraisal of "touching" or "moving" entertainment offerings that induce tender and ambivalent emotional states and leave viewers contemplating life's meaning. More specifically, Oliver and Bartsch (2010) defined appreciation as "an experiential state that is characterized by the perception of deeper meaning, the feeling of being moved, and the motivation to elaborate on thoughts and feelings inspired by the experience" (p. 76). Studies by Oliver and Bartsch (2010) showed that many types of movies may be capable of evoking appreciation responses in viewers, including even more sophisticated thriller movies or heartwarming comedies, but that appreciation is especially triggered by more serious content that is typical in drama, classics, or documentaries.

In this line of research, meaningfulness is generally thought to form the core cognitive underpinning of viewers' appreciation response. Users characterize movies that they appreciate as particularly moving and thought-provoking (Oliver & Bartsch, 2010). These qualities are also strongly linked to the finding that viewers report that such entertainment tends to result in long-lasting impressions (Oliver & Bartsch, 2010). Characteristics such as "thought-provoking" or "long-lasting impression" suggest that meaningful movies cognitively challenge their viewers and urge them to cope with partly distressful information or insights. The frequently troubling insights provided by meaningful movies often tap into fundamental principles of life (e.g., that all life is fleeting; that everybody has only one life; Oliver & Bartsch, 2011; Oliver & Hartmann, 2010). Very similar to the way people cope with existential crises such as fatal illnesses (Schwarzer & Knoll, 2003), movie viewers seem to cope with distressful information about life by engaging in sense-making activities, cognitive restructuring, and an integration of the distressful information into broader cognitive frameworks such as their worldview (Koltko-Rivera, 2004; Park & Folkman, 1997). This search for meaning may persist beyond the actual movie. To the extent that this search for meaning is successful, the negative affective valence associated with the distressful information may be reframed with positive thoughts and feelings. Accordingly, viewers may actively generate meaning to cope with distressful information, with their cognitive elaborations eventually making a movie meaningful. Meaningfulness,

then, implies a broadening of viewers' understanding of the self and the world. In this sense, meaningfulness also implies that viewers become wiser from the experience and, thus, psychologically grow into more mature persons (Allport, 1961; King, 2001).

This line of research also argues that viewers find entertainment meaningful that inspires them to contemplate about human poignancies and meaningful life questions. Movies such as tragedies or drama typically present distressing information about life. Coping with this information seems to trigger a search for meaning in viewers that often leads to the recognition of fundamentally beautiful aspects of life. As Schwarzer and Knoll (2003) noted, "By understanding the cause of an event, one may appraise its significance and what it symbolizes about one's life, often leading to existential reappraisals of life and one's appreciation for it" (Schwarzer & Knoll, 2003, p. 403). Although systematic content analyses are missing to date, it seems reasonable to argue that this pattern is also greatly supported by the narratives of most meaningful movies. Although they often lack a happy ending, meaningful movies do not portray the world as entirely bad and life as entirely pointless but refer to the beauty of life and the human condition as well (e.g., by portraying exemplars of moral excellence; Oliver, Hartmann, & Woolley, 2012). In a study by Oliver and Hartmann (2010), viewers were asked to freely recall important insights they gained from watching either their favorite pleasurable or meaningful movie. The study found that most viewers in the pleasurable-film condition struggled to identify insights they found very important, whereas viewers in the meaningful-film condition reported that the movie made them aware of the uniqueness and beauty of life, recalled important (prosocial) values and human virtues, and highlighted the importance of keeping faith despite the deficiencies of life. In a similar approach, Wirth et al. (2012) adapted Ryff and Singer's (2004) model of eudaimonic well-being to explore viewers' experiences of meaningful movies. Their study found support for five different types of meaningful insights that viewers derive from movies, including a sense of purpose in life and self-acceptance, insights about autonomy, competence and personal growth, relatedness, and the activation of central values. Despite the fact that the authors applied a sad-movie stimulus in their study (*Hotel Rwanda*), participants reported primarily positive meaningful insights about life that they attained from watching the movie.

If meaningfulness is the core cognitive underpinning of the appreciation response, ambivalent affective states and mixed emotions have been found to be its characteristic affective aspects. Although meaningful experiences frequently entail sadness, they are also associated with the simultaneous experience of positive emotions such as joy or happiness (Ersner-Hershfield, Mikels, Sullivan, & Carstensen, 2008; Larsen, McGraw, &

Cacioppo, 2001). Accordingly, viewers of meaningful movies can feel happy and sad at the same time (Larsen & McGraw, 2011). In a series of studies, Larsen and colleagues (Larsen & McGraw, 2011; Larsen et al., 2001) found that participants reported mixed emotions of happiness and sadness after watching the tragicomedy *Life Is Beautiful*. Likewise, Oliver, Limperos, Tamul, and Woolley (2009) reported that viewers' meaningful responses (e.g., moved, tender, contemplative) to entertainment media were associated with the experiencing of both happy and sad affect simultaneously (see also Oliver & Bartsch, 2010; Oliver & Hartmann, 2010; Oliver, Hartmann, & Woolley, 2012).

Illuminating the discrete emotions underlying mixed affective states of viewers of meaningful movies is a more tedious—and to date not fully accomplished—empirical task. Meaningful experiences of viewers and related contemplative, introspective, or meditative states seem to be accompanied frequently by a complex blend of poignant and tender emotions and a general sense of being moved or touched (Oliver, 2008; Oliver & Raney, 2011). These features closely resemble what Fosha (2000) describes as "healing affects" in a therapeutical context. Fosha introduces the term to address positive therapeutical experiences of patients who "feel moved, touched, and strongly emotional, on the one hand, and love, gratitude, and tenderness on the other" (p. 171). The striking similarity between the affective connotations of the appreciation response and healing affects suggests that meaningful movies have a cathartic or therapeutic effect on their viewers (Scheele & DuBois, 2006). Feeling "moved" and "touched" appear to be two specific sensations of the cathartic or therapeutic experience.

One discrete emotion that has received particular attention in the context of meaningful entertainment is elevation (Oliver, Ash, & Woolley, 2012; Oliver, Hartmann, & Woolley, 2012). Elevation belongs to a class of other-praising affective states and is elicited in response to witnessing acts of moral excellence or "manifestation[s] of humanity's higher or better nature" (Haidt, 2003). Algoe and Haidt (2009) showed that elevation is associated with concrete physiological symptoms such as feelings of warmth and openness in one's chest, but also chills and goosebumps. Further, when feeling elevated, people are more inclined to follow prosocial behavioral tendencies. The narratives of most meaningful movies, such as *Hotel Rwanda*, address struggles of exemplars of moral excellence in a mean-spirited or life-denying world. Accordingly, many movies that induce meaningful affect in viewers may also hold the potential to elevate viewers. A recent study by Oliver, Hartmann, & Woolley (2012) examined this assumption and found that portrayals of moral virtue in films indeed elicited meaningful affect and physiological symptoms associated with elevation among viewers and also resulted in prosocial motivational outcomes.

An important yet to date understudied question is why viewers of

meaningful entertainment experience mixed affect. One explanation is that meaningful entertainment causes viewers to confront distressing information about life that induces negative affect. Viewers may successfully cope with these insights by turning them into meaningful information and thus may experience parallel positive affect. The same mechanism, accompanied by similar blends of mixed affective states, has been observed among individuals coping with a major real-life crisis, for example, a serious illness (Spiegel, 1998). An alternative explanation for the mixed affect experienced by viewers grows out of theorizing concerning the experience of poignancy, a mixed emotional experience that occurs in the face of "no longer having something that one once had" (Ersner-Hershfield et al., 2008). From this perspective, viewers may derive the uplifting insight from meaningful entertainment that their lives are unique, special, if not beautiful—but at the same time finite. The awareness that life is fleeting may trigger mixed affective states. A related explanation is that meaningful movies such as *Hotel Rwanda* often contrast the portrayal of an ill-spirited or life-denying world with exemplars of human beauty or virtue. Thus meaningful movies may not only induce negative affect such sadness or grief but may also evoke parallel layers of uplifting emotions such as elevation or hope. Future research is necessary, however, to fully understand the precise mechanisms underlying the mixed affect of viewers' appreciation response.

In summary, the proposed concept of appreciation broadens the perspective on media entertainment and provides another plausible solution to the sad-movie paradox. According to the approach, users may not enjoy sad movies, but they appreciate meaningful movies that focus on the human condition. Viewers' affective responses to meaningful movies are complex, and sadness may be just one voice in the concert of mixed affect that viewers of meaningful movies experience. Many meaningful movies, especially dramas or tearjerkers, confront viewers with inconvenient truths about life in general and the "self in the world." These insights may induce negative affect that viewers need to cope with. They may do so by searching for meaning and integrating their insights into general meaning structures. Meaningful movies usually assist viewers' search for meaning by portraying exemplars of human beauty that may elicit hope and elevation. Together, these factors may explain why mixed affect, tender affective states, and uplifting emotions such as elevation are typical affective states reported by viewers of meaningful movies.

ADDITIONAL QUESTIONS REGARDING THE USE OF TRAGIC AND MEANINGFUL ENTERTAINMENT

The idea that the *enjoyment* of *sad entertainment* may be frequently reconceptualized in terms of the *appreciation* of *meaningful entertainment* is a

potentially fruitful way of addressing seeming paradoxes noted in extant research. However, this particular approach to understanding media entertainment is arguably only newly recognized—at least among media psychologists. As a result, this approach requires a great deal of additional research to better explicate the experience of meaningful-entertainment consumption. This final section considers three potential avenues that future scholarship may find fruitful in the examination of both tragic and meaningful content: (1) the conditions that may heighten the appreciation of tragic and meaningful entertainment; (2) the outcomes that may occur as a result of these experiences; and finally (3) the implications of a rapidly changing media landscape for opportunities to engage with meaningful content.

What Gives Rise to the Appreciation of Tragic and Meaningful Entertainment?

We note that the diversity of media entertainment illustrates that there is considerable variation in entertainment preferences. Of course, this variation implies that not all individuals appreciate meaningful entertainment to the same extent or that they even perceive a given entertainment offering as meaningful to the same degree. Importantly, too, in addition to variations that may reflect individual differences or more stable, trait-like characteristics, variations in media preferences also undoubtedly reflect state-like preferences, with a given individual more interested in sad or meaningful entertainment at one given moment than at another. We believe that these variations are worthy of our research attention, not only because they provide one means by which measures of entertainment preferences can be validated but also because they encourage the expansion and development of theory that may be important in our understanding of how media entertainment and meaningfulness intersect.

Trait-Like Predictors of Entertainment Preference

The list of potential individual characteristics that predict entertainment preferences is seemingly endless (for a review, see Krcmar, 2009). However, sad films, or tearjerkers in particular, seem to readily suggest some potentially important predictors, albeit ones that may reflect stereotypical assumptions. In particular, sad films and more sentimental dramas are so strongly associated with female viewers that the phrase "chick flicks" is commonly employed to identify this particular class of entertainment. Although this phrase may signify a hint of condescension or dismissiveness, it does seem to capture what appears to be an enduring preference among females for entertainment that focuses on the sorrowful or even tragic plights of characters that are frequently (though not always) female

(e.g., *Steel Magnolias*, *The Notebook*, *Love Story*). The specific reasons that these films hold greater appeal for females than for males is not completely understood. One possible explanation previously mentioned in this chapter is that displays of sadness are generally less acceptable for male than female viewers, and hence male viewers ultimately come to associate entertainment in this genre with social sanctions (Oliver, 1993). An alternative possibility is that male viewers would actually appreciate these types of films were they to feature situations that were relevant to them. Consistent with this argument, Oliver, Weaver, and Sargent (2000) found that gender differences in reported interest in sad films was nonexistent for films described as portraying characters in contexts such as sporting competitions. Consequently, although existing research points to gender as an important predictor of preference for sad films, this conclusion should be tempered to acknowledge that male viewers may actually also find sad films gratifying if the narrative is relevant or *meaningful* to them (e.g., *Brian's Song*, *Platoon*, *Saving Private Ryan*).

In addition to demographic-like characteristics that serve to predict entertainment preferences, individuals' dispositional traits also undoubtedly play important roles. For example, meaningful entertainment, particularly when it is relevant to the self, likely provides viewers with the opportunity to make greater connections between entertainment narratives and issues or questions about life meanings that may be particularly salient. Of course, not all individuals may find gratification in contemplating meaning-in-life questions but instead may take comfort in ignoring such issues or in focusing their attention on issues that may be more hedonically positive. In contrast, other individuals may find gratification in grappling with life questions, even if such contemplations may be associated with melancholia or even existential angst. Consistent with this reasoning, Oliver and Raney (2011) reported a host of individual-difference variables associated with greater eudaimonic motivations for entertainment consumption. For example, eudaimonic motivations were associated with higher levels of need for cognition, a finding suggesting that meaningful entertainment may be particularly cognitively challenging and/or thought-provoking. Similarly, greater tendencies to search for meaning in life and higher levels of reflectiveness were associated with eudaimonic entertainment preferences—suggesting that viewers can turn to entertainment as a means of contemplating questions of life's purpose. Finally, higher levels of need for affect were associated with interest in meaningful media—suggesting that viewers' responses to these forms of entertainment have an important affective component.

Of course, the study of trait-like dispositions that predict greater appreciation of meaningful entertainment has examined only a very small slice of the variables that undoubtedly play consequential roles in viewers'

responses. Future scholarship that examines additional variables such as age, culture, life experiences, or even moral values, would undoubtedly provide a clearer and more complete picture.

State-Like Predictors of Entertainment Preference

It is important to note that entertainment preferences not only vary *between* individuals but also *within* individuals at different points in time. That is, a given person may prefer to watch a comedy at one time but a tragedy at another. As a consequence, examining the intraindividual variances in preferences for sad and/or meaningful entertainment may help to provide a greater understanding of how these experiences function for individuals in their day-to-day lives.

Perhaps the most frequently studied state-like predictor of entertainment preference is mood or affect. As mentioned previously, mood-management theory has generally suggested that mood is a consequential predictor, as individuals will select entertainment that will serve the hedonistic goals of terminating negative moods or enhancing positive moods (Zillmann, 2000).

In contrast, how mood functions in the preference for more *meaningful* entertainment consumption is not adequately studied at this point. However, some recent and emerging research points to the idea that affective variables may play important roles in predicting the desire to consume entertainment that is more somber or poignant. For example, Oliver (2008) reported that feelings of tenderness (e.g., tenderness, sympathy, compassion) were associated not only with the desire to view sad films or tragedies but also with a desire to view any more serious entertainment that featured storylines pertaining to human drama. In subsequent research, Oliver and her colleagues argued that prior research suggesting that sadness gives rise to preferences for sad entertainment might be better described in terms of mixed-affective states (e.g., tenderness, compassion, poignancy) that give rise to a desire to view entertainment that elicits similar mixed-affective responses (Oliver et al., 2009).

Although the scant research that has been conducted on affective predictors points to their importance in the selection of meaningful entertainment, this research has failed to fully consider the circumstances that give rise to the affective predictors in the first place. As such, although affect may be the most proximate predictor of entertainment choice, more distal predictors may provide greater explanation and theoretical depth. For example, some research from a terror-management perspective (Greenberg, Solomon, & Pyszczynski, 1997) implies that mortality salience may be potentially fruitful variable to explore. Consistent with this reasoning, Goldenberg, Pyszczynski, Johnson, Greenberg, and Solomon (1999)

reported that priming thoughts of mortality led to greater emotional responses to tragic literary excepts. These authors interpreted their findings as suggesting that tragedy helps individuals confront their own fears of death. Although such an interpretation is plausible, measures of fear or anxiety were not accessed in this study. Consequently, additional interpretations may be possible. For example, thoughts of one's own death may be associated with feelings of greater reflection, poignancy, or tenderness, with these feelings giving rise to appreciation of tragic drama. Given the relative dearth of research examining the role of media in addressing feelings of existential angst, much more work is clearly warranted. The apparent frequency with which individuals turn to media such as music, poetry, films, and so forth in times of tragic reflection makes this direction of research particularly valuable.

What Are the Outcomes Associated with Entertainment Consumption?

The previous discussion of how tragic or meaningful media may help address individuals' fears or viewers' questions regarding life meanings implies that the consumption of this form of content may have effects that go well beyond responses experienced only during the time of viewing itself. In this regard, we suggest that meaningful entertainment may have a host of important potential outcomes, some of which may pertain to viewers' thoughts and feelings about their own lives and some of which may pertain to viewers' perceptions of and behavior toward others.

In terms of the self, one possible effect of meaningful-media consumption is a heightened sense of reflection, introspection, or deliberation. The fact that higher levels of reflectiveness predict greater eudaimonic entertainment preferences is consistent with this argument. Further, popular notions of entertainment as "therapeutic" imply similar reasoning (Peske & West, 1999). Likewise, Zillmann (2000) employed the term *telic hedonism* to refer to the idea that viewers may be willing to experience negative affect from entertainment in the short run for the purposes of some future goal, including goals such as greater information or insight that may ultimately prove to be helpful (if not comforting) to viewers. However, systematic research on the mental health outcomes associated with entertainment is sorely lacking, though it appears to be gaining increasing acceptance among some therapists (Fleming & Bohnel, 2009). Certainly, research that tests for this particular type of outcome would be a valuable addition to media psychology.

Additional outcomes pertaining to perceptions of others have garnered much more study and are associated with greater empirical support.

Specifically, research on the role of elevation in eliciting feelings that humanity is generally "good," in heightening desires to help others, and in actually engaging in altruistic behaviors all point to the idea that meaningful media may have a particularly strong impact on individuals' interactions with other people (Algoe & Haidt, 2009; Schnall, Roper, & Fessler, 2010). It is worth noting that extant research growing out of media effects scholarship has traditionally examined the role of media (in particular television) in creating impressions of society as "mean and dangerous"—a phenomenon referred to as the "mean-world syndrome" (Gerbner & Gross, 1976). However, the potential for inspiring or meaningful entertainment—including sad or tragic entertainment—to facilitate feelings of greater connectedness and closeness to others suggests that some forms of media may do the opposite and, instead, result in effects that may stress perceptions of goodness and compassion—what may be aptly called a "kind-world syndrome."

Finally, we note that the potential for media portrayals to create greater connection with others may be a fruitful means of addressing pressing social harms. For example, campaigns designed to address issues such as bullying, abuse, or stigmatization may find it fruitful to contextualize their messages in narrative media that are particularly adept at eliciting feelings of elevation or compassion, even if such portrayals may simultaneously arouse negative emotions such as sadness or sympathy that frequently accompany meaningful affective responses. Although such reasoning has received some empirical support (Oliver, Dillard, Bae, & Tamul, 2012), additional research would provide a much clearer picture of the many mechanisms that play consequential roles and that may therefore be effectively harnessed for purposes of social good.

Implications of Newer Media

Throughout this chapter we have made reference to a variety of entertainment formats, including music, films, novels, and television. Though these media forms may likely represent the most typical types of entertainment for many people, we believe we would be remiss not to acknowledge that the media landscape is rapidly changing and thus presenting individuals with opportunities to engage with entertainment that may be substantially different than in the ancient and contemporary past.

First, we believe it is important to note that recent technological changes have not only increased the sheer number of entertainment opportunities but also changed the nature of the entertainment experience itself. Video games are perhaps the most obvious example of such changes, with almost half of all U.S. households owning at least one gaming console

(Entertainment Software Association, 2012). Although video games share many similarities with other forms of entertainment in terms of their ability to elicit enjoyment and to be used as a means of managing moods (Reinecke et al., 2012; Tamborini, Bowman, Eden, & Grizzard, 2010), they are qualitatively different from more traditional forms of entertainment in a variety of ways, including the degree of user interactivity that they require, as well as the types of emotions that they may elicit (e.g., guilt).

Whereas we may not be ready to fully endorse Roger Ebert's declaration that video games can never be considered high art (Ebert, 2010), we are intrigued with related questions posed by gamers and the gaming industry, such as "Can a video game make you cry?" The popularity of action, shooter, and sports games suggests that although video games may be able to elicit tears, the games that are played most frequently rarely do so. On the other hand, we also think it is interesting to consider how the technological variables unique to games (e.g., interactivity, presence) may play consequential roles in the extent to which games may have an enhanced opportunity to create meaningful experiences, including experiences that may elicit sadness in their portrayals of tragedy, in ways that surpass traditional forms of entertainment (Tamborini et al., 2010). Further, the growing popularity of video games that employ narrative formats, such as *Heavy Rain* or *Mass Effect*, may imply a greater movement toward video games that are as meaningful and moving to viewers as more traditional forms of entertainment, such as films or novels. Further, there is an emerging genre of educational games or "serious games," including titles such as *Darfur Is Dying*, that are designed to engage users with serious or even tragic aspects of reality in an interactive way (cf. Vorderer & Ritterfeld, 2009). Given the extent to which games represent an increasing share of the entertainment experience, we believe this direction of investigation is particularly timely and important.

An additional, new form of entertainment that may be particularly relevant concerns user-generated content (UGC). Unlike traditional forms of media entertainment, such as books, films, or television programs, UGC is not only created by users but also typically invites viewers or readers to share their reactions, to create their own written or video response, and to share the content with others. Hundreds of forms of UGC undoubtedly exist, including blogs, wikis, and discussion boards, among others, though perhaps the most salient example is YouTube—a video-sharing website that now hosts billions of videos (*www.youtube.com*). Although many of the videos available on YouTube reflect content taken from traditional media, such as television programs or films, many of the videos are created by amateur users who produce videos on topics ranging from music to comedy to narrative fiction.

There are several reasons why we believe that UGC may be a fruitful area of exploration for scholars interested in meaningful media or in content that may arouse tears. First, although many of the videos uploaded on YouTube are undoubtedly silly or banal, there are many notable examples of videos that are heartfelt and inspiring, if not moving or even tragic. Importantly, these videos appear to strike a chord with viewers, as many of them have gone "viral"—that is, have become very popular through the process of users sharing links via e-mail or social-networking sites. For example, the heartbreaking video by Ben Breedlove, a Texas teenager with a fatal heart condition, posted approximately a week before his death has generated upward of 7 million views, with individuals expressing their sorrow, condolences, feelings of inspiration, and shedding of tears (see *www.youtube.com/watch?v=tmlTHfVaU9o*). We believe that videos such as this, as well as many additional meaningful types of UGC (e.g., the "free hugs" campaign; see *www.youtube.com/watch?v=vr3x_rrjdd4*) may have the potential to be particularly powerful via user engagement, as users can participate by uploading their own video responses, by corresponding with other users regarding their reactions, or by creating their own, new postings that mimic, critique, or elaborate upon the content or the message. For example, the "It Gets Better" project, designed to provide support and hope to lesbian, gay, bisexual, and transgender (LGBT) youth, has generated thousands of user-generated video responses from individuals all over the world (*www.itgetsbetter.org*), many of which depict the suffering that numerous youths confront but that simultaneously provide messages of hope and optimism. Ultimately, because this new medium is widely used, quickly shared, and collaborative in design, we believe it holds promise of being a particularly interesting avenue of research among scholars of meaningful media, including media that feature messages of inspiration, sorrow, or questions regarding the human condition.

CONCLUSION

In thinking of media entertainment that elicits negative emotional responses, perhaps sad or tragic examples come to mind most readily. We recognize the importance of tragedy as an esteemed form of entertainment throughout human history. However, we also believe that the value that tragic entertainment holds for many people lies not only in its stories of heartbreak or sorrow but also in the insights it provides about questions concerning the human spirit. By recognizing the interplay between *sad* and *meaningful* entertainment, we hope that we have positioned ourselves not only to address many of the seeming paradoxes in extant theorizing but

also to shed light on opportunities to explore how meaningful entertainment may ultimately provide its users with insight into the human condition and our poignant yet fragile understanding of life's purpose.

REFERENCES

Algoe, S. B., & Haidt, J. (2009). Witnessing excellence in action: The "other-praising" emotions of elevation, gratitude, and admiration. *Journal of Positive Psychology, 4*(2), 105–127.

Allport, G. W. (1961). *Pattern and growth in personality.* New York: Holt, Rinehart & Winston.

Aristotle. (1961). *Poetics* (S. H. Butcher, Trans.). New York: Hill & Wang.

Bartsch, A., Appel, M., & Storch, D. (2010). Predicting emotions and meta-emotions at the movies: The role of the need for affect in audiences' experience of horror and drama. *Communication Research, 37,* 167–190.

Bartsch, A., Vorderer, P., Mangold, R., & Reinhold, V. (2008). Appraisal of emotions in media use: Toward a process model of meta-emotion and emotion regulation. *Media Psychology, 11,* 7–27.

Bryant, J., & Miron, D. (2002). Entertainment as media effect. In J. Bryant & D. Zillmann (Eds.), *Media effects: Advances in theory and research* (2nd ed., pp. 549–582). Mahwah, NJ: Erlbaum.

Bryant, J., & Miron, D. (2003). Excitation-transfer theory and three-factor theory of emotion. In J. Bryant, D. Roskos-Ewoldsen, & J. Cantor (Eds.), *Communication and emotion: Essays in honor of Dolf Zillmann* (pp. 31–59). Mahwah, NJ: Erlbaum.

Ebert, R. (2010, April 16). Video games can never be art. *Chicago Sun Times.* Retrieved from *http://blogs.suntimes.com/ebert/2010/04/video_games_can_never_be_art.html.*

Entertainment Software Association. (2012). *Essential facts about the computer and videogame industry.* Retrieved from *www.theesa.com.*

Ersner-Hershfield, H., Mikels, J. A., Sullivan, S. J., & Carstensen, L. L. (2008). Poignancy: Mixed emotional experience in the face of meaningful endings. *Journal of Personality and Social Psychology, 94,* 158–167.

Festinger, L. (1954). A theory of social comparison processes. *Human Relations, 7,* 117–140.

Fleming, M., & Bohnel, E. (2009). Use of feature film as part of psychological assessment. *Professional Psychology: Research and Practice, 40,* 641–647.

Fosha, D. (2000). *The transforming power of affect: A model of accelerated change.* New York: Basic Books.

Gerbner, G., & Gross, L. (1976). The scary world of TV's heavy viewer. *Psychology Today, 9*(11), 41–45.

Gibson, R., Aust, C. F., & Zillmann, D. (2000). Loneliness of adolescents and their choice and enjoyment of love-celebrating versus love-lamenting popular music. *Empirical Studies of the Arts, 18,* 43–48.

Goldenberg, J. L., Pyszczynski, T., Johnson, K. D., Greenberg, J., & Solomon, S.

(1999). The appeal of tragedy: A terror management perspective. *Media Psychology, 1*, 313–329.

Greenberg, J., Solomon, S., & Pyszczynski, T. (1997). Terror management theory of self-esteem and cultural worldviews: Empirical assessments and conceptual refinements. In M. P. Zanna (Ed.), *Advances in experimental social psychology* (Vol. 29, pp. 61–139). San Diego, CA: Academic Press.

Haidt, J. (2003). The moral emotions. In R. J. Davidson, K. R. Scherer, & H. H. Goldsmith (Eds.), *Handbook of affective sciences* (pp. 852–870). Oxford, UK: Oxford University Press.

King, L. A. (2001). The hard road to the good life: The happy, mature person. *Journal of Humanistic Psychology, 41*, 51–72.

Knobloch, S., Weisbach, K., & Zillmann, D. (2004). Love lamentation in pop songs: Music for unhappy lovers? *Zeitschrift für Medienpsychologie, 16*, 116–124.

Knobloch-Westerwick, S. (2006). Mood management: Theory, evidence, and advancements. In J. Bryant & P. Vorderer (Eds.), *Psychology of entertainment* (pp. 239–254). Mahwah, NJ: Erlbaum.

Koltko-Rivera, M. E. (2004). The psychology of worldviews. *Review of General Psychology, 8*, 3–58.

Krcmar, M. (2009). Individual differences in media effects. In R. L. Nabi & M. B. Oliver (Eds.), *Sage handbook of media processes and effects* (pp. 237–250). Thousand Oaks, CA: Sage.

Larsen, J. T., & McGraw, A. P. (2011). Further evidence for mixed emotions. *Journal of Personality and Social Psychology, 100*, 1095–1110.

Larsen, J. T., McGraw, A. P., & Cacioppo, J. T. (2001). Can people feel happy and sad at the same time? *Journal of Personality and Social Psychology, 81*, 684–696.

Lazarus, R. S. (1991). *Emotion and adaptation*. Oxford, UK: Oxford University Press.

Mares, M. L., & Cantor, J. (1992). Elderly viewers' responses to televised portrayals of old age: Empathy and mood management versus social comparison. *Communication Research, 19*, 459–478.

Mayer, J. D., & Gaschke, Y. N. (1988). The experience and meta-experience of mood. *Journal of Personality and Social Psychology, 55*(1), 102–111.

Mills, J. (1993). The appeal of tragedy: An attitude interpretation. *Basic and Applied Social Psychology, 14*(3), 255–271.

Nabi, R. L., Finnerty, K., Domschke, T., & Hull, S. (2006). Does misery love company?: Exploring the therapeutic effects of TV viewing on regretted experiences. *Journal of Communication, 56*, 689–706.

Oliver, M. B. (1993). Exploring the paradox of the enjoyment of sad films. *Human Communication Research, 19*(3), 315–342.

Oliver, M. B. (2003). Mood management and selective exposure. In J. Bryant, D. Roskos-Ewoldsen, & J. Cantor (Eds.), *Communication and emotion: Essays in honor of Dolf Zillmann* (pp. 85–106). Mahwah, NJ: Erlbaum.

Oliver, M. B. (2008). Tender affective states as predictors of entertainment preference. *Journal of Communication, 58*(1), 40–61.

Oliver, M. B., Ash, E., & Woolley, J. K. (2012). The experience of elevation: Responses to media portrayals of moral beauty. In R. Tamborini (Ed.), *Media and the moral mind* (pp. 93–108). New York: Taylor & Francis.

Oliver, M. B., & Bartsch, A. (2010). Appreciation as audience response: Exploring entertainment gratifications beyond hedonism. *Human Communication Research, 36*(1), 53–81.

Oliver, M. B., & Bartsch, A. (2011). Appreciation of entertainment: The importance of meaningfulness via virtue and wisdom. *Journal of Media Psychology: Theories, Methods, and Applications, 23*(1), 29–33.

Oliver, M. B., Dillard, J. P., Bae, K., & Tamul, D. J. (2012). The effect of narrative news format on empathy for stigmatized groups. *Journalism and Mass Communication Quarterly, 89*, 205–224.

Oliver, M. B., & Hartmann, T. (2010). Exploring the role of meaningful experiences in users' appreciation of "good movies." *Projections, 4*(2), 128–150.

Oliver, M. B., Hartmann, T., & Woolley, J. K. (2012). Elevation in response to entertainment portrayals of moral virtue. *Human Communication Research, 38*, 360–378.

Oliver, M. B., Limperos, A., Tamul, D., & Woolley, J. (2009, May). *The role of mixed affect in the experience of meaningful entertainment.* Paper presented at the annual meeting of the International Communication Association, Chicago.

Oliver, M. B., & Raney, A. A. (2011). Entertainment as pleasurable *and* meaningful: Identifying hedonic and eudaimonic motivations for entertainment consumption. *Journal of Communication, 61*, 984–1004.

Oliver, M. B., Weaver, J. B., & Sargent, S. L. (2000). An examination of factors related to sex differences in enjoyment of sad films. *Journal of Broadcasting and Electronic Media, 44*(2), 282–300.

Park, C. L., & Folkman, S. (1997). Meaning in the context of stress and coping. *Review of General Psychology, 1*, 115–144.

Peske, N. K., & West, B. (1999). *Cinematherapy: The girl's guide to movies for every mood.* New York: Dell.

Postman, N. (1986). *Amusing ourselves to death.* New York: Penguin Books

Raney, A. A. (2003). Disposition-based theories of enjoyment. In J. Bryant, D. Roskos-Ewoldsen, & J. Cantor (Eds.), *Communication and emotion: Essays in honor of Dolf Zillmann* (pp. 61–84). Mahwah, NJ: Erlbaum.

Raney, A. A., & Bryant, J. (2002). Moral judgment and crime drama: An integrated theory of enjoyment. *Journal of Communication, 52*, 402–415.

Reinecke, L., Tamborini, R., Grizzard, M., Lewis, R., Eden, A., & Bowman, N. D. (2012). Characterizing mood management as need satisfaction: The effects of intrinsic needs on selective exposure and mood repair. *Journal of Communication, 62*(3), 437–453.

Ryan, R. M., & Deci, E. L. (2001). On happiness and human potentials: A review of research on hedonic and eudaimonic well-being. *Annual Review of Psychology, 52*, 141–166.

Ryff, C. D. (1989). Happiness is everything, or is it?: Explorations on the meaning of psychological well-being. *Journal of Personality and Social Psychology, 57*, 1069–1081.

Ryff, C. D., & Singer, B. (2004). Ironies of the human condition: Well-being and health on the way to mortality. In L. G. Aspinwall & U. M. Staudinger (Eds.),

A psychology of human strengths: Fundamental questions and future directions for a positive psychology (3rd ed., pp. 271–287). Washington, DC: American Psychological Association.

Schachter, S., & Singer, J. (1962). Cognitive, social, and physiological determinants of emotional state. *Psychological Review, 69,* 379–399.

Scheele, B., & DuBois, F. (2006). Catharsis as a moral form of entertainment. In J. Bryant & P. Vorderer (Eds.), *Psychology of entertainment* (pp. 405–422). Mahwah, NJ: Erlbaum.

Scherer, K. R. (2001). Appraisal considered as a process of multilevel sequential checking. In K. R. Scherer, A. Schorr, & T. Johnstone (Eds.), *Appraisal processes in emotion* (pp. 92–120). New York: Oxford University Press.

Schnall, S., Roper, J., & Fessler, D. M. T. (2010). Elevation leads to altruistic behavior. *Psychological Science, 21*(3), 315–320.

Schramm, H., & Wirth, W. (2010). Exploring the paradox of sad-film enjoyment: The role of multiple appraisals and meta-appraisals. *Poetics, 38,* 319–335.

Schwarzer, R., & Knoll, N. (2003). Positive coping: Mastering demands and searching for meaning. In S. J. Lopez & C. R. Snyder (Eds.), *Positive psychological assessment: A handbook of models and measures* (pp. 393–409). Washington, DC: American Psychological Association.

Spiegel, D. (1998). Getting there is half the fun: Relating happiness to health. *Psychological Inquiry, 9,* 66–68.

Tamborini, R., Bowman, N. D., Eden, A. L., & Grizzard, M. (2010). Defining media enjoyment as the satisfaction of intrinsic needs. *Journal of Communication, 60,* 758–777.

Vorderer, P., & Ritterfeld, U. (2009). Digital games. In R. L. Nabi & M. B. Oliver (Eds.), *Sage handbook of media processes and effects* (pp. 455–467). Thousand Oaks, CA: Sage.

Waterman, A. S. (1993). Two conceptions of happiness: Contrasts of personal expressiveness (eudaimonia) and hedonic enjoyment. *Journal of Personality and Social Psychology, 64,* 678–691.

Weber, R., Tamborini, R., Lee, H. E., & Stipp, H. (2008). Enjoyment of daytime soap operas: A longitudinal test of affective disposition theory. *Media Psychology, 11,* 462–487.

Wirth, W., Hofer, M., & Schramm, H. (2012). Beyond pleasure: Exploring the eudaimonic entertainment experience. *Human Communication Research, 38,* 406–428.

Zillmann, D. (1980). Anatomy of suspense. In P. Tannenbaum (Ed.), *The entertainment functions of television* (pp. 133–163). Hillsdale, NJ: Erlbaum.

Zillmann, D. (1988). Mood management through communication choices. *American Behavioral Scientist, 31,* 327–340.

Zillmann, D. (1998). Does tragic drama have redeeming value? *Siegener Periodikum für Internationale Literaturwissenschaft, 16,* 1–11.

Zillmann, D. (2000). Mood management in the context of selective exposure theory. In M. E. Roloff (Ed.), *Communication yearbook* (Vol. 23, pp. 103–123). Thousand Oaks, CA: Sage.

Zillmann, D., & Bryant, J. (1986). Exploring the entertainment experience. In

J. Bryant & D. Zillmann (Eds.), *Perspectives on media effects* (pp. 303–324). Hillsdale, NJ: Erlbaum.

Zillmann, D., & Cantor, J. R. (1977). Affective responses to the emotions of a protagonist. *Journal of Experimental Social Psychology, 13,* 155–165.

Zillmann, D., Hezel, R. T., & Medoff, N. J. (1980). The effect of affective states on selective exposure to televised entertainment fare. *Journal of Applied Social Psychology, 10,* 323–339.

11

The Right Tool for the Job

Functional Analysis
and Evaluating Positivity/Negativity

JULIE K. NOREM

Marcia Ball is an American zydeco/blues singer and piano player. She and her band perform a rollicking version of a song called "The Right Tool for the Job" (author unknown). The lyrics to the first verse are:

> When I go to eat my dinner/I reach for my spoon and fork/When it's time to cut my steak/I make sure my knife is sharp./And if I need to hang a picture/I reach for a hammer and nails./And when I got to clean that floor/I get out a mop and pail./I don't like to waste my time/I make sure I got/The right tool for the job.

I can enthusiastically recommend the excellent piano and guitar work in Ball's recordings of this song. In the present context, however, my focus is on the ways in which the ideas in the song resonate with the purpose of this edited volume. The most obvious point in the song is that the appropriate tool varies according to the task at hand. The "right tool" metaphor is useful, because it points to questions concerning affect that our theories need to encompass. Specifically, given substantial evidence that both positive and negative affect can have both positive and negative effects, how do we understand when, where, and for whom different effects will occur?

In this chapter, I consider a specific approach to anxiety regulation—the strategy of defensive pessimism. This strategy involves combining the negative cognitive processes of pessimistic expectations and negative thinking with the negative affect of anxiety. Although it may seem counterintuitive, evidence supports the claim that defensive pessimism is an example of "the right tool" for those who are anxious and whose challenges include conflicting approach and avoidance motivations. Defensive pessimism is a coherent and effective tool that helps these individuals pursue their goals.

More generally, defensive pessimism illustrates how a functional approach to the study of affect and related processes and structures can highlight questions about the boundary conditions for the effects we study. Looking at what people are trying to accomplish and how a specific process functions toward those ends across different contexts reinforces our awareness that different goals are relevant for different individuals. Positive thinking does not help those who typically use defensive pessimism, and positive affect is not their highest priority outcome (Tamir, 2009; see Tamir & Bigman, Chapter 9, this volume). Positivity is not the right tool for them.

FUNCTIONAL VERSUS HEDONIC FOCI IN THE STUDY OF AFFECT

Though we may not always consciously use it in the same way that we swing a hammer or saw a board, in the context of evolutionary history and our current lives, affect is a tool that is integral to our adaptation. When it comes to specifics, there are different foci and points of contention among those who take a functionalist approach to affect; but, at their core, all functional perspectives emphasize that affect *does* something: affect has purpose or function (e.g., Gable & Harmon-Jones, 2010; Fridja, 1986; Panksepp, 2010; Parrott, 2002; Snyder & Cantor, 1998). It provides a signal, information, or input, or it may infuse our thinking in more subtle ways (Forgas, 1995). It influences the intensity and direction of our motivations (Gable & Harmon-Jones, 2010). Intra-and interpersonally, it is a defining part of the contexts and situations that we navigate in daily life.

Hedonic perspectives on affect—perspectives that focus on the motivational and behavioral implications of how emotions *feel*—tend to treat affect as an outcome; that is, as the result of a particular way of thinking or acting (e.g., Diener & Biswas-Diener, 2008; Eid & Larsen, 2008). That focus does not entirely ignore the function of affect, but it does emphasize affect as an end in itself. As well, it emphasizes efforts to avoid or decrease negative, "bad" affect and approach or increase positive, "good" affect. Yet the "right tool for the job" metaphor reminds us that the status of a given affect as "good" or "bad" cannot be known without taking into account

"the job"—and where it is being done, by and with whom, for what reason. In other words, a functionally oriented approach does not assume that experiencing positive affect is necessarily or exclusively good nor that experiencing negative affect is categorically bad. Instead, the implications and evaluations of both kinds of experiences are assumed to go beyond (and sometimes even be the opposite of) their hedonic value and to encompass other outcomes and dimensions of experience (Parrott, 1993; Tamir & Gross, 2011).

The specific chapters in this volume describe compelling research and important arguments about positive aspects of negative affect, as well as laudable nuance about the function of affect more generally. Beyond the significance of its individual parts, however, the volume as a whole represents an important counterweight to an overly hedonic focus. That counterweight—arriving as a critical mass in this book, rather than diffused across isolated instances—has been a long time coming.

SOME RECENT HISTORICAL CONTEXT FOR THE CONSIDERATION OF POSITIVE AND NEGATIVE AFFECT

American cultural sensibilities have long provided fertile ground for arguments about the benefits of positivity. Psychological research on optimism, positive illusions, self-enhancement, and positive coping were important foundations for what Forgas calls the "cult of positivity" (Chapter 1, this volume; see also Held, 2002). By the mid-1980s, work on both attributional[1] and dispositional optimism was already going strong (Peterson et al., 1982; Scheier & Carver, 1985). In addition, influential papers were published in which prominent researchers argued for the importance and universality of processes that protect the self from negative information (Greenwald, 1980) and the necessity of positive illusions to maintain self-esteem and buffer against depression (Taylor & Brown, 1988). Stress and coping research and health psychology were enjoying boom times. Negative affect (mild dysphoria and anxiety in particular) was viewed primarily as a risk factor or an outcome to be ameliorated or avoided.

There were, of course, voices protesting different aspects of what became a dominant position. Colvin and Block (1994), for example, argued vehemently that neither the progression of argument nor the evidence cited (and subsequently published) supported Taylor and Brown's (1988) proposition that positive illusions were fundamental in maintaining mental health. They rejected the assumption that "illusory" processes induced with specific laboratory tasks represented real-world processing and outcomes. They reviewed the contradictory evidence from available studies and discussed problems with some of the operational definitions used for

the terms *accurate, optimistic,normal,* and *healthy* (e.g., contrasts between the cognition of depressed psychiatric patients and the less accurate but more positive cognition of nondepressed psychiatric patients as evidence that positive illusions contribute to mental health; or a mean of 1.9 on a scale from negative expectations (1) to positive expectations (5) presented as "optimism").

There were some fascinating exchanges surrounding these basic propositions over the next few years (Block & Colvin, 1994; Colvin, Block & Funder, 1995; Taylor & Brown, 1994a, 1994b). In addition, some researchers continued to warn of the dangers of *unrealistic* optimism: Most notably, Weinstein (1980) and colleagues showed the negative health effects associated with that particular brand of positivity (see also Doan & Gray, 1992). Others challenged the idea of depressive realism, which had achieved status as a truism (e.g., Dunning & Story, 1991; Coyne & Gotlib, 1983). Nevertheless, these efforts seem to have had minimal impact on the belief, at least among social psychologists, that most nondepressed individuals use self-deception, self-enhancement, unrealistic optimism, and positive illusions to maintain self-esteem and a generally positive outlook and that the presence of those processes is essentially a sign of mental health.

Most of the debate that did occur concerned definitions and criteria for judging accuracy and the role of accurate self-perception in adaptation across contexts (e.g., John & Robins, 1994). The assumption that positivity in general was *a* "good" and that positive affect and positive thinking are "good" (healthy, normal, indicative of appropriate adaptation) was seldom questioned.

Into this context (ironically, it seemed to some of us) came the positive psychology movement (Seligman & Csikszentmihalyi, 2000). As widely promoted by then-American Psychological Association President Martin Seligman, need for the movement was justified by the claim that psychology as a field was overly focused on the negative—negative affect, negative thinking, and addressing the ills of individuals and society—as opposed to promoting virtues, strengths, health, and growth. Affective science—and particularly affective neuroscience—took off during roughly this same period. Fueled by both the energy of the positive psychology movement and the burgeoning interest in affect generally, the late 1990s and 2000s have seen an explosion of research on (and publication outlets for) positive affect and positivity (e.g., Frederickson, 2001).

Defensive Pessimism: How Many Negatives Does it Take to Make a Positive?

In this context, research on the concept of defensive pessimism began in the mid-1980s. In Nancy Cantor's lab at the University of Michigan, the

dominant theoretical perspective was a social-cognitive focus on how individual differences in ways of thinking about the self and situations would influence goal pursuit in daily life (Cantor, 1990; Cantor, Norem, Niedenthal, Langston, & Brower, 1987). One of the prototypical patterns that emerged from observation and interviews was called *defensive pessimism*. The label developed from the observation of pessimistic expectations among those who were doing well; for example, people who seemed pessimistic in order to guard against disappointment or otherwise motivate themselves as opposed to those who were pessimistic based on past negative experiences in a particular domain or a generally dour way of being. More colloquially, we looked around and saw a lot of salient examples of successful, likable people who were notably pessimistic about their own anticipated outcomes. Despite extensive published research proclaiming the advantages of optimism and the dangers of self-fulfilling prophecies among those who hold negative expectations, successful pessimists did not seem in short supply. That was interesting, and we began to study the operation and function of their brand of pessimism.

What Makes a Strategy?

Defensive pessimism is a motivated cognitive strategy (Norem, 1989; Showers & Cantor, 1985). Strategies describe coherent patterns of responses that unfold over time; that is, they describe processes rather than states or structures. In using the term *strategy*, we assumed that the patterns we observed served some function and that their coherence came from their relevance to an individual's goals.

Assuming function and coherence as part of a strategy does not require assuming that a strategy is effective. In thinking about this, we were inspired by research on self-handicapping, which revealed the "sense" in that strategy (Berglas & Jones, 1978). Self-handicapping is not coherent because it is necessarily effective; indeed, it can often be detrimental to performance, reputation, and health, especially over the long term. It does make sense, however, in the context of the goal of distancing oneself from the most negative implications of a poor performance. Preemptive self-handicapping provides less damaging alternatives to attributions of lack of ability, intelligence, or skill (or so those using the strategy appear to believe), and thus "makes sense" if the self-handicapper's goal is to avoid particularly damning conclusions that otherwise might be drawn from a poor showing.

People using defensive pessimism feel anxious as they anticipate a particular performance, task, or type of situation. Defensive pessimism is typically measured using the Defensive Pessimism Questionnaire–Revised (DPQ-R; see Norem, 2001, for psychometric, reliability, and validity information),[2] a 12-item self-report measure. The questions focus on

both expectations and the tendency to reflect on possible outcomes before approaching a goal. They can be tailored to a specific kind of task or domain of endeavor to generate domain-specific scores, and there is moderate domain specificity, with defensive pessimism scores averaging correlations of about .30 across domains. The DPQ-R correlates moderately and positively with trait and state measures of anxiety and less strongly but positively with more general measures of negative affective tendencies, such as Big Five neuroticism (e.g., Norem & Cantor, 1986a, 1986b; Norem, 2001; Wilson, Raglin, & Pritchard, 2002; see Perkins & Corr, Chapter 2, this volume, for other aspects of anxiety).

People using defensive pessimism are typically motivated both to approach success and to avoid failure (Cantor et al., 1987; Elliot & Church, 2003; Maatta, Nurmi, & Stattin, 2007; Yamawaki, Tschanz, & Feick, 2004). They are typically pessimistic about how they will do, often despite positive past outcomes in similar situations.[3] Following their negative expectations, they mentally rehearse negative possible outcomes prior to an event (Norem & Illingworth, 1993; Sanna, 1996). Thus the strategy begins with anxiety and motivational conflict, proceeds to pessimism, and then to negative mental simulations, or what we eventually called *reflectivity*. We hypothesized that defensive pessimism functions to help people harness their anxiety in productive ways. Mentally simulating possible negative outcomes involves a specific and concrete focus on what might happen, which in turn facilitates thinking about how (and working in order) to prevent negative outcomes.

Defensive Pessimism and Strategic Optimism

Initially, to explore the possible functions and coherence in defensive pessimism, we were most interested in contrasting those using defensive pessimism with people doing the "opposite." Drawing from research on optimism and self-protective attributions, we coined the term *strategic optimism*[4] to describe people who were optimistic and not anxious prior to a performance, task, or situation. We hypothesized that these individuals would not engage in thinking about possible negative outcomes prior to a particular situation[5] but would protect themselves after the fact from negative outcomes that could threaten their self-esteem by attributing them to bad luck or lack of control and enhance their self-esteem by claiming control over positive outcomes.

An early paper showed that people prescreened for use of defensive pessimism, who were indeed anxious and pessimistic, performed as well on laboratory tasks as people using strategic optimism (Norem & Cantor, 1986a). To us, this lack of performance difference was important in and of itself, because we interpreted the literature on expectations as strongly

predicting that those with more pessimistic expectations would, on average, perform more poorly.

In that same study, after their performance, we gave randomly assigned false-positive or false-negative performance feedback to our participants and found that people using defensive pessimism gave after-the-fact ratings of control and effort that did not differ by feedback condition, whereas those using strategic optimism reported more effort and more control in the positive feedback condition than in the negative feedback condition. The results for the strategic optimists, in other words, conformed to descriptions of self-serving biases that were supposed to be important to maintaining mental health among nondepressives (Miller & Ross, 1982). The defensive pessimists, however, did not show this self-serving attributional pattern (see also Newman, Nibert, & Winer, 2009).

Doomed by Negativity?

Given the focus at this time on research contrasting depressive with "normal" cognition, our results immediately raised the question of whether, despite their performance, people using defensive pessimism were "depressives in waiting." Given their lack of cognitive illusions to protect against negative feedback, surely they would eventually succumb under the triple threat of their negative affect (anxiety), negative expectations, and negative reflectivity. Further research showed, however, that the detailed, specific, and future-oriented negative reflections characteristic of defensive pessimism were notably different from the past-focused, repetitive, negative ruminations characteristic of depressives (Sanna, 1996; Showers, 1988; Showers & Ruben, 1990).

Our research goals were to show how defensive pessimism was different from strategic optimism and how defensive pessimism functioned with respect to the defensive pessimist's goals. The data showed that people using defensive pessimism performed as well as those using strategic optimism, did not use self-protective attributional maneuvers, yet did not seem to be at particular risk of depression—that is, that defensive pessimism was neither related to poor performance nor just another example of depression-related cognition. Simply differentiating defensive pessimism from strategic optimism and depressive or depressogenic cognition, however, does not greatly illuminate the function of defensive pessimism itself. That function can be more clearly seen by manipulating key features of the strategy.

Function of the Triple Threat: Anxiety, Pessimism, and Negative Thinking

Studies by multiple investigators have addressed each of the key negative features of defensive pessimism: anxiety, pessimism, and negative

reflectivity. These studies demonstrated that it was possible to put those using defensive pessimism into a positive mood, or to get them to be more optimistic in their expectations, or to get them to think more positively, or to distract them from thinking negatively about what would happen. In each case, however, doing so led to worse performance.

Encouraging those who use defensive pessimism raises their expectations, but they subsequently perform more poorly than those who are not encouraged and remain pessimistic (Norem & Cantor, 1986b). Experiments using mood inductions show that "cheering up" those who use defensive pessimism leads to less negative reflectivity but poorer performance and that naturally occurring negative mood is positively related to performance for those who use defensive pessimism (del Valle & Mateos, 2008; Norem & Illingworth, 2004; Sanna, 1998). Similarly, getting those who use defensive pessimism to think about positive possible outcomes instead of negative ones or exposing them to inductions meant to either relax or distract them also leads to performance decrements (Norem & Illingworth, 1993; Sanna, 1996; Showers, 1992; Spencer & Norem, 1996).

For example, Spencer and Norem (1996) randomly assigned defensive pessimists and strategic optimists to listen to one of three kinds of imagery tapes prior to a dart-throwing task: coping imagery, mastery imagery, or relaxation imagery. In the coping-imagery condition, participants listened to a description of the process of throwing a dart, during which problems arise: for example, the dart misses the board. The mastery-image tape, in contrast, described a series of perfect dart throws in fine detail. The relaxation-imagery tape was a prototypical description of slow, deep breathing and pleasurable sensations, unrelated to dart throwing. After listening to their imagery tapes, all participants played a dart-throwing game. Across conditions, there was no overall difference in performance between defensive pessimists and strategic optimists in this study. There was a significant interaction between imagery condition and strategy, however. Defensive pessimists scored highest in the coping-imagery condition, which was meant to mimic and thus accommodate or even facilitate their typical strategy. Their scores were significantly lower in the relaxation condition. Strategic optimists, in contrast, scored highest in the relaxation condition and significantly lower in the coping condition. Both groups scored lowest in the mastery condition; interestingly, this is the condition that most closely mimics general "positive thinking." Tomaya (2005) found a conceptually similar pattern in a study of Japanese junior high students: Defensive pessimists who did not use avoidant thinking performed better than those who did, whereas strategic optimists performed better when they used avoidant thinking (see also Gasper, Lozinski, & LeBeau, 2009).

Norem and Illingworth (1993) found a similar pattern in an experiment in which participants prescreened for use of defensive pessimism or strategic optimism were randomly assigned to either a reflectivity condition or a distraction condition prior to an arithmetic task. Participants in the reflectivity condition completed a thought-listing questionnaire that asked them to generate negative outcome scenarios for the upcoming task, whereas participants in the distraction condition were given an attention-demanding clerical task so that they would not be able to think about the upcoming task. All participants then worked on a set of arithmetic problems. There were no overall differences between the strategy groups in performance across conditions. Defensive pessimists, however, scored significantly higher in the reflectivity condition than in the distraction condition, whereas strategic optimists scored higher in the distraction condition than in the reflectivity condition. Further analyses showed that anxiety mediated these effects.

In a conceptual replication of this effect, an experience-sampling study of graduate nursing students showed that being prompted to think about the progress they were making toward their goals was related to reports of greater progress on important life tasks among defensive pessimists but reports of less progress among strategic optimists (Norem & Illingworth, 1993, Study 2).

These studies, then, demonstrate that the negativity of defensive pessimists is not incidental to what they are doing but integral to how they prepare or "psych up." Further evidence supports the argument that defensive pessimists are able to "harness"—that is, effectively use—their anxiety, at least on some tasks in some situations. Seery, West, Weisbuch, and Blascovich (2008) used physiological measures indicative of challenge versus threat appraisals to test defensive pessimists during task performance under different conditions. Following Spencer and Norem (1996), they assigned defensive pessimists and controls[6] to negative, positive, or control imagery conditions, using varying written prompts that required participants to elaborate on "what the experience would be like and what would happen" (Seery et al., 2008, p. 517). They found that defensive pessimists in the negative imagery condition had more correct attempts (a performance measure that gets at guessing strategies) relative to the other two conditions (with a nonsignificant reversal of that pattern among controls). In addition, cardiovascular changes among defensive pessimists indicated patterns more consistent with threat among those in the negative-imagery condition relative to defensive pessimists in the positive- or control-imagery conditions. Mediation analyses supported the "harnessing" hypothesis that increased threat appraisal following negative thinking led to use of an accuracy-focused performance strategy among defensive pessimists.

Defensive Pessimism as a Tool

In other words, defensive pessimism appears to function by amplifying and then channeling anxiety toward a particular problem-solving approach (one favoring accuracy over speed) under time-limited conditions. Seery and colleagues (2008) discuss the possibility that the physiological changes associated with threat appraisal may take a serious toll on health over time, a point to which I return later in this chapter.

They also emphasize that accuracy-oriented and speed-oriented approaches can lead to similar outcomes in some situations and that the efficacy of either approach will be a function of the task, as well as other parameters, which could include both situational and person factors. They are careful to note that their study, along with most experimental investigations of defensive pessimism, offered no opportunity for actual task-related preparation such as practice prior to the task performance.

Indeed, extant experimental research says relatively little about how defensive pessimism might influence specific preparatory behaviors over longer time courses. There is research, however, on "real-life" goal pursuit that shows that defensive pessimists tend to appraise their goals differently than more optimistic, less anxious individuals. As in laboratory settings, they are more anxious, feel less in control, and perceive more conflict among their goals than strategic optimists (Cantor et al., 1987; Eronen, Nurmi, & Salmela-Aro, 1998; Norem, 1989; Norem & Illingworth, 1993, Study 2; Norem & Andreas Burdzovic, 2007). In other words, defensive pessimists' appraisals of personally relevant goals in the context of daily life are similar to their appraisals in laboratory contexts.

Intriguing research also suggests that defensive pessimism may help anxious individuals prepare in real-world contexts. For example, defensive pessimists actively engaged in more preventative behavior prior to a predicted SARS outbreak in Singapore (Chang & Sivam, 2004). Schoneman (2002) found that socially anxious individuals who used defensive pessimism were more likely to approach real-world social interaction opportunities than socially anxious individuals who were more optimistic. African American students at predominantly white institutions who used defensive pessimism had significantly higher retention rates than other African American students at those institutions, according to a large-scale study of retention rates (Brower & Ketterhagen, 2004). A Finnish study found that, over a 2-year period, defensive pessimism was positively associated with academic achievement (Eronen et al., 1998). Garcia (1995) found that seventh graders who use defensive pessimism were significantly higher in volitional self-control than other students. Norem and Andreas Burdzovic (2007) found that over their years in college, female defensive pessimists showed significant increases in self-esteem relative to equally anxious women who

did not use defensive pessimism. Ntoumanis, Taylor and Standage (2010) found that defensive pessimism predicted intentions to pursue self-improvement in physical education, and Wilson and colleagues (2002) found that defensive pessimism predicted better performance among college track and field athletes at actual track meets.

Comparing Strategies: Different Tools for Different Jobs

Several studies have found that people using defensive pessimism achieve better outcomes than those using self-handicapping (Elliot & Church, 2003; Eronen et al., 1998; Martin, Marsh, & Debus, 2001, 2003; Rodriguez, Cabanach, Valle, Nuñez, & Gonzalez-Pienda, 2004). Results comparing people using defensive pessimism with those using self-handicapping are particularly revealing because both strategies are used by individuals who are situationally or dispositionally anxious (and equivalently so). Defensive pessimism and self-handicapping represent alternative strategies, but they provide tools for different aspects of the job of managing anxiety, and they vary in how effective they are relative to performance goals versus short-term hedonic goals. Those using defensive pessimism show stronger approach tendencies than those using self-handicapping; for example, although both groups fear failure, defensive pessimists have stronger performance approach goals, whereas self-handicappers have stronger performance avoidance goals (Elliot & Church, 2003). They are also more engaged in their achievement efforts (Maatta et al., 2007). This difference is important because anxiety can tempt people to avoid the situations that make them anxious, and if one cannot approach—that is, actively try to be involved with a task or situation—opportunities to improve are few. They can avoid diagnostic negative feedback, but their uncertainty and consequent tendency to avoid are likely to persist in an ongoing cycle. Given their stronger engagement and approach tendencies, it is not surprising that objective achievement (e.g., grade-point average) is also higher for defensive pessimists than for self-handicappers. On the other hand, self-handicappers may "succeed" in the sense that they protect themselves from undiluted negative feedback (by devising preemptive excuses) and avoid the acute anxiety of the fully engaged defensive pessimists, which may be especially intense as defensive pessimists engage in negative thinking about possible outcomes.

Comparing the function of defensive pessimism and other strategies relative to different kinds of goals reveals patterns of costs and benefits characteristic of each strategy. People using defensive pessimism typically perform well compared with other individuals. They do better than those using self-handicapping specifically and than other anxious individuals generally. The majority of studies show that defensive pessimists perform

as well as strategic optimists overall. Each group performs best in situations that accommodate their preferred strategy and worse in situations that interfere with that strategy. Thus each group is potentially vulnerable, in terms of performance, to situations or "jobs" for which their preferred tools are not well suited. For defensive pessimists, those situations might include times when there is no opportunity for preperformance preparation and they are thus unable to control and direct the arousal related to their anxiety; for example, if a boss drops by for a surprise visit and asks for an impromptu progress report. For strategic optimists, unexpected situations that arouse unfamiliar anxiety may be especially challenging—for example, if a boss insists on troubleshooting possible negative outcomes prior to an important meeting, strategic optimists may become anxious but be unable to rely on their usual distractions to calm themselves.

When Chang and Sivam (2004) found that defensive pessimists were especially likely to engage in preventative behavior in the face of a possible SARS outbreak in Singapore, they may have been studying a context particularly well designed to highlight the potential advantages of defensive pessimism. The authors reported that traditional or heritage values in the population they studied predicted use of defensive pessimism. They describe a cultural context in which self-confidence and optimism are not necessarily regarded as virtues, suggesting that expressions of worry and pessimism may not meet with the same negative social reactions everywhere as they do in the United States. The heritage values of prudence, industry, and civic responsibility may also help to buffer those who do take precautions from others' teasing or scorn if those precautions turn out not to have been necessary. More generally, Chang argues that defensive pessimism fits particularly well with East Asian cultural sensibilities (Chang, 1996; Norem & Chang, 2002).

In addition, defensive pessimism may work especially well to motivate people when there are effective precautions one can take but when they are facing an unfamiliar or *potential* threat, when the extent to which it may apply to them personally is unclear, and when it is likely that some people will remain uninfected because of chance or unknown physical conditions that strengthen resistance. The anxiety aroused in such a situation may be diffuse and hard to direct, except for those who are used to using defensive pessimism: that is, the experts.

Brower and Ketterhagen's (2004) findings that defensive pessimism predicted better retention of African American students at predominantly white institutions suggests that there are cultural contexts in which anxiety may be hard to avoid. Stereotype threat is likely to be pervasive for African American students in such a setting, with performance demands throughout the semester in a variety of classes and contexts, all of which represent the possibility not just of personal failure but of failure that could

incriminate one's entire group (Steele & Aronson, 1995). Students who have developed defensive pessimism have a tool ready to use in those situations. This interpretation is bolstered by research showing that women using defensive pessimism perform better on a math test under stereotype threat conditions (Perry & Skitka, 2009).

The Hedonic Failure of Defensive Pessimism

Defensive pessimism looks like an effective tool when it comes to performance outcomes. It looks markedly less effective from a hedonic perspective, however. Those who use defensive pessimism are not depressed (or, at least, defensive pessimism does not seem to cause depression). Nevertheless, they do consistently report more negative affect (although not necessarily less positive affect) than those who use strategic optimism (e.g., Cantor et al., 1987; Norem & Illingworth, 1993, 2004). Moreover, defensive pessimism does not "work" as an anxiety management strategy by decreasing anxiety; rather, it harnesses that anxiety and may exacerbate it. Put simply, there is no evidence to suggest that defensive pessimism is fun. Even worse, as Seery et al. (2008) suggest, it may be that the repeated experiences of hypothalamic–pituitary–adrenal (HPA) activation associated with threat appraisals among defensive pessimists have negative effects on health over time.

On the other hand, available evidence suggests that anxiety cannot be wished away for the defensive pessimists. It is wrapped up in the package of their experience and understanding of situations, and they have developed a way to use it, largely to their advantage. Comparing their hedonic experience with that of people who are not anxious is somewhat missing the point. Comparing their hedonic experience with that of those who are anxious but do not use defensive pessimism makes the potential costs of defensive pessimism seem worth it, at least in many situations.

Of course, it is important to examine the potential costs of a strategy, but it is also important to do so with awareness of the broader context of those costs and with consideration of whether there are realistic alternatives. As important, we cannot simply assume that an alternative that does not result in a particular cost (in a particular situation) has no potential other costs. For example, self-handicapping *may* blunt the physiological costs of acute anxiety, but it is likely to have significant performance costs over the long term, which in turn may exacerbate anxiety, loneliness, and performance problems (Maatta et al., 2007). Strategic optimism may not exact the costs of repeated or chronic threat appraisals and may facilitate avoidance of some negative affect. It does not follow that it is cost-free, however. Strategic optimism was significantly less successful in experimental situations in which those using it had to reflect on negative possibilities.

It did not render those using it invulnerable to situational influences, and it does not seem a great stretch to suggest that there may be real-life situations in which it is important—even if hedonically unpleasant—to be able to think through negative possible outcomes without impairing one's performance. More generally, the ability to tolerate the experience of negative affect without needing to suppress it or distract oneself is crucial to delay of gratification, a key life skill. When one thinks in terms of long-term costs, Segerstrom's (2006) research suggests that the short-term increases in immune functioning associated with optimism can turn into impaired functioning over time when there are chronic stressors.

Finally, at some point it is important to acknowledge the validity of individual differences in appraisals, the reality that there are rarely no-cost solutions to difficult situations in real life, and the probability that no single strategy will fit every situation and task (Bohart, 2002). Not to do so risks serious misunderstanding of the complexity of human experience (Norem, 2008). It would be disrespectful (at best!) to fail to acknowledge that African American students at predominantly white institutions (or women in traditionally male-dominated fields, or the impoverished vs. the comfortable across situations, etc.) are in a different situation than are white students at those institutions and may need to use different strategies to meet their goals in that context.

As another example, at least two studies have found significant advantages to more negative appraisals among older adults, and one found that pessimism during this life stage was associated with better health outcomes (Isaacowitz & Seligman, 2001; Lang, Weiss, Gerstorf & Wagner, 2013). Strategies that foster health during adolescence or young adulthood (i.e., times of robust health on average) may not fit well with changes in health associated with aging.

A hedonic perspective on emotion reflects the uncontroversial observation that positive emotions feel good and negative emotions feel bad. There is nothing inherently wrong with a hedonic perspective, of course, and it would be foolish to ignore the fundamental observations upon which it is based. It transcends species and evolutionary time, and it has compelling implications for motivation. The problem with a hedonic perspective is the ease with which it creates something akin to a halo effect; it is terribly tempting to assume that feelings that *feel* good *are* good. This happens despite evidence that there are negative sides to positive emotion (e.g., Forgas & East, 2008; Gruber, Mauss, & Tamir, 2011) and that willingness to tolerate negative affect is an important part of personal growth (Adler & Hershfield, 2013; Mauss et al., 2012; Pomerantz, Saxon, & Oishi, 2000; Ryff & Singer, 1998; Shallcross, Troy, Boland, & Mauss, 2010). With further, subtle elision, it is a very short step to complete the equation that success at feeling good is equivalent to success at *being* good—if not morally,

then at least in terms of living successfully. In other words, hedonic perspectives can create an essentially stereotypical, unnuanced conception of adaptation in which those who experience more positive emotions are considered to be better adapted and those who are better adapted in this way are better people.

Whatever problems result—and there are several—from assuming that happier people are better people, there are bigger problems associated with the view that people who experience negative emotions have somehow failed or, worse, are "bad" people. Yet descriptions of people who experience more positive affect can become prescriptive (as gender stereotypes are; see Fiske & Stevens, 1993). They not only describe the characteristics of people who experience more positive affect, but they also imply that those characteristics describe how people *should* be.

I frequently receive e-mail or letters from people who have come across the concept of defensive pessimism, usually in a newspaper or magazine article. They recognize themselves in the description of the concept, and they are often delighted to have a name for what they do and some research-based validation that it is a viable approach. They are happy and relieved because they feel the pressure of prescriptive optimism (in the United States) without knowing how to push back. One correspondent generated a particularly poignant description of such pressure:

> I tested out to be a Defensive Pessimist . . . the surprise came when I realized that it wasn't wrong for me to be the pessimist that I am, and that realization has changed my life almost over night, because I have put aside the notion that I need to look on the bright side of everything. . . . I made copies of the article and passed it out to my Wife, and some overly optimistic people that I have had continued conflict with at work. . . . My wife loved the article because now she understands me better than she ever did, and that will help our relationship to grow even stronger. Now I know I don't have to change into someone I'm not, and that is a huge stress reliever for me. I think if you were to ask the pessimistic people, if they feel they need to change and look on the bright side of everything the way the optimist does in order to cope in the work place, or even at home, you might find that there is a lot of stress being placed on these people to change. . . . There is a lot of emphasis placed on the power of positive thinking in the work place . . . it is unfair to the pessimist because they are taking on the problems associated with the task at hand and also the task of trying to appear positive even when they do not have that feeling.

Expanding our understanding of the function of affect and strategies for managing it may help to counteract, or at least avoid further contributions to, cultural prescriptions that assume that there is one good,

positive way to appraise, respond, feel, and behave (see also Hosogoshi, 2009). Closer examination of the range of costs and benefits associated with different affects and strategies can help us to understand the boundary conditions that influence the fit among strategies, goals, contexts, and individuals.

Exploring Costs, Benefits, and Boundary Conditions

What makes a given tool the right tool for the job? Characteristics of the tool, characteristics of the job, the context in which the job needs to be done, and characteristics of the individual using the tool all contribute. Defensive pessimism is a good tool for managing anxiety if the goal is good performance, but less good if the goal is to feel calm or happy. It may work better in situations or cultural contexts in which there is less pressure to be "upbeat" or to appear confident; for example, people who use defensive pessimism may want to keep their strategy covert during a job interview if they can see that the interviewer has a particularly "gung-ho" style.

Although we know that strategies can change (Martin et al., 2003; Maatta et al., 2007), it is unlikely that someone picking up a new tool for the first time will experience the same results as someone who has used it over years. Evidence from experiments in which people are induced to use strategies different from their own suggests that the effects of a strategy are not necessarily automatically or instantaneously realized.

Other individual differences are likely to influence the likelihood of developing a strategy, the effectiveness of strategy use, and the effects of different affects. Just as taller people will have an easier time swinging a sledgehammer than shorter people, individuals are likely to find specific strategies easier or harder to implement, and their experiences with those strategies may vary. Differences in the effects of emotional expressions provide a striking (no pun intended) example of this. Lewis (2000) reports that when male managers express anger when something goes wrong, it increases their employees' perceptions of their competence relative to when they express sadness, but the same is not true for female managers (see Hess, Chapter 3, this volume, for further discussion). When there are important variations in who is expected or *allowed* to feel and express specific emotions in particular situations, or to pursue particular goals, those contextual and cultural constraints influence strategy options and effectiveness (see Chentsova-Dutton, Senft, & Ryder, Chapter 7, this volume).

Frequency and intensity of affective experiences and strategy use change their meaning and are thus likely to influence their consequences. An explosion of anger from someone who chronically throws tantrums is likely to have different kinds of causes and effects than a sudden expression of anger from someone who is usually calm and composed (even if

there are similarities in neural activation across these instances; Carver & Harmon-Jones, 2009). The former may induce in the audience the tendency to get away until it blows over, whereas the latter may be interpreted as a sign that something is very wrong and lead to solicitous responses. For those experiencing the anger, an eruption also has different implications. Feeling and expressing anger, for someone who often does so, is likely to signal that things are relatively normal. For someone who is rarely angry, however, that feeling and expression may be at odds with their understanding of themselves and create embarrassment or other discomfort; they may see it as a sign that they have let things go too far and need to take action.

In a similar vein, Grant and Schwartz (2011) remind us that there can be too much of any good thing and that the beneficial effects of "positive" characteristics are often not evenly distributed across the range of those characteristics. For example, high levels of optimism and self-esteem are related, respectively, to riskier health behaviors (Milam, Richardson, Marks, Kemper, & McCutchan, 2004) and to poorer relationships (Baumeister, Campbell, Krueger, & Vohs, 2003), whereas more moderate levels tend to be associated with more positive outcomes.

Personality traits such as extraversion and neuroticism, motivational sensitivities represented in the behavioral inhibition and behavioral activation systems (BIS/BAS), and positive and negative affective tendencies all describe consistent individual differences in characteristic affective experiences (Larsen & Augustine, 2008) that are likely to moderate the fit between individuals and strategies. They are also likely to influence, via their effects on accumulated experiences, the development, content, and structure of self-knowledge (Tamir, 2005). Both self-knowledge and stable tendencies, in turn, will influence the goals an individual pursues and thus the strategies that are likely to provide the best fit.

THE RIGHT TOOL FOR THE JOB

Tools can be blunt or sharp, or otherwise vary in strength and precision. There are a number of sensible and informative ways to categorize tools: for example, tools for putting things together versus tools for taking things apart, or categories such as hammers and screwdrivers. As much as the category "hammer" may make sense, though, ball peen hammers do not work as well as sledgehammers to take down a wall, and knowing how to use the former effectively may not help much the first time one wields the latter. As anyone who has tried to screw in a Phillips-head screw with a flathead screwdriver can testify, one cannot necessarily consider tools within a category to be interchangeable. Importantly, it also matters who is using a particular tool. Power tools can be dazzlingly efficient in the hands

of an expert and frighteningly destructive when used by the inexperienced. (Trust me.) Those who work on the same kinds of tasks over time typically develop habits and particular ease or expertise in using their tools, as is clearly seen by watching how different cooks rely relatively more on serrated knives or chef's knives for tasks that accommodate either.

At the risk of mangling my metaphor beyond recognition, there are analogies one can make between some of the important points to remember about tools and some of the important points to remember about affect. Affect includes both diffuse moods and discrete emotions (discrete, at least, as experienced), and both can vary in intensity. Affect can be categorized in a variety of theoretically interesting and useful ways—for example, positive or negative; social or nonsocial; self-conscious or non-self-conscious; approach-related or avoidance-related; pre–goal attainment or post–goal attainment (Gable & Harmon-Jones, 2010, 2011; Tracy, Robins, & Tangney, 2007; Watson, Wiese, Vaidya & Tellegen, 1999). The categories that have explanatory and predictive power at one level of analysis, however, will not necessarily work well at another (e.g., those that best capture felt experience are unlikely to be isomorphic with those describing patterns of neural activation or motivational tendencies). Nor will the positive or negative effects observed at one level of analysis necessarily translate across levels, as when hormonal processes that produce positive affect also lead to risky behavior. Affects within a category do not necessarily have the same influence on other processes and outcomes: for example, anger and sadness have typically different effects.

Finally, although it can be informative to talk about basic processes, average effects, and typical functions, it does matter *who* is feeling what in a particular situation: for example, the onset of performance anxiety in someone who typically does not experience that kind of anxiety may have very different effects than the anxiety an experienced performer may routinely feel. The same affect does not necessarily function in the same way for all individuals, as is aptly illustrated by the different reactions to male and female expressions of anger. Similarly, a given affect may show different developmental trajectories and may be felt by different people in response to different objective or subjective situations, including cultural context (Crystal, Parrott, Okazaki & Watanabe, 2001).

Research in psychology seems increasingly translational. Researchers are under pressure to "give away" their results and knowledge to the public, whose taxes help support it. Members of the public, in turn, are eager consumers of advice on how to be happier and live well, particularly if that advice is based on "the latest research." I suspect that the latter trend especially has been accelerated by the widespread media presence of the positive psychology movement: Ample funding, prominent leaders, and a vocal and enthusiastic membership, organized into a movement to

promote individual and societal transformation, makes for a potent cultural phenomenon.

Scientific progress, of course, needs always to include understanding of boundary conditions; indeed, one can hardly claim much understanding at all if those boundaries are not thoroughly investigated. In the context of research that will be disseminated to the public, however, researchers in psychology bear additional burdens. We are responsible for knowing the side effects of anything we "prescribe" and the conditions that may limit or facilitate the processes we recommend. In particular, we need to be wary of "feel-good" (literally, in the sense of recommendations designed to make people feel happier) solutions that, despite their appeal, are not well suited to particular situations, tasks, or individuals. Before we assume we have found the right tool for the job, we need to have thoroughly explored the job, the tool, the person who will be using it, and conditions under which it will be used. Only then can we sing lustily along with Marcia Ball and her band: (last verse) "We all need someone[7] who knows how to do the things that please/. . . . "

NOTES

1. The label for attributional style evolved over the years from *explanatory style* to *attributional style*. At some point when it was called *attributional style*, the modifiers *optimistic* and *pessimistic* were attached; later, the *attributional style* part of the label was often dropped, and what was formerly an optimistic attributional style was simply called *optimism*.

2. Publications prior to about 1990 use a shorter, earlier version of the scale, but the two versions correlate above .70, so they are quite comparable. The DPQ-R has a clearer factor structure and higher internal consistency than the original measure. Two correlated factors are represented in the scale—pessimism and reflectivity—but all the items also load on a single, unrotated factor with loadings high enough to justify a single-factor solution using conventional factor analytic standards.

3. Defensive pessimism shows small to moderate positive correlations (.20–.35) with dispositional pessimism, as measured by the Life Orientation Test (Scheier, Carver, & Bridges, 1994), and small positive correlations with the internality, stability, and globality dimensions of the Attributional Style Questionnaire used to measure the attributional style described as pessimistic (Peterson et al., 1982). See Norem (2001) for reliability and validity information on the Defensive Pessimism Questionnaire (DPQ).

4. If I could go back in time, I would change the term *defensive pessimism* to *reflective pessimism*, as opposed to nonreflective optimism. *Defensive* carries the burden of too many additional potential meanings from the psychoanalytic literature and other sources. By choosing *defensive* to label the pessimistic strategy we were studying but *strategic* to label the optimistic counterpart, we

inadvertently implied that there was something better (i.e., more "strategic") about strategic optimism compared with defensive pessimism before we had gathered any data. Perhaps that is evidence of the pervasive influence of the positivity zeitgeist I describe—or validation for my decision not to go into advertising.

5. Originally we thought these individuals might focus on thinking about positive possible outcomes, but the correlations among items on the DPQ suggested, and subsequent research confirmed (e.g., Sanna, 1996), that they do not typically mentally simulate either positive or negative possible outcomes prior to entering a situation.

6. There are some questions about the extent to which the DPQ consistently and reliably assesses the optimistic part of strategic optimism, so some investigators prefer to contrast defensive pessimists with "controls," defined as those not using defensive pessimism. There are a number of interesting conceptual and psychometric issues here (e.g., whether and when optimism–pessimism can be considered as one bipolar dimension vs. whether or when we should consider two unipolar dimensions, from "pessimistic" to "not pessimistic" and from "optimistic" to "not optimistic"), and they deserve further consideration. I do not think they are directly relevant to the functional interpretation of defensive pessimism that is the focus in this chapter, however, and as space limitations preclude a thorough discussion, they are left for other venues.

7. I took the liberty of changing the original words from "A woman needs a man to know . . . ," so they would be more inclusive.

REFERENCES

Adler, J. M., & Hershfield, H. E. (2013) Mixed emotional experience is associated with and precedes improvements in psychological well-being. *PLOS ONE*, *7*(4), e35633.

Baumeister, R. F., Campbell, J. D., Krueger, J. I., & Vohs, K. D. (2003). Does high self-esteem cause better performance, interpersonal success, happiness or healthier lifestyles? *Psychological Science in the Public Interest, 4*, 1–44.

Berglas, S. J., & Jones, E. E. (1978). Drug choice as a self-handicapping strategy in response to noncontingent success. *Journal of Personality and Social Psychology, 36*, 405–417.

Block, J., & Colvin, C. R. (1994). Positive illusions and well-being revisited: Separating fiction from fact. *Psychological Bulletin, 116*, 28.

Bohart, A. C. (2002). Focusing on the positive, focusing on the negative: Implications for psychotherapy. *Journal of Clinical Psychology, 58*, 1037–1043.

Brower, A. M., & Ketterhagen, A. (2004). Is there an inherent mismatch between how black and white students expect to succeed in college and what their college expects from them? *Journal of Social Issues, 60*, 95–116.

Cantor, N. (1990). From thought to behavior: "Having" and "doing" in the study of personality and cognition. *American Psychologist, 45*, 735–750.

Cantor, N., Norem, J. K., Niedenthal, P. M., Langston, C. A., & Brower, A.

(1987). Life tasks, self-concept ideals, and cognitive strategies in a life transition. *Journal of Personality and Social Psychology, 53*, 1178–1191.

Carver, C. S., & Harmon-Jones, E. (2009). Anger is an approach-related affect: Evidence and implications. *Psychological Bulletin, 135*, 183–204.

Chang, E. C. (1996). Cultural differences in optimism, pessimism, and coping: Predictors of subsequent adjustment in Asian American and Caucasian American college students. *Journal of Counseling Psychology, 43*, 113–123.

Chang, W. C., & Sivam, R. W. (2004). Constant vigilance: Heritage values and defensive pessimism in coping with severe acute respiratory syndrome in Singapore. *Asian Journal of Social Psychology, 7*, 35–53.

Colvin, C. R., & Block. J. (1994). Do positive illusions foster mental health?: An examination of the Taylor and Brown formulation. *Psychological Bulletin, 116*, 3–20.

Colvin, C. R., Block, J., & Funder, D. C. (1995). Overly positive self-evaluations and personality: Negative implications for mental health. *Journal of Personality and Social Psychology, 68*, 1152–1162.

Coyne, J. C., & Gotlib, I. H. (1983). The role of cognition in depression: A critical appraisal. *Psychological Bulletin, 94*, 472–505.

Crystal, D. S., Parrott, W. G., Okazaki, Y., & Watanabe, H. (2001). Examining relations between shame and personality among university students in the United States and Japan: A developmental perspective. *International Society for the Study of Behavioral Development, 25*, 113–123.

del Valle, C. H. C., & Mateos, P. M. (2008). Dispositional pessimism, defensive pessimism and optimism: The effect of induced mood on prefactual and counterfactual thinking and performance. *Cognition and Emotion, 22*, 1600–1612.

Diener, E., & Biswas-Diener, R. (2008). *The science of optimal happiness*. Boston: Blackwell.

Doan, B. D., & Gray, R. E. (1992). The heroic cancer patient: A critical analysis of the relationship between illusion and mental health. *Canadian Journal of Behavioural Science, 24*, 253–266.

Dunning, D., & Story, A. L. (1991). Depression, realism, and the overconfidence effect: Are the sadder wiser when predicting future actions and events? *Journal of Personality and Social Psychology, 61*, 521–532.

Eid, M., & Larsen, R. J. (2008). *The science of subjective well-being*. New York: Guilford Press.

Elliot, A. J., & Church, M. A. (2003). A motivation analysis of defensive pessimism and self-handicapping. *Journal of Personality, 71*, 369–396.

Eronen, S., Nurmi, J. E., & Salmela-Aro, K. (1998). Optimistic, defensive–pessimistic, impulsive and self-handicapping strategies in university environments. *Learning and Instruction, 8*, 159–177.

Fiske, S. T., & Stevens, L. E. (1993). What's so special about sex?: Gerder stereotypes and discrimination. In S. Oskamp & M. Costanzo (Eds.), *Gender issues in contemporary society* (pp. 173–196). Thousand Oaks, CA: Sage.

Forgas, J. P. (1995). Mood and judgment: The affect infusion model (AIM). *Psychological Bulletin, 116*, 39–66.

Forgas, J. P., & East, R. (2008). On being happy and gullible: Mood effects on skepticism and the detection of deception. *Journal of Experimental Social Psychology, 44*, 1362–1367.

Frederickson, B. L. (2001). The role of positive emotions in positive psychology: The broaden-and-build theory of positive emotions. *American Psychologist, 56*, 218–226.

Frijda, N. (1986). *The emotions.* Cambridge, UK: Cambridge University Press.

Gable, P. A., & Harmon-Jones, E. (2010). The effect of low versus high approach-motivated positive affect on memory for peripherally versus centrally presented information. *Emotion, 10*, 599–603.

Gable, P. A., & Harmon-Jones, E. (2011). Attentional consequences of pregoal and postgoal positive affects. *Emotion, 11*, 1358–1367.

Garcia, T. (1995). The role of motivational strategies in self-regulated learning. In P. R. Pintrich (Ed.), *New directions for teaching and learning* (Vol. 63, pp. 29–42). San Francisco: Jossey-Bass.

Gasper, K., Lozinski, R. H., & LeBeau, L. S. (2009). If you plan, then you can: How reflection helps defensive pessimists pursue their goals. *Motivation and Emotion, 33*, 203–216.

Grant, A. M., & Schwartz, B. (2011). Too much of a good thing: The challenge and opportunity of the inverted U. *Perspectives on Psychological Science, 6*, 61–76.

Greenwald, A. G. (1980). The totalitarian ego: Fabrication and revision of personal history. *American Psychologist, 35*, 603–618.

Gruber, J., Mauss, I. B., & Tamir, M. (2011). A dark side of happiness?: How, when and why happiness is not always good. *Perspectives on Psychological Science, 6*, 222–233.

Held, B. S. (2002). The tyranny of the positive attitude in America: Observation and speculation. *Journal of Clinical Psychology, 58*, 965–992.

Hosogoshi, H. K. M. (2009). Accepting pessimistic thinking is associated with better mental and physical health in defensive pessimists. *Shinrigaku Kenkyu, 79*, 542.

Isaacowitz, D. M., & Seligman, M.E. P. (2001). Is pessimism a risk factor for depressive mood among community dwelling older adults? *Behavior Research and Therapy, 39*, 255–272.

John, O. P., & Robins, R. W. (1994). Accuracy and bias in self-perception: The role of individual differences in self-enhancement and narcissism. *Journal of Personality and Social Psychology, 66*, 206–219.

Lang, F. R., Weiss, D., Gerstorf, D., & Wagner, G. G. (2013). Forecasting life satisfaction across adulthood: Benefits of seeing a dark future? *Psychology and Aging, 428*, 249–261.

Larsen, R. J., & Augustine, A. A. (2008). Basic personality dispositions related to approach and avoidance: Extraversion/neuroticism, BAS/BIS, and positive/negative affectivity. In A. Elliot (Ed.), *Handbook of approach and avoidance motivation* (pp. 151–164). Hoboken, NJ: Psychology Press.

Lewis, K. M. (2000). When leaders display emotion: How followers respond to negative emotional expression of male and female leaders. *Journal of Organizational Behavior, 21*, 221–234.

Maatta, S., Nurmi, J.-E., & Stattin, H. (2007). Achievement orientations, school adjustment and well-being: A longitudinal study. *Journal of Research on Adolescence, 17*(4), 789–812.

Martin, A. J., Marsh, H. W., & Debus, R. L. (2001). Self-handicapping and defensive pessimism: Exploring a model of predictors and outcomes from a self-protection perspective. *Journal of Education Psychology, 93*, 87–102.

Martin, A. J., Marsh, H. W., & Debus, R. L. (2003). Self-handicapping and defensive pessimism: A model of self-protection from a longitudinal perspective. *Contemporary Educational Psychology, 28*, 1–36.

Mauss, I. B., Savino, N. S., Anderson, C. L., Weisbuch, M., Tamir, M., & Laudenslager, M. L. (2012). The pursuit of happiness can be lonely. *Emotion, 12*, 908–912.

Milam, J. E., Richardson, J. L., Marks, G., Kemper, C. A., & McCutchan, A. (2004). The roles of dispositional optimism and pessimism in HIV disease progression. *Psychology and Health, 19*, 167–181.

Miller, D. T., & Ross, M. (1982). Self-serving biases in the attribution of causality: Fact or fiction? *Psychological Bulletin, 82*, 213–225.

Newman, L. S., Nibert, J. W., & Winer, E. S. (2009). Mnemic neglect is not an artifact of expectancy: The moderating role of defensive pessimism. *European Journal of Social Psychology, 38*, 477–486.

Norem, J. K. (1989). Cognitive strategies as personality: Effectiveness, specificity, flexibility and change. In D. M. Buss & N. Cantor (Ed.), *Personality psychology: Recent trends and emerging directions* (pp. 45–60). New York: Springer-Verlag.

Norem, J. K. (2001). Defensive pessimism, optimism, and pessimism. In E. C. Chang (Ed.), *Optimism and pessimism: Implications for theory, research and practice* (pp. 77–100). Washington, DC: American Psychological Association.

Norem, J. K. (2008). Defensive pessimism, anxiety, and the complexity of evaluating self-regulation. *Social and Personality Psychology Compass, 2*, 121–134.

Norem, J. K., & Andreas Burdzovic, J. A. (2007). Understanding journeys: Individual growth analysis as a tool for studying individual differences in change over time. In A. D. Ong & M. V. Dulmen (Eds.), *Handbook of methods in positive psychology* (pp. 477–486). London: Oxford University Press.

Norem, J. K., & Cantor, N. (1986a). Anticipatory and post hoc cushioning strategies: Optimism and defensive pessimism in "risky" situations. *Cognitive Therapy and Research, 10*, 347–362.

Norem, J. K., & Cantor, N. (1986b). Defensive pessimism: Harnessing anxiety as motivation. *Journal of Personality and Social Psychology, 51*, 1208–1217.

Norem, J. K., & Chang, E. C. (2002). The positive psychology of negative thinking. *Journal of Clinical Psychology, 58*, 993–1001.

Norem, J. K., & Illingworth, K. S. S. (1993). Strategy-dependent effects of reflecting on self and tasks: Some implications of optimism and defensive pessimism. *Journal of Personality and Social Psychology, 65*, 822–835.

Norem, J. K., & Illingworth, K. S. S. (2004). Mood and performance among defensive pessimists and strategic optimists. *Journal of Research in Personality, 38*, 351–366.

Ntoumanis, N., Taylor, I. M., & Standage, M. (2010). Testing a model of

antecedents and consequences of defensive pessimism and self-handicapping in school physical education. *Journal of Sports Sciences, 28,* 1515–1525.

Panksepp, J. (2011). The primary process affects in human development, happiness, and thriving. In K. M. Sheldon, T. B. Kashda, & M. F. Steger (Eds.), *Designing positive psychology: Taking stock and moving forward* (pp. 51–88). New York: Oxford University Press.

Parrott, W. G. (1993). Beyond hedonism: Motives for inhibiting good moods and maintaining bad moods. In D. M. Wegner & J. W. Pennebaker (Eds.), *Handbook of mental control* (pp. 278–305). Upper Saddle River, NJ: Prentice Hall.

Parrott, W. G. (2002). The functional utility of negative emotions. In L. F. Barrett & P. Salovey (Eds.), *The wisdom in feeling: Psychological processes in emotional intelligence* (pp. 341–359). New York: Guilford Press.

Perry, S. P., & Skitka, L. J. (2009). Making lemonade?: Defensive coping style moderates the effect of stereotype threat on women's math test performance. *Journal of Research in Personality, 43,* 918–920.

Peterson, C., Semmel, A., von Baeyer, C., Abramson, L. Y., Metalsky, G. I., & Seligman, M. E. P. (1982). The Attributional Style Questionnaire. *Cognitive Therapy and Research, 6,* 287–299.

Pomerantz, E., Saxon, J. L., & Oishi, S. (2000). The psychological trade-offs of goal investment. *Journal of Personality and Social Psychology, 79,* 617–630.

Rodríguez, S., Cabanach, R. G., Valle, A., Nuñez, J. C., & Gonzalez-Pienda, J. A. (2004). Differences in use of self-handicapping and defensive pessimism and its relation with achievement goals, self-esteem and self-regulation strategies. *Psicothema, 16,* 625–631.

Ryff, C. D., & Singer, B. (1998). The contours of positive human health. *Psychological Inquiry, 9,* 1–28.

Sanna, L. J. (1996). Defensive pessimism, optimism, and stimulating alternatives: Some ups and downs of prefactual and counterfactual thinking. *Journal of Personality and Social Psychology, 71,* 1020–1036.

Sanna, L. J. (1998). Defensive pessimism and optimism: The bitter-sweet influence of mood on performance and prefactual and counterfactual thinking. *Cognition and Emotion, 12,* 635–665.

Scheier M. F., & Carver, C. S. (1985). Optimism, coping and health: Assessment and implications of generalized outcome expectancies. *Health Psychology, 4,* 219–247.

Scheier, M. F., Carver, C. S., & Bridges, M. W. (1994). Distinguishing optimism from neuroticism (and trait anxiety, self-mastery, and self-esteem): A reevaluation of the Life Orientation Test. *Journal of Personality and Social Psychology, 67,* 1063–1078.

Schoneman, S. W. (2002). The role of the cognitive coping strategy of defensive pessimism within the social-evaluative continuum. *Dissertation Abstracts International, 63,* 3024.

Seery, M. D., West, T. V., Weisbuch, M., & Blascovitch, J. (2008). The effects of negative reflection for defensive pessimists: Dissipation or harnessing of threat? *Personality and Individual Differences, 45,* 515–520.

Segerstrom, S. C. (2006). How does optimism suppress immunity?: Evaluation of three affective pathways. *Health Psychology, 25,* 653–657.

Seligman, M. E. P., & Csikszentmihalyi, M. (2000). Positive psychology [Special issue]. *American Psychologist, 55*.

Shallcross, A. J., Troy, A. S., Boland, M., & Mauss, I. B. (2010). Let it be: Accepting negative emotional experiences predicts decreased negative affect and depressive symptoms. *Behaviour Research and Therapy, 48*, 921–929.

Showers, C. J. (1988). The effects of how and why thinking on perceptions of future negative events. *Cognitive Therapy and Research, 12*, 225–240.

Showers, C. J. (1992). The motivational and emotional consequences of considering positive or negative possibilities for an upcoming event. *Journal of Personality and Social Psychology, 63*, 474–484.

Showers, C., & Ruben, C. (1990). Distinguishing defensive pessimism from depression: Negative expectations and positive coping mechanisms. *Cognitive Therapy and Research, 14*, 385–399.

Snyder, M., & Cantor, N. (1998). Understanding personality and social behavior: A functionalist strategy. In D. T. Gilbert, S. T. Fiske, & G. Lindzey (Eds.), *The handbook of social psychology* (pp. 635–679). New York: McGraw-Hill.

Spencer, S. M., & Norem, J. K. (1996). Reflection and distraction: Defensive pessimism, strategic optimism, and performance. *Personality and Social Psychology Bulletin, 22*, 354–365.

Steele, C. M., & Aronson, J. (1995). Stereotype threat and the intellectual test performance of African-Americans. *Journal of Personality and Social Psychology, 65*, 797–811.

Tamir, M. (2005). Don't worry, be happy?: Neuroticism, trait-consistent affect regulation and performance. *Journal of Personality and Social Psychology, 89*, 449–461.

Tamir, M. (2009). What do people want to feel and why?: Pleasure and utility in emotion regulation. *Current Directions in Psychological Science, 18*, 101–105.

Tamir, M., & Gross, J. J. (2011). Beyond pleasure and pain?: Emotion regulation and positive psychology. In K. M. Sheldon, T. B. Kashda, & M. F. Steger (Eds.), *Designing positive psychology: Taking stock and moving forward* (pp. 89–100). New York: Oxford University Press.

Taylor, S. E., & Brown, J. D. (1988). Illusion and well-being: A social psychological perspective on mental health. *Psychological Bulletin, 103*, 193–210.

Taylor, S. E., & Brown, J. D. (1994a). Illusions and well-being revisited: Separating fact from fiction. *Psychological Bulletin, 116*, 21–27.

Taylor, S. E., & Brown, J. D. (1994b). "Illusion" of mental health does not explain positive illusions. *American Psychologist, 49*, 972–973.

Tomaya, M. (2005). Influence of cognitive strategies on test coping strategies and academic achievement: Defensive pessimism and strategic optimism. *Japanese Journal of Educational Psychology, 53*, 220–229.

Tracy, J. L., Robins, R. W., & Tangney, J. P. (Eds.). (2007). *The self-conscious emotions: Theory and research*. New York: Guilford Press.

Watson, D., Wiese, D., Vaidya, J., & Tellegen, A. (1999). The two general activation systems of affect: Structural findings, evolutionary considerations, and psychobiological evidence. *Journal of Personality and Social Psychology, 76*, 820–838.

Weinstein, N. D. (1980). Unrealistic optimism about future life events. *Journal of Personality and Social Psychology, 39,* 806–820.

Wilson, G. S., Raglin, J. S., & Pritchard, M. E. (2002). Optimism, pessimism, and precompetition anxiety in college athletes. *Personality and Individual Differences, 32,* 893–902.

Yamawaki, N., Tschanz, B. T., & Feick, D. L. (2004). Defensive pessimism, self-esteem instability and goal strivings. *Cognition and Emotion, 18,* 233–249.

12

Feeling, Function, and the Place of Negative Emotions in a Happy Life

W. GERROD PARROTT

The dominant approach to emotion in contemporary Western cultures places a high value on positive emotions and a low value on negative emotions. Happiness, optimism, and cheerfulness characterize attitudes that are considered desirable; sadness, pessimism, anger, and fear exemplify attitudes that are thought to be unhelpful and best avoided (Held, 2002; Kotchemidova, 2005; McMahon, 2006). At its root, this perspective combines two beliefs—one that emotions are principally pleasant or unpleasant feelings, the other that a person's goal in life is to experience pleasure and contentment. The preference for positive emotions extends to many realms: social roles, personal relationships, moral thinking, the workplace, and the health clinic are among the aspects of culture that have been shaped by the preference for positive emotions and (their close relative) positive thinking (Bruckner, 2000; Ehrenreich, 2009; Stearns, 1994). Even academic psychology has spawned an approach called "positive psychology" (Seligman & Csikszentmihalyi, 2000).

These cultural values are apparent in reports I have collected from American undergraduate students. When I ask students to write about an emotion they have recently had, to describe its effects, and to rate the ways

in which these effects were functional or dysfunctional, they tend to rate pleasant emotions as functional and unpleasant emotions as dysfunctional regardless of the emotion's actual consequences. In the students' judgments, their emotion's pleasantness overrides all other factors in determining the overall benefit or harm of the emotion. Feeling good is the outcome that matters most.

The dominant Western model is not the only way to approach emotion. Consider the perspectives that were contrasted in a classic episode of the television program *Star Trek* ("This Side of Paradise," first broadcast in 1967). Crew members from the starship *Enterprise* beam down to a planet where all members of a small agricultural colony appear to be blissfully happy and, despite lethal radiation levels, in perfect health. The colonists have been infected by the spores of a local flower, which provides immunity to the radiation, as well as feelings of all-encompassing love and peace of mind—Mr. Spock likens the spores to a "happiness pill." When the *Enterprise* crew members are infected by the spores, they cheerfully mutiny, abandon their starship, and join the colony, where they relax, play, and enjoy a paradise of health, happiness, and love. Even Spock falls in love and spends his day nuzzling, hanging upside down from trees, finding shapes in clouds, and sipping mint juleps. In this episode, the colonists and *Enterprise* crew express contemporary Western culture's prevailing view: Paradise would be continual happiness, without want or need.

Throughout the episode, the dissenting voice is that of Captain Kirk, who rejects the others' vision of paradise and argues that dissatisfaction is what drives achievement and that people will stagnate without challenges and ambitions that instill a desire for self-improvement. Kirk contradicts both tenets of the culturally dominant approach to emotions. He values emotions not on the basis of how they feel but on the basis of what they motivate a person to do. For Kirk, the purpose of emotions is to serve some goal that lies beyond the emotion itself; feelings, per se, are beside the point.

The turning point in the episode occurs when Kirk, alone on the *Enterprise*, also becomes infected. As he gathers some belongings in preparation for joining the colony he comes upon a medal that he had been awarded, and this symbol of achievement triggers a powerful angry response that frees him from the spores' influence and sparks an idea that allows him to cure the colonists and his crew. The episode clearly signals which philosophy is considered superior: At the moment when the leader of the colony breaks free of the spores, he looks around and realizes that he and the other colonists have accomplished nothing during the 3 years they have been on the planet; they have wasted their time, making no progress toward building a colony or making the planet a garden as they set out to do.

This episode of *Star Trek* captures several important themes that recur in this volume: that negative emotions serve valuable functions; that in

many circumstances they are more effective than positive emotions; that negative emotions involve much more than feelings; and that even aversive feelings can be welcome and meaningful. Captain Kirk's defense of negative emotions probably slights the value of positive emotions—he seems to think of belonging, play, happiness, and love as mere recreation or distraction—but his role in this episode is to remind the viewer of what the prevailing assumptions are missing.

The present chapter aims to examine how these themes contribute to a general understanding of both positive and negative emotions. At the simplest level, the belief that negative emotions are undesirable rests on two assumptions: that emotions are feelings, and that people are hedonists; that is, that people would never want to feel bad if there was a way to feel good. But neither of these assumptions is consistent with what psychologists know. Emotions are not merely feelings, and people's desires and choices involve more than merely what will be most pleasant—emotions, both positive and negative, can serve many functions and can help achieve goals. They can also be quite dysfunctional, and the factors that determine whether an emotion is useful or harmful in any particular instance are numerous and subtle. Westerners live in a culture that values cheerfulness and positive attitude, so they have trouble recognizing the benefits of negative emotions. Nevertheless, they do seek negative emotions when they have utility, they do watch sad entertainments that provide insights into the human condition, and they do accept negative emotions as part of a full and meaningful life.

EMOTIONS ARE NOT MERELY FEELINGS

The idea that emotions are primarily feelings is relatively recent. I can't find much evidence for it until the 18th century. Prior to that time, emotion concepts such as *passion* emphasized not feelings but forces of desire and aversion that overcome the mind and body, guiding thoughts and actions in ways that can be difficult to control (James, 1997). But in the 18th century, German faculty psychologists developed the idea that the mind has three aspects—*thought*, the *will*, and *feeling*. This idea was further developed by Kant and adopted by early psychologists such as Alexander Bain; it became central to 19th-century thinking about emotion (Hilgard, 1980). When the term *emotion* was first adopted, around 1820, as a secular replacement for the theologically tinged term *passion*, the idea of feeling was central to its definition (Dixon, 2003). Early psychological researchers used newly developed medical instruments to investigate whether emotional feelings corresponded to physiological changes in the body (Dror, 1999). That emotion had become virtually synonymous with feelings can be seen from William

James's (1884) theory, which stated that emotion is nothing more than the perception of bodily changes. This theory makes no sense except as an account of where emotional feelings come from; perceiving bodily changes says nothing about why those bodily changes occurred and not some others, or about what functions those changes have in people's lives (Dewey, 1894). It seems fair to say that, during the late 18th and most of the 19th centuries, the word *emotion* was often treated as synonymous with feelings.

During the 20th century, however, the idea that emotions are primarily feelings became obsolete. It lives on among laypersons, but among psychological researchers feelings have come to be considered but one aspect of emotions, and possibly not an essential one at that. Early biological researchers discovered that physiological changes did not correspond with subjective feelings, and their research methods increasingly focused on animals who could not report on feelings, so their conception of emotion shifted from feelings to physiology. Behaviorism made investigation of feelings seem unscientific and focused attention on emotional behaviors such as aggression and escape, and its replacement by the mid-century cognitive revolution awakened interest not in feelings but in perception, interpretation, memory, attention, and decision making. Research during the 19th century on facial expressions by Duchenne and Darwin was rediscovered by 20th-century psychologists such as Ekman and Izard, whose work helped ignite interest in emotions, leading to the modern study of emotion that began in the 1970s and continues to the present.

The psychological theories that have most influenced contemporary emotion research (e.g., Frijda, 1986; Scherer, 1984) largely abandoned the emphasis on feelings. Psychologists now conceive of emotions as involving a cluster of components, only one of which is conscious feeling and none of which is absolutely necessary. In addition to feelings, emotions include inclinations to think and behave in certain ways (*action tendencies*), ways of construing the situation at hand (*appraisals*), ways of signaling one's action tendencies and appraisals to others (*expressions*), and ways of modulating these reactions (*self-regulation*). These components can be studied on different levels of analysis, so they can be examined in terms of biology, individual psychological processes, and social and cultural processes (Parrott, 2007). Although all of these components are typical of emotional states, none of them is absolutely essential, which means not only that emotions are not equivalent to feelings but also that emotions do not necessarily involve feelings at all. An unconscious emotion is conceivable, such as when a person is judged by others to be angry but isn't aware of being angry him- or herself.

This expanded understanding of what emotions are like provides one fundamental justification for the idea that negative emotions can be

positive: negative emotions *aren't* just feelings. There's much more to them. The modern multicomponential approach, by linking emotional states to action tendencies, appraisals, self-regulation, and social signals, provides a multitude of additional ways in which emotions can have consequences (Frijda, 1986). Emotions can prepare a person to flee, confront, be friendly, acquire information, control others' actions, or enter a variety of other modes of action readiness. Expressions of emotion can alert others about a person's interpretations of events and about the actions a person is likely to take; they can affect other people's emotions. The effects of emotions range from the hormonal to the sociological. Emotions modify heart rate and brain activity; they direct attention and thinking; they alter perception and memory; they motivate antagonism or affection; they intimidate or pacify others; they ostracize or solicit assistance from others; they promote trust or suspicion; they unify or demoralize groups; they challenge or accept the social order. The multicomponent approach underlies the approach known as *functionalism*, the dominant approach to contemporary psychological research on emotion (Fischer & Manstead, 2008; Keltner, Haidt, & Shiota, 2006; Oatley & Jenkins, 1992).

NEGATIVE EMOTIONS CAN HAVE ADAPTIVE FUNCTIONS

The most common form of functionalism is the evolutionary approach, which considers emotions to have a genetic basis that resulted from natural selection (Nesse & Ellsworth, 2009). The presumption therefore is that emotions must have beneficial effects, or at least that they once did, otherwise they would not exist. Emotions, including negative emotions, are understood as having evolved in order to maximize the chances of an individual's genes being passed on to subsequent generations. Most chapters in this volume allude to negative emotions as resulting from natural selection of responses that increase an animal's ability to meet challenges that have recurred over the course of evolution.

In the case of humans, this evolutionary functionalism must be expanded to accommodate our species' cultural variability. Simply put, different emotions don't necessarily work the same way in one culture as they do in another. The reasons for this functional variability are numerous. The rules for how to relate to other people vary among cultures, so whereas an aggressive response might be advantageous in one culture, it might be highly ineffective in another. Cultural variability in attitudes toward an emotion might change how an emotion feels and how it is self-regulated. Cultures have different scripts regarding how emotions ought to occur, when they should occur, and how others should react to them. Cultures

may conceive of emotions differently and thereby influence what aspects people pay attention to and what effects they expect. A culture's assumptions about interpersonal relationships can change the meaning that an emotion has. For such reasons, the way an emotion functions will depend on the culture in which it occurs (Chentsova-Dutton, Senft, & Ryder, Chapter 7, this volume; Sundararajan, Chapter 8, this volume).

When functionalist theorists refer to "different emotions" or to "a particular emotion," they are dividing emotions into discrete categories such as anger, happiness, shame, pride, fear, envy, and sadness. Discrete categories are not the only way to describe the variety of emotions; some theorists rely on a small number of dimensions, such as valence and activation, to describe continuous variation in emotional quality in what has been called "core affect" (Russell, 2003). It is significant that dimensional theories focus on feelings more than on the other components of the modern conception of emotion. But, as noted by several authors in this volume, the categorical approach has predominated in analyses of emotional functionality because it seems better able to capture the particular consequences of emotional appraisals, signals, and action tendencies (Henniger & Harris, Chapter 4, this volume; Van Kleef & Côté, Chapter 6, this volume). Dimensional conceptions, such as core affect, specify only the degree of an emotion's negativity or positivity and its activation or deactivation, and this information does not provide sufficiently rich data about the nature of its appraisal and action tendencies to account for the way that it functions. For example, fear and anger are fairly similar in both their degree of negativity and their degree of activation, but they can have quite different functions.

Discrete categories of emotion can be said to serve different functions. Each emotion's expression and action tendencies provide information about the effects the emotion is likely to have on a person's physiology, behavior, and social companions. Each emotion's appraisal makes it likely that the emotion occurs under circumstances in which the expression and action tendencies are likely to be useful. Self-regulation helps to fine-tune these responses to work under those immediate circumstances. Information about appraisals, action tendencies, expression, and self-regulation makes it possible to characterize the functions that an emotion may serve and to infer how they might aid in coping with types of threat or opportunity that are common evolutionarily and culturally (Chentsova-Dutton et al., Chapter 7, this volume; Nesse & Ellsworth, 2009).

One goal that is shared by all the authors of this book is to describe the effects of negative emotions and how they can be beneficial under the right circumstances. Thus Perkins and Corr (Chapter 2, this volume) describe research showing how reactions characteristic of fear and anxiety are adaptive under particular circumstances: Fear mobilizes flight and rivets attention on a present threat that must be monitored, evaded, or confronted;

anxiety, in contrast, broadens attention, increases distractibility, promotes worry and perception of threat, and energizes back-and-forth movements that maximize detection of unknown threats that seem probable. Anxiety's social benefits may be seen in the context of long-term relationships, in which expressions of anxiety increase understanding and intimacy and solicit support and assistance (Baker, McNulty, & Overall, Chapter 5, this volume).

Anger also can have beneficial effects. Anger is aroused in situations characterized by a goal obstruction, and it functions well when that situation can confidently be construed as unjust, as someone else's fault, and as something one has the authority and power to confront (Hess, Chapter 3, this volume). Anger facilitates removal of the obstruction by providing the determination, energy, and attention to address the problem. Its benefits include not only the possibility of fixing the problem but also that of being perceived by others as willing to stand up for oneself, for friends, or for principle. Socially, expressions of anger signal the angry person's displeasure with another person's behavior, as well as signaling the determination not to tolerate it. As Van Kleef & Côté point out (Chapter 6, this volume), negotiators tend to offer greater concessions to opponents who get angry at an offer than to opponents who seem happy. As Baker et al. point out (Chapter 5, this volume), expressions of anger toward one's partner in a close romantic relationship give the partner an opportunity to make adjustments that reduce conflict within the relationship.

Sadness can also be good for you, as the title of Forgas's chapter (Chapter 1, this volume) states. Forgas's research on sad moods is consistent with these moods displaying a style of thinking that is distinct from that which characterizes happy moods. Whereas happy moods employ thinking that blithely assumes that the world is consistent with one's preexisting conceptions of it, sad moods engage a style of thinking that is more carefully attentive to the specific details of the world as it actually is. Each style has its strengths and weaknesses, but there are certainly times when the sad style is superior. Forgas's evidence suggests that thinking in a sad frame of mind promotes greater accuracy of memory for details, makes one's assertions more persuasive by lacing them with vivid examples, and increases one's ability to detect deception; it makes one less likely to apply negative stereotypes to strangers from stigmatized groups and makes one more likely to follow social norms for fairness and cooperation when one might wish to act selfishly. In addition to these cognitive action tendencies studied by Forgas, sadness also signals need to others, and Van Kleef and Côté (Chapter 6, this volume) describe research showing that its expression increases cooperation, helping, and support from others.

One might think that embarrassment is an emotion that no one would ever want to have, but what if it turned out that people are fonder of an

embarrassed person than of an unembarrassed one? They are, because they perceive embarrassment as a sign that a person is aware of social norms and is motivated to maintain them. As Henniger and Harris (Chapter 4, this volume) report, embarrassment also motivates the embarrassed person to restore his or her social standing and to monitor how others respond. Guilt and shame have similar adaptive effects (Stearns & Parrott, 2012). Henniger and Harris describe research that suggests that jealousy directs attention to preserving important relationships and that envy motivates people to compete for higher social standing.

As previously noted, a particular type of emotion can have beneficial effects in one culture but not in another. Cultures determine major aspects of the environment in which emotions occur, as well as the rules and norms to which they must conform. This volume provides many excellent examples of negative emotions with effects that vary across human cultures. As Chentsova-Dutton et al. describe in Chapter 7, Russian and American cultures have very different attitudes toward sadness and happiness. Consequently, sadness is a more negative experience for Americans (who perceive it as a sign of weakness or failure) than for Russians (who perceive it as a valuable experience and an appropriate response to stress). The cheerful demeanor that is normative in the United States would be decidedly odd in Russia, thereby having quite different social effects. To cite another example, Chinese culture places high value on emotional connections between people and places relatively low emphasis on individualism (see Sundararajan, Chapter 8, this volume). In consequence, sadness on behalf of others is highly valued by the Chinese because it is viewed as a symptom of love, and mild shaming can be used to teach children to be generous and committed within their social relationships.

The cultural relativity of the effects of anger are apparent in the research on negotiation reported by Van Kleef and Côté in Chapter 6. Anger can be socially appropriate in negotiation settings in European and European American cultures, where it is quite effective in eliciting favorable offers from negotiation partners; anger is generally inappropriate in these contexts in Japan, where it proves to be an ineffective tactic. Chentsova-Dutton et al. (Chapter 7) argue that the frequency with which an emotion occurs in a culture can influence its effect. If negative emotions are either very rare or very common, they may not have much informational value. An emotion's frequency is influenced by many factors, including the objective circumstances of the environment and the types of behavior that a culture encourages, as well as the types of emotion that the culture values. As examples, Chentsova-Dutton et al., in Chapter 7, propose that expressions of sadness are less informative in cultures in which solemnity is the norm than in those in which cheerfulness is the norm and that fear expressions are more likely to lead to widespread anxieties in cultures in

which real dangers are quite uncommon then in cultures in which danger is moderately common.

As a final piece of evidence that negative emotions can be beneficial, it's worth noting that psychiatric disorders exist that are characterized by a *lack* of certain negative emotions. For example, people with psychopathy (a type of antisocial personality disorder) exhibit a pattern of behavior that is malicious, ruthless, cruel, or criminal; they disregard social norms and take chances without concern for danger. Research has found that criminal offenders diagnosed with psychopathy show a striking lack of fear in response to images of bodily injury and violent scenes (Herpertz et al., 2001). The deficit of fear in this disorder suggests that fear plays important functions in the everyday lives of healthy individuals.

The research reviewed in this section focuses on negative emotions' useful effects, which include motivation and behavior (providing energy and determination), cognition (guiding attention, memory, and thought), and social interaction and relationships (signaling behavioral intentions and values, soliciting cooperation and support, improving relationships and social standing). These benefits emphasize the pragmatic benefits of negative emotions and provide the most straightforwardly persuasive arguments against the view that negative emotions are uniformly undesirable. Yet useful functions are not the only attraction that negative emotions have to offer. Negative emotions have meanings that provide symbolic and informational value quite apart from their practical utility (Parrott, 1993). One's sadness about a relative's death signifies one's love, one's agitation about a friend's troubles or a distant nation's war provides proof of the centrality of one's cares and loyalty. One's guilt about a transgression that cannot be undone can restore one's self-image and public reputation by demonstrating that one's remorse is nevertheless real or by leading to some form of self-punishment (Nelissen & Zeelenberg, 2009; Stearns & Parrott, 2012). In some cultures, negative emotions signify humility, the absence of hubris, or a lack of complacency about future adversity (Parrott, 1993). Cultures can also instill negative emotions with spiritual value (Tamir & Bigman, Chapter 9, this volume).

In summary, a profound implication of the multicomponent approach is that emotions have ample means through which to be functional. If emotions were to consist of nothing more than feelings, they would have limited means of making a practical difference in everyday life. Yes, they could motivate people to seek pleasantness or avoid unpleasantness, although here emotion could work only by affecting motivation. And, yes, they could provide consciousness with information about a person's evaluations of circumstances, although here emotion could work only by affecting beliefs. In contrast, multicomponent emotions involve all three aspects of the 18th-century tripartite theory of mind: not only *feelings* but also *thought* (in the

form of appraisals) and the *will* (in the form of motivated tendencies toward certain types of action and thought). Furthermore, multicomponent emotions extend the 18th-century mental trilogy to social interactions, communication, social relationships, and culture. This conceptualization permits a *functionalist* approach to emotions. The most central question about an emotion is no longer "How does it feel?" but rather "What does it do?" And, as the chapters in this volume make abundantly clear, negative emotions do many things that are very beneficial under the right circumstances.

Despite all the ways in which negative emotions can be functional, they obviously can sometimes be dysfunctional. It is easy to think of examples of envy and resentment that eroded a relationship, of anger that resulted in a trivial event being blown out of proportion, of anxiety that harmed performance, of embarrassment that only made a situation more awkward than it already was, of irrational shame that caused dysfunctional low self-esteem. And those are just the normal everyday examples; negative emotions lie at the heart of many mental disorders, including depression, phobia, posttraumatic stress, and intermittent explosive disorder. There needs to be an account of what makes emotions that are ostensibly functional sometimes horribly dysfunctional. Before attempting such an account, however, it is important to consider that this issue is not unique to negative emotions.

POSITIVE EMOTIONS ALSO CAN BE FUNCTIONAL AS WELL AS DYSFUNCTIONAL

The analysis applied to negative emotions applies to positive emotions as well. Positive emotions are not merely pleasant feelings. They also entail appraisals, mental and behavioral action tendencies, expressions, and self-regulation. They have effects that are biological, cognitive, social, and cultural. And they can have effects that are either beneficial or harmful.

Functions of Positive Emotions

Because positive emotions feel good, it seems less urgent to provide any further justification for them, but a deeper understanding of what positive emotions do is essential to appreciate how they can be both functional and dysfunctional. Ironically enough, it is actually more difficult to identify the beneficial functions of positive emotions than of negative emotions.

Negative emotions occur when people encounter a problem, when they dislike something, or when they face a threat, a setback, or a loss. For this reason, their action tendencies tend to be fairly specific: attacking, escaping, withdrawing, pacifying, becoming vigilant, making reparations, expelling, pushing back, giving up. Positive emotions, in contrast, occur

when people like what happens and when things seem to be problem-free or at least getting better. So what are their action tendencies? It required some intellectual work to realize that positive emotions do have action tendencies but that they are less specific than those of negative emotions.

The action tendencies associated with positive emotions are ones that allow a person to take advantage of safety, success, and opportunity, and these turn out to be rather open-ended: exploration, sociability, friendliness, playfulness, creativity, savoring, or a general readiness to engage with whatever the world happens to offer. Fredrickson (2001) discerned two common denominators across this assortment of nonspecific tendencies and coined the name "broaden and build" to characterize them. The functions of positive emotions, she theorized, are to broaden the scope of thought and actions and to build up physical, intellectual, and social resources.

The usefulness of positive emotions isn't restricted to a context of safety and success, however. These emotions can provide benefits even under conditions of threat and loss. Positive emotions can assist in coping with stress, and successful grieving, for example, involves a mixture of positive and negative emotions (Moskowitz, 2001). In these contexts, positive emotions promote resilience, facilitate drawing on social support, and assist in recovery from negative emotions (Fredrickson, Tugade, Waugh, & Larkin, 2003).

One way that positive emotions function is by projecting a positive attitude, even an element of self-deception, that leads to optimism, persistence, and discovery of opportunities that exist even in negative situations. Some of the benefits of positive emotions may therefore reflect a tendency to interpret events in an optimistic and confident manner.

The Negative Side of Positive Emotions

Positive emotions are capable of being dysfunctional, just as negative emotions are. Many examples can be found simply by reversing the reasons already provided for negative emotions being beneficial, which were largely based on favorable comparisons with positive emotions. Thus the cognitive effects of happiness and sadness that are reviewed by Forgas (Chapter 1, this volume) each can be beneficial, but under different conditions. For example, when accurate and detailed memory is needed, being in a happy mood is significantly inferior to being in a sad mood. Happiness can increase creativity, but it also makes people prone to ethnic stereotyping, as well as more gullible.

Likewise for the effects of happiness when compared with other negative emotions discussed in this volume. In tough negotiations, expressions of happiness often yield poorer results than do expressions of anger (Van Kleef & Côté, Chapter 6, this volume). When a threat arises, a happy

person will be slower to notice it than will an anxious person (Perkins & Corr, Chapter 2, this volume). When giving one's long-term friend a final ultimatum to change an insulting behavior lest you sever your friendship, a loving tone may fail to communicate one's resolve, whereas an angry tone will more likely succeed in making the threat seem real, and a sad tone might succeed in inducing guilt, pity, and a motivation to relieve one's suffering (Baker et al., Chapter 5, this volume). In a culture that values sadness, such as in Russia, a cheerful expression in a business context will not make the good impression it does in the United States; the cheerfulness will convey foolishness, not optimism and self-confidence, whereas a somber expression will convey seriousness, not weakness (Chentsova-Dutton et al., Chapter 7, this volume).

Even when positive emotions are well-matched to the situation, they can cause problems by being excessively strong or by not being combined with some beneficial negative emotions. An analysis of several large datasets found that, on average, people who are very happy make less money, get lower grades, and obtain less education than do people who are only moderately happy. The researchers hypothesized that too much happiness leads to complacency and erodes feelings of dissatisfaction that motivate striving, achievement, and self-improvement (Oishi, Diener, & Lucas, 2007). If correct, these findings suggest that dissatisfaction has some benefits compared with satisfaction and contentment.

Positive thinking may also hurt motivation more than it helps. Self-help guides often suggest imagining oneself succeeding in reaching a desired goal as a way of making it happen, but research suggests otherwise. People who imagine getting a good job, doing well on an exam, or having a successful outcome to surgery actually have poorer outcomes than those who do not engage in positive fantasies, and experimental research suggests that such fantasies create a great amount of relaxation and contentment that actually decreases the amount of energy devoted to achieving the goal (Barry Kappes & Oettingen, 2011). As Captain Kirk suspected, there is risk in approaching a task in a mood of blissful self-confidence if it leads to anticipating the rewards of success rather than in motivating mental focus and hard work.

Although positive emotions can support perseverance, resourcefulness, and social influence, there is a risk that such optimistic interpretations will result in perceiving an illusory world that is a distortion of reality (Baumeister, 1989). It has been suggested that several large-scale failures during the administration of U.S. President George W. Bush might have been partly due to that president's insistence on maintaining optimism and discouraging his advisers from expressing anxiety, worry, or doubt (e.g., Ehrenreich, 2009). When planning the invasion and occupation of Iraq, or when evaluating reports that New Orleans' levees could not withstand the

storm surge from a major hurricane, more anxiety and worry might have had beneficial effects in drawing attention to the possibility that everything might not happen as well as was hoped.

Positive emotions are associated with mental disorders, just as negative emotions are. Bipolar disorder typically involves episodes of heightened positive emotion known as mania. The positive emotions involved in manic episodes are usually those related to reward and achievement, such as joy and pride, and their occurrence and persistence is related to pervasive problems in emotion regulation (Gruber, 2011). Episodes of intense happiness and pride often lead to very bad outcomes: extreme self-confidence, certainty, and racing thoughts and impulses promote grandiosity, distractibility, risk taking, financial recklessness, and ill-advised sexual encounters. The consequences can range from bankruptcy and unemployment to lost friendships and divorce.

WHAT DETERMINES WHETHER EMOTIONS FUNCTION ADAPTIVELY?

The straightforward implication of this research on the nature and functions of negative and positive emotions is that both types of emotion have their purposes and can be very beneficial under the right circumstances. This understanding of emotions is much superior to believing that positive emotions are good and negative emotions are bad. It is not trivial to have realized that the choice between positive and negative emotions involves much more than choosing between feeling good and feeling bad. Emotions have the potential to be useful, but whether this potential is realized requires a variety of skills and intelligence in order to produce the right emotion in the right manner (Parrott, 2002). The trick, as Norem (Chapter 11, this volume) aptly puts it, is to find the right tool for the job.

Norem's metaphor is instructive, both for what it captures and for what it doesn't. Choosing a tool, such as when selecting a saw to cut wood, requires a degree of awareness about the properties of the tools (e.g., coping saws, crosscut saws, rip saws) and about the job (cutting a straight line or an intricate curve; cutting with the grain of the wood or across it), as well as an ability to match the properties of the tool to the demands of the job. This latter requirement is straightforward if one tool is perfect for the job, but if none is, it requires recognizing each tool's drawbacks, as well as its advantages, and doing a sort of cost–benefit calculation to choose the best available tool. In some circumstances choosing an emotion is very similar to choosing a tool—when the situation is familiar (the "job") and when the person has experience with how various emotions (the "tools") work for him or her in that type of situation. Sometimes these requirements are met.

For example, many athletes know how various emotions help or hurt them in their sport, and they practice techniques of emotion regulation to try to induce their preferred emotion and keep it at the optimal intensity during competition (Hanin, 2000). Artists develop a sense of how various emotional states affect their creativity and technique. For example, William Blake wrote a letter in 1800 that described how he had tried drawing in both good moods and bad and had figured out that, although he completed the work sooner in a bad mood, the result was not as good (Keynes, 1969, p. 807). Even college professors, with much practice in lecturing, develop a sense of just what emotional state is optimal for most effective teaching. Examples such as these are about as close as emotions get to being tools that can be deliberately chosen for a particular job. Particularly in situations that recur and are predictable, a person can gain experience with the effects of different emotions by trial and error and can develop a sense of the advantages and disadvantages of each and strive to self-regulate emotions so as to choose the right tool for the job.

Most of the time, however, one or more elements of the tool-choosing metaphor are not present, so tool choosing is less straightforward. Many situations ("jobs") are not as familiar or as predictable as the ones just described, so we may not know what frame of mind will work best in them. Many people may be unaware of the ways in which their emotions ("tools") are useful and so may not take advantage of them. For example, what emotional state makes people better at detecting deception: happiness or sadness? People who have very good intuitions about the effects of happiness and sadness or a lot of experience judging deception with feedback about their accuracy will know the answer, but many others will not be sure unless they know about the research conducted by Forgas (Chapter 1, this volume) showing that people who just watched a sad film about dying of cancer were better able to detect lies than were people who watched an amusing comedy film or a neutral nature documentary (Forgas & East, 2008).

The way in which we "choose" our emotions can be quite different from the way we choose our tools. Although the athletes, artists, and professors described earlier develop considerable control over their emotions, that control requires extensive practice and is never quite the same as reaching for a screwdriver from the toolbox. We often are unaware of the role we are playing in choosing and shaping our emotions, and, in many situations, our emotions arise without much choice at all. A frequent goal of psychological therapy, for example, is to make patients aware that there are alternatives to their natural interpretations of events (Novaco, 1975). Even low-level neural organization allows context and expectations to guide emotional responding (Parrott & Schulkin, 1993). It would be as if our claw hammer were to fly off its hook and land in our hand. In cases in

which "choosing" is not what determines our emotion, then, what does? The answer is "appraisal."

Appraisal is frequently automatic, not a deliberate choice. It is shaped by experience, socialization, and even deliberate training, but the result is something akin to how a person perceives an ambiguous figure following exposure to an unambiguous version of one of the two alternatives—people are not at all aware that there exists any interpretation other than the one that effortlessly pops to mind. As a result, whether we use the right emotion for the situation at hand depends on the accuracy of the appraisal of that situation. If the appraisal is accurate and realistic, then it likely gives rise to an emotion that is well suited to that situation. Mistaken appraisals are an important source of dysfunctional emotions (Parrott, 2001, 2002). Appraising a high risk of sexual infidelity in a faithful and trustworthy partner gives rise to jealousy that is unlikely to strengthen the relationship; feeling morally responsible for injustices over which one's only involvement is living on the same planet yields dysfunctional guilt; failing to realize that a friend's demands are inconsiderate will fail to generate anger that might well have led to changes in that friend's behavior. In short, not only are "jobs" and "tools" often different for tools and emotions, but so also is "choosing."

One critical ingredient that has been neglected so far is that choosing the right tool for the job is only the beginning—one then has to use the tool correctly! With skill and finesse, the right tool will do a lovely job, but in the wrong hands, even the most perfectly chosen tool can utterly ruin the project it was selected for. The same is true for emotions. Emotion words such as *anger, jealousy,* or *cheerfulness* refer to a general category of appraisal and action tendency, not to a fixed behavioral reaction, so there are many ways in which any type of emotion can manifest itself. The way in which a type of emotion is adapted to its circumstances influences its usefulness just as much as the selection of the right type of emotion. The right emotion may nevertheless bring disaster if is deployed inappropriately, and there are many ways an emotion can be poorly deployed (Parrott, 2001). The emotion's intensity must be neither too strong nor too mild. The emotion must be allowed to have its effect and not be ignored, dismissed, or repressed. And, most nuanced of all, the emotion must be adapted to its particular circumstances. The highly effective uses of anger described by Hess (Chapter 3, this volume) and by Van Kleef and Côté (Chapter 6, this volume) are the result of more than merely selecting anger rather than sadness or awe; they are the result of well-calibrated intensities and skillfully modulated expressions, and if they had resulted in other expressions of anger—for example, loud cursing, spluttering inarticulateness, throwing furniture, or inscrutable sulking—they would not have had their useful effects. If anger is expressed with a strength that is disproportional to

the offense or without clearly specifying what the problem is or about a situation that cannot be changed, then the anger will more likely hurt the relationship than help it. A related set of findings shows that expressions of anger are effective in situations (such as negotiations) in which assigning blame is appropriate but are harmful in situations (such as soliciting donations to a charity) in which assigning blame is inappropriate (Van Kleef & Côté, Chapter 6). The ways in which negative emotions may be ineffectively deployed in the context of close relationships are surveyed by Baker et al. (Chapter 5, this volume).

People can vary with respect to which tools work best for them. One source of variability is one's sex—Hess (Chapter 3) reviews research showing that expressions of anger can affect onlookers very differently depending on whether the angry person is male or female. Another source of individual differences is practice and skill with a particular emotion. For example, one person may be a master of embarrassment and can act flustered and self-deprecating in an amusing way that generates sympathy and trivializes his or her offense, whereas another person may become so flustered that the situation becomes even more awkward for everyone present. Other individual differences may be less liable to modification by practice. As Norem (Chapter 11, this volume) argues, although some people may be able to avoid some needless anxiety by using "strategic optimism," not everyone is able to stop their anxiety, so for them the "best" emotion is not an option at all. Defensive pessimism is a strategy that works well for such people. People's control over their emotions is not absolute, so people must work within their natural repertoire. Realistically, the best tool for the job at hand must be one that is actually in the toolbox.

WHAT DO PEOPLE REALLY WANT?

Emotions arise when a situation is appraised as affecting a person's goals, desires, strivings, cares, or needs. Nico Frijda (2007) uses the term *concerns* to cover this range of concepts, and he supplies a subtle analysis of whether pleasure is the ultimate goal or whether pleasure is a guide toward goals but not the goal itself. The question of whether people would want to experience a negative emotion hinges on this question of motivation. Do people strive to experience pleasure and avoid pain and choose their activities and goals according to their expectation of the feelings they will provide? If so, they act according to *hedonism* (Weijers, 2011). Alternatively, do people strive for objects and goals that they value for reasons other than the pleasure they experience when they obtain them? If so, people act according to motivational *hormism*, to use the term proposed by Duncker (1941). If emotions were nothing more than feelings, and positive and

negative emotions differed only in whether they felt pleasant or unpleasant, then hormism would not be relevant to emotional preferences because there would be nothing upon which to value emotions other than their hedonic quality. However, for the reasons summarized in this chapter, emotions can be valued on the basis of much more: the ways in which they modify thought and action, the effects they have on other people, the ways in which they conform to the norms of our society, the meanings they have.

Contemporary Western cultures, especially European American culture, approach emotions in a manner that is predominantly hedonistic. The predominant idea is that emotions are good if they feel pleasant, and otherwise they are bad. This perspective results from centuries of cultural change, including the Renaissance transition from an otherworldly to a more worldly orientation, as well as the conditions of freedom and equality that arose in America (McMahon, 2006). Contrasting earlier eras with the present yields a striking sense of just how exceptional a hedonistic orientation is. For example, Europeans during the Middle Ages and the Renaissance considered sadness to have sufficient benefits that it was cultivated despite its unpleasant feelings and physical lethargy. In 1586, Timothy Bright observed that melancholy causes people "to be more exact and curious in pondering the very moments of things" (p. 130). Even in 1776, when Thomas Jefferson included "the pursuit of happiness" among the inalienable rights of man in the Declaration of Independence, he referred not to pleasant feelings but rather to a fulfilling and meaningful existence that served the collective public good (Wills, 1978). As recently as the mid-19th century, American culture valued emotional intensity as the source of a full life and considered all emotions to be potentially useful; some emotions were considered to be dangerous and in need of control, but all could benefit society if directed toward an appropriate target (Stearns, 1994). The key historical transition occurred during the first half of the 20th century. The distinction between pleasant and unpleasant emotions, not a central concern of the Victorians, came to the fore, and positive emotions came to be treated very differently from their negative counterparts. Intensity itself came to be seen as risking loss of control. Most negative emotions were to be avoided (such as fear, anger, and jealousy), and milder emotions, such as embarrassment, were promoted as substitutes for stronger ones such as guilt and shame. A cheerful demeanor became the norm, and happiness became a sign of success. Stearns (1994), who documents this transition, suggests that these changes likely resulted from the rise of the service economy, consumerism, secularism, and concerns about how emotions affected health.

This *culture of cheerfulness* has generated something of a backlash in recent years. Critics have pointed out the shortcomings of continual happiness and criticized the intolerance of sadness, anxiety, and regret (e.g.,

Burkeman, 2012; Ehrenreich, 2009; Horwitz & Wakefield, 2007; Norem, 2001; Landman, 1996; Wilson, 2008). A frequent complaint is that happiness is considered not just desirable but mandatory and that unhappy people are inferior to happy ones (Held, 2002; Norem, Chapter 11, this volume). This attitude was originally distinctly American, but no longer is that true. In 1959, Viktor Frankl could write that "to the European, it is a characteristic of the American culture that, again and again, one is commanded and ordered to 'be happy'" (p. 140). Just 40 years later, in France no less, Pascal Bruckner (2000, p. 46) observed that "we are moving from happiness as a right to happiness as an imperative." Positive psychology in its early years was a target of this backlash as well (e.g., Held, 2004), although recently it has demonstrated more acceptance of negative emotions and has generated important critiques of and alternatives to hedonism (Seligman, 2002; Sheldon, Kashdan, & Steger, 2011).

Nevertheless, academic psychologists in Western cultures, even those who study emotions, clearly show the influence of their culture's emphasis on cheerfulness. One illustration of this influence comes from my own experience—actually, it is what originally sparked my interest in the positive side of negative emotions. I was doing research on "mood-congruent recall," the tendency for people to be more likely to remember happy events when they are happy than when they are sad and more likely to remember sad events when they are sad than when happy (Blaney, 1986). In a series of experiments I found the opposite of mood-congruent recall under some conditions. I proposed that people recall "mood-incongruent memories" when they want to regulate their emotions to become less sad or less happy (Parrott & Sabini, 1990). Yet I encountered strong resistance to this explanation; psychologists accepted that sad people might be motivated to recall pleasant memories to cheer themselves, but they strongly resisted the complementary proposal that happy people might be motivated to recall unpleasant memories to rid themselves of their cheerful state of mind. The resistance of academic psychologists motivated my investigation of the multitude of motives people have for fostering negative emotions and avoiding positive ones (Parrott, 1993). (Just for the record, there is now more evidence in support of the self-regulation explanation. Mood-incongruent memory is most likely to occur in situations in which positive or negative emotions are unhelpful or inappropriate; it is also most likely to occur in the sort of people one would expect to engage in such emotion regulation, namely those with strong tendencies toward self-regulation and emotional awareness; for a summary, see Parrott & Spackman, 2000.)

A second illustration of how hedonistic assumptions pervade academic psychology is provided by the history of research on why people seek out theater, film, and stories that depict sad events, a phenomenon that is summarized by Oliver, Bartsch, and Hartmann in Chapter 10 (this volume).

Social scientists' label for this phenomenon—the "paradox of tragedy"—itself demonstrates their hedonistic assumptions, as do their theories of why people seek out negative emotions. One such theory proposes that sad entertainment provides distractions or alleviates boredom, thereby resulting in a net increase in pleasure. Other hedonically oriented theories include the suggestion that sad entertainment evokes pleasure at the depiction of justice, that negative emotions somehow boost the intensity of subsequent positive emotions, and that some people associate sad emotions with positive appraisals. What is striking is the lengths to which theorists have gone to avoid concluding that people sometimes choose negative emotions for reasons unrelated to feeling good. Oliver et al. (Chapter 10) show that these theories do not account for the facts concerning people's enjoyment of tearjerkers and other entertainments that evoke negative emotions.

In the face of such powerful cultural forces, what is really impressive is that people not only continue to have negative emotions but actually choose to do so. Swedish college students, who prefer to feel pleasant emotions as a general rule, express a preference for negative emotions in contexts in which such emotions will have a useful function (Vastfjall & Garling, 2006). German adults who are prompted by mobile phone to report their current emotions and whether they wanted to enhance, maintain, or dampen them reported 15% of the time that they wanted to feel less of a positive emotion or more of a negative emotion (Riediger, Schmiedek, Wagner, & Lindenberger, 2009). And, in a remarkable series of laboratory experiments by Maya Tamir and her colleagues, American college students have been shown to try to increase the intensity of their negative emotions when they believe that these emotions will be useful and when the benefits of the emotion's utility exceed the burden of the emotion's unpleasantness (for a review, see Tamir & Bigman, Chapter 9, this volume). Apparently, Western culture's hedonistic ideology has not prevented people from learning the instrumental value of negative emotions.

Even so, it seems likely that the culture of cheerfulness has some bad consequences. The largest effect may be that Westerners are unaware of what they implicitly know about negative emotions and how to use them. The Western appreciation of negative emotions is therefore stunted, and Westerners are only aware of the value of negative emotions in certain contexts (Kashima & Haslam, 2007). The degree to which negative emotions' potential usefulness is underutilized in Western cultures is yet to be determined. The cultural bias is likely to be most evident with regard to how people explain their actions, just as people in individualistic cultures provide individualistic reasons for doing such collectivistic things as caring for sick parents (Bellah, Madsen, Sullivan, Swidler, & Tipton, 1985). One effect that Western culture may have is to encourage negative emotions about having negative emotions—such emotions can be termed

metaemotions (see Oliver et al., Chapter 10, this volume). One final drawback of hedonism deserves mention: By setting up positive feelings as the goal of life, the culture of cheerfulness actually makes happiness more difficult to achieve by setting people up for disappointment (Mauss, Tamir, Anderson, & Savino, 2011). As John Stuart Mill put it in the 19th century, "Ask yourself whether you are happy, and you cease to be so. The only chance is to treat, not happiness, but some end external to it, as the purpose of life" (Mill, 1873/1989, p. 117).

There is a deeper reason that feeling good makes a poor goal for living a good life: It supplants other purposes that transcend the self, that are connected to values, and that therefore are more richly rewarding. In trying to understand why people choose to view tearjerkers and tragedies, Oliver et al. (Chapter 10) proposed that *meaningfulness* provides a better account than does pleasure. One does not enjoy a tragedy so much as one finds it gratifying, thought-provoking, or moving. In taking this approach, Oliver and colleagues tap into a long-standing debate about whether satisfaction with one's life is best defined in terms of momentary experiences of positive emotion or in terms of an overall sense of finding meaning, purpose, and fulfillment (Baumeister, Vohs, Aaker, & Garbinsky, 2013; Ryff, 1989). Some psychologists measure life satisfaction by counting positive emotions (e.g., Kahneman, 1999), others by measuring meaningfulness (Ryff, 1989); and in actuality both methods account for some aspects of human life satisfaction and often operate in tandem (Kashdan, Biswas-Diener, & King, 2008). But hedonism cannot convincingly account for why people choose to view tragedies that do not provide pleasure but do spur reflection, personal growth, and perspective. The goal is not to feel good but to find meaning.

Similarly, real-life emotions can be enjoyed as a hedonic experience, but most of the time the ultimate goal that people strive for is not pleasure but rather something that is valued apart from any hedonic effect (Frijda, 2007). There is an important sense in which striving for pleasantness puts the hedonic cart before the purposive horse. Experiencing negative emotions that have utility for achieving nonhedonic goals is part of meaningful striving; negative emotions' relation to nonhedonic concerns give them meaning. To find emotions meaningful allows one to look beyond the present and connect one's current situation with one's past and future (Baumeister et al., 2013).

Struggles, frustrations, and suffering can be a valuable part of a meaningful life, despite being unpleasant, because they reflect one's commitment to a valued cause. To live life fully inevitably means to experience misfortune, disappointment, betrayal, and loss. To avoid negative emotions under such conditions would require disengagement or denial, whereas to engage passionately with all aspects of life gives rise to negative emotions that

will be meaningful because they are connected to commitments and goals that are treasured (Sundararajan, 2005; Chapter 8, this volume). A well-lived life reflects one's aspirations and values, regardless of whether that life consists of contentment and satisfaction or of suffering, frustration, and struggle (Solomon, 2007). Captain Kirk was right: Negative emotions have an important place in a fulfilling and meaningful life.

REFERENCES

Barry Kappes, H., & Oettingen, G. (2011). Positive fantasies about idealized futures sap energy. *Journal of Experimental Social Psychology, 47,* 719–729.

Baumeister, R. F. (1989). The optimal margin of illusion. *Journal of Social and Clinical Psychology, 8,* 176–189.

Baumeister, R. F., Vohs, K. D., Aaker, J. L., & Garbinsky, E. N. (2013). Some key differences between a happy life and a meaningful life. *Journal of Positive Psychology, 8,* 505–516.

Bellah, R. N., Madsen, R., Sullivan, W. M., Swidler, A., & Tipton, S. M. (1985). *Habits of the heart: Individualism and commitment in American life.* Berkeley: University of California Press.

Blaney, P. H. (1986). Affect and memory: A review. *Psychological Bulletin, 99,* 229–246.

Bright, T. (1586). *A treatise of melancholie.* London: Vautrolier.

Bruckner, P. (2000). *Perpetual euphoria: On the duty to be happy* (S. Rendall, Trans.). Princeton, NJ: Princeton University Press.

Burkeman, O. (2012). *The antidote: Happiness for people who can't stand positive thinking.* New York: Faber & Faber.

Dewey, J. (1894). The theory of emotion: I. Emotional attitudes. *Psychological Review, 1,* 553–569.

Dixon, T. (2003). *From passions to emotions: The creation of a secular psychological category.* Cambridge, UK: Cambridge University Press.

Dror, O. E. (1999). The scientific image of emotion: Experience and technologies of inscription. *Configurations, 7,* 355–401.

Duncker, K. (1941). On pleasure, emotion and striving. *Philosophy and Phenomenological Research, 1,* 391–430.

Ehrenreich, B. (2009). *Bright-sided: How positive thinking is undermining America.* New York: Picador.

Fischer, A. H., & Manstead, A. S. R. (2008). Social functions of emotion. In M. Lewis, J. M. Haviland-Jones, & L. Feldman Barrett (Eds.), *Handbook of emotions* (3rd ed., pp. 456–468). New York: Guilford Press.

Forgas, J. P., & East, R. (2008). On being happy and gullible: Mood effects on skepticism and the detection of deception. *Journal of Experimental Social Psychology, 44,* 1362–1367.

Frankl, V. E. (1959). *Man's search for meaning: An introduction to logotherapy* (I. Lasch, Trans.). Boston: Beacon Press.

Fredrickson, B. L. (2001). The role of positive emotions in positive psychology:

The broaden-and-build theory of positive emotions. *American Psychologist,* *56,* 218–226.

Fredrickson, B. L., Tugade, M. M., Waugh, C. E., & Larkin, G. R. (2003) What good are positive emotions in crises? A prospective study of resilience and emotions following the terrorist attacks on the United States on September 11th, 2001. *Journal of Personality and Social Psychology, 84,* 365–376.

Frijda, N. H. (1986). *The emotions.* Cambridge, UK: Cambridge University Press.

Frijda, N. H. (2007). *The laws of emotion.* Mahwah, NJ: Erlbaum.

Gruber, J. (2011). A review and synthesis of positive emotion and reward disturbance in bipolar disorder. *Clinical Psychology and Psychotherapy, 18,* 356–365.

Hanin, Y. L. (2000). Individual zones of optimal functioning (IZOF) model. In Y. L. Hanin (Ed.), *Emotions in sport* (pp. 65–89). Champaign, IL: Human Kinetics.

Held, B. S. (2002). The tyranny of the positive attitude in America: Observation and speculation. *Journal of Clinical Psychology, 58,* 965–992.

Held, B. S. (2004). The negative side of positive psychology. *Journal of Humanistic Psychology, 44,* 9–46.

Herpertz, S. C., Werth, U., Lucas, G., Qunaibi, M., Schuerkens, A., Kunert, H., et al. (2001). Emotion in criminal offenders with psychopathy and borderline personality disorders. *Archives of General Psychiatry, 58,* 737–745.

Hilgard, E. R. (1980). The trilogy of mind: Cognition, affection, and conation. *Journal of the History of the Behavioral Sciences, 16,* 107–117.

Horwitz, A. V., & Wakefield, J. C. (2007). *The loss of sadness: How psychiatry transformed normal sorrow into depressive disorder.* New York: Oxford University Press.

James, S. (1997). *Passion and action: The emotions in seventeenth-century philosophy.* Oxford, UK: Oxford University Press.

James, W. (1884). What is an emotion? *Mind, 9,* 188–205.

Kahneman, D. (1999). Objective happiness. In D. Kahneman, E. Diener, & N. Schwarz (Eds.), *Well-being: The foundations of hedonic psychology* (pp. 3–25). New York: Russell Sage.

Kashdan, T. B., Biswas-Diener, R., & King, L. A. (2008). Reconsidering happiness: The costs of distinguishing between hedonics and eudaimonia. *Journal of Positive Psychology, 3,* 219–233.

Kashima, Y., & Haslam, N. (2007). Explanation and interpretation: An invitation to experimental semiotics. *Journal of Theoretical and Philosophical Psychology, 27–28,* 234–256.

Keltner, D., Haidt, J., & Shiota, M. N. (2006). Social functionalism and the evolution of emotions. In M. Schaller, J. A. Simpson, & D. T. Kenrick (Eds.), *Evolution and social psychology* (pp. 115–142). New York: Psychology Press.

Keynes, G. (Ed.). (1969). *Blake: Complete writings.* London: Oxford University Press.

Kotchemidova, C. (2005). From good cheer to "Drive-by Smiling": A social history of cheerfulness. *Journal of Social History, 39*(1), 5–37.

Landman, J. (1996). Social control of "negative" emotions: The case of regret. In

R. Harré & W. G. Parrott (Eds.), *The emotions: Social, cultural and biological dimensions* (pp. 89–116). London: Sage.

Mauss, I. B., Tamir, M., Anderson, C. L., & Savino, N. S. (2011). Can seeking happiness make people unhappy? Paradoxical effects of valuing happiness. *Emotion, 11*, 807–815.

McMahon, D. M. (2006). *Happiness: A history.* New York: Atlantic Monthly Press.

Mill, J. S. (1989). *Autobiography* (J. M. Robson, Ed.) New York: Penguin. (Original work published 1873)

Moskowitz, J. T. (2001). Emotion and coping. In T. J. Mayne & G. A. Bonanno (Eds.), *Emotions: Current issues and future directions* (pp. 311–336). New York: Guilford Press.

Nelissen, R. M. A., & Zeelenberg, M. (2009). When guilt evokes self-punishment: Evidence for the existence of a Dobby effect. *Emotion, 9*, 118–122.

Nesse, R. M., & Ellsworth, P. C. (2009). Evolution, emotions, and emotional disorders. *American Psychologist, 64*, 129–139.

Norem, J. K. (2001). *The positive power of negative thinking.* New York: Basic Books.

Novaco, R. (1975). *Anger control: The development and evaluation of an experimental treatment.* Lexington, MA: Heath.

Oatley, K., & Jenkins, J. M. (1992). Human emotions: Function and dysfunction. *Annual Review of Psychology, 43*, 55–85.

Oishi, S., Diener, E., & Lucas, R. E. (2007). The optimum level of well-being: Can people be too happy? *Perspectives on Psychological Science, 2*, 346–360.

Parrott, W. G. (1993). Beyond hedonism: Motives for inhibiting good moods and for maintaining bad moods. In D. M. Wegner & J. W. Pennebaker (Eds.), *Handbook of mental control* (pp. 278–305). Englewood Cliffs, NJ: Prentice-Hall.

Parrott, W. G. (2001). Implications of dysfunctional emotions for understanding how emotions function. *Review of General Psychology, 5*, 180–186.

Parrott, W. G. (2002). The functional utility of negative emotions. In L. F. Barrett & P. Salovey (Eds.), *The wisdom in feeling: Psychological processes in emotional intelligence* (pp. 341–359). New York: Guilford Press.

Parrott, W. G. (2007). Components and the definition of emotion. *Social Science Information, 46*, 419–423.

Parrott, W. G., & Sabini, J. (1990). Mood and memory under natural conditions: Evidence for mood incongruent recall. *Journal of Personality and Social Psychology, 59*, 321–336.

Parrott, W. G., & Schulkin, J. (1993). Neuropsychology and the cognitive nature of the emotions. *Cognition and Emotion, 7*, 43–59.

Parrott, W. G., & Spackman, M. (2000). Emotion and memory. In M. Lewis & J. Haviland-Jones (Eds.), *Handbook of emotions* (2nd ed., pp. 476–490). New York: Guilford Press.

Riediger, M., Schmiedek, F., Wagner, G. G., & Lindenberger, U. (2009). Seeking pleasure and seeking pain: Differences in prohedonic and contra-hedonic motivation from adolescence to old age. *Psychological Science, 20*, 1529–1535.

Russell, J. A. (2003). Core affect and the psychological construction of emotion. *Psychological Review, 110,* 145–172.

Ryff, C. D. (1989). Happiness is everything, or is it? Explorations on the meaning of psychological well-being. *Journal of Personality and Social Psychology, 57,* 1069–1081.

Scherer, K. R. (1984). On the nature and function of emotion: A component process approach. In K. R. Scherer & P. Ekman (Eds.), *Approaches to emotion* (pp. 293–317). Hillsdale, NJ: Erlbaum.

Seligman, M. E. P. (2002). *Authentic happiness.* New York: Free Press.

Seligman, M. E. P., & Csikszentmihalyi, M. (2000). Positive psychology: An introduction. *American Psychologist, 55,* 5–14.

Sheldon, K. M., Kashdan, T. B., & Steger, M. F. (Eds.). (2011). *Designing positive psychology: Taking stock and moving forward.* Oxford, UK: Oxford University Press.

Solomon, R. C. (2007). *True to our feelings: What our emotions are really telling us.* Oxford, UK: Oxford University Press.

Stearns, D. C., & Parrott, W. G. (2012). When feeling bad makes you look good: Guilt, shame, and person perception. *Cognition and Emotion, 26,* 407–430.

Stearns, P. N. (1994). *American cool: Constructing a twentieth-century emotional style.* New York: New York University Press.

Sundararajan, L. (2005). Happiness donut: A Confucian critique of positive psychology. *Journal of Theoretical and Philosophical Psychology, 25,* 35–60.

Vastfjall, D., & Garling, T. (2006). Preference for negative emotions. *Emotion, 6,* 326–329.

Weijers, D. (2011). Hedonism. In J. Fieser & B. Dowden (Eds.), *The Internet encyclopedia of philosophy* (updated August 10, 2011). Retrieved from *www.iep.utm.edu/hedonism*

Wills, G. (1978). *Inventing America: Jefferson's Declaration of Independence.* Garden City, NY: Doubleday.

Wilson, E. G. (2008). *Against happiness: In praise of melancholy.* New York: Sarah Crichton Books.

Index

An *f* following a page number indicates a figure; an *n* following a page number indicates a note.

DI210284